OXFORD MEDICAL PUBLICATIONS

Analysing Health Systems

Analysing Health Systems

A Modular Approach

AVI YACAR ELLENCWEIG

*Department of Medical Ecology,
School of Public Health and Community
Medicine, Hebrew University-Hadassah
Faculty of Medicine, Jerusalem*

Oxford New York Tokyo
OXFORD UNIVERSITY PRESS

This book has been printed digitally and produced in a standard specification in order to ensure its continuing availability

OXFORD
UNIVERSITY PRESS

Great Clarendon Street, Oxford OX2 6DP

Oxford University Press is a department of the University of Oxford.
It furthers the University's objective of excellence in research, scholarship, and education by publishing worldwide in

Oxford New York

Auckland Cape Town Dar es Salaam Hong Kong Karachi
Kuala Lumpur Madrid Melbourne Mexico City Nairobi
New Delhi Shanghai Taipei Toronto

With offices in

Argentina Austria Brazil Chile Czech Republic France Greece
Guatemala Hungary Italy Japan South Korea Poland Portugal
Singapore Switzerland Thailand Turkey Ukraine Vietnam

Oxford is a registered trade mark of Oxford University Press in the UK and in certain other countries

Published in the United States by Oxford University Press Inc., New York

Reprinted 2011

ISBN 978-0-19-262085-9

Printed and bound in Great Britain by CPI Antony Rowe, Chippenham and Eastbourne

TO

Esthi, Nathali, Ben, and Or

Preface

When John Smith of Hope, British Columbia, Canada, needs to see a doctor, he would be likely to contact his family practitioner to set an appointment over the phone. He would also report his Medical Services Plan number. If the scheduled appointment resulted in prescription of drugs, Mr Smith would probably bear the full cost of medicines purchased in a commercial pharmacy. When Moshe Drori of Haifa, Israel, needs to see a doctor, he would probably line up in a 'Kupat Holim' clinic until his unscheduled appointment with the doctor. If drugs are prescribed, Mr Drori would apply to the clinic's pharmacy and receive the drugs nearly free of charge, except for a small co-payment. Both Mr Smith and Mr Drori are entitled to free doctor care since they paid the prepaid premiums to their respective insurers—a provincial Ministry of Health in Canada and a voluntary sick fund in Israel. When John O'Kupte of Nairobi, Kenya, needs to see a doctor, his needs would be satisfied differently. Mr O'Kupte might apply to a private practitioner and would bear the full cost of consultation and medicines. Otherwise, he might line up for hours or even days in a government out-patient clinic.

These three examples illustrate the striking variety of health systems and how different they are from each other. With these differences in mind, three principal questions are suggested by Victor Sidel (see also Chapter 1).

- Why should we compare health systems?
- Who are the people making comparisons?
- How can such comparisons be carried out?

The first question concerns the rationale of comparing different systems. There are several reasons for making such comparisons. To mention just a few, comparing health systems internationally can help to raise questions about one's own system. In addition, looking at other systems can furnish alternative ideas and help establish new models of care. Furthermore, studying other systems can help us to avoid pitfalls already experienced by professionals working in those other systems. The efforts of other societies in their health systems can inspire in us an openmindedness for change, a value that is often lacking in traditional planning and decision making.

Regarding the second question, the people comparing health systems are the very people who may be reading this book. These readers may include professionals of many kinds, like a hospital director interested in variations of hospital use across regions or a national director of health concerned with health policy at large. They may independently study and evaluate various aspects of international comparisons. Cross-comparisons are also of interest to health statisticians of all levels from that of a local health agency where vital data of several counties are compared, to the managerial team of National Statistics where forecasting trends in a multisystem perspective are evaluated. Planners, too, should make cross comparisons since they not only ought to avoid others' mistakes but also replicate their successes. The book may be useful to scholars and students studying and analysing case studies. They might find it useful for forecasting future trends, raising questions about the existing system, and suggesting alternatives for better care. More broadly, almost all modern health professionals share some decision-making responsibility and should be interested to learn from the accumulation of international knowledge and experience. This book, then, is as much for the general audience of health practitioners, clinicians, nurses, and others, as for the executors, planners, scholars, and students in administration, public health and international health, all of whom may be active in comparing health systems.

As for the third question, addressing methodological issues in international comparisons of health services is a very complex process. This book is mostly intended to be a thorough effort to review existing methods and approaches for comparisons, and to suggest ways to make this task easier.

This focus determines the scope of the book but leaves open the choice between two options. The first is a rigorous methodological textbook in which *methods* are discussed in depth rather than their applications and case studies. The second consists of a more practical text mostly based on empirical findings. This second option is thus less demanding in methodological scrutiny than the first one. Here, the second option is used for three reasons. First, because the issue of international comparisons is very important for decision-makers and administrators. A thorough methodological text might have been discouraging to non-scholars. Second, rigorous methodology is available in other texts: for instance, rather than discussing the concept of measurement in depth, appropriate references are recommended to the reader throughout the text. Third, because comparisons of health systems are not, in most part, soundly based methodologically, several topics are discussed empirically based on many case studies.

As a result, this book has the following objectives. The first objective is to improve the usability and increase the use of cross-comparisons of health systems by health professionals whose health care systems would thus benefit. It would also be particularly helpful for those who could profit from the implementation of successful models. Beyond the immediate application of cross-comparisons, there is the longer range need to build the cumulative scientific basis from which cross-comparisons of health systems can be derived and tested. The second objective of this book is to provide means to reach that end. This can be by bridging the several existing models in comparative health into an inclusive model for the study and analysis of health systems.

The chapters are presented in three parts. In Part I, cross-comparisons of health systems are placed in a conceptual and contextual perspective. Here we seek to answer the following questions: What is a health system? What are health system dynamics? and How were health systems compared in previous studies?

In Chapter 1 the theoretical concepts of health systems and of the systems' approach are reviewed with a brief overview of their historical developments. Having clarified these concepts and their uses we provide a concise methodological overview on the operationalization of concepts. We review topics relating to measurement including quantification and scales, unidimensionality, validity, reliability, and sensitivity. Finally, we present the instruments for measurement, that is the indicators and their characteristics. Chapter 2 deals with approaches in comparative health. First the attributes of health systems are discussed. Then models in the literature, based on these various approaches, are reviewed and the pros and cons of each are weighed. Three principal approaches are considered:

(1) the health services approach;

(2) the case study approach;

(3) the health policy approach.

Finally, the modular approach is presented as a possible solution for the difficulties in comparing health systems. Here we answer the questions: How can we examine and compare several different health systems at once? How can we overcome the problems of unreliable or scanty information? What can be done when some of our information is suspect?

In Part II the modular approach is presented in depth. Each topic is discussed first at the conceptual level and then at the operational level. Here the concepts and methods reviewed in the conceptual overview in Part I are applied to the selection of measurement instruments. In Chapter 3 health systems are examined from the perspective of the consumer leading to an analysis of population needs. Several questions related to needs assessment are reviewed from a comparative perspective. The different solutions presented are the single indicator approach, the compound method, and qualitative methods for comparisons. Finally, specific indicators for each method are presented. In Chapter 4 the inputs of a health system are examined. First, tangible resources are considered, including manpower, physical resources, and financial assets. Then external influences affecting the system are analysed including the general economic conditions, the political process, and the cultural attributes in a given area or country.

In Chapter 5 we ask: How can inputs be organized in health systems to provide health care? What are the components pertinent to the implementation of the process of care? The structural characteristics of the system, the availability and accessibility of resources, and the appropriateness of the arrangements are analysed as well as issues of co-ordination, equity, and the accountability of the health system. There is also a cross-comparison of the planning processes and reimbursement in several health systems. In Chapter 6 the process of care is considered and the direct and indirect attributes related to the process of care are distinguished. In the first part of the chapter descriptive studies on the utilization of health services at cross-national and cross-regional levels are reviewed. Then, analytical instruments for comparative utilization are suggested. Next, accessibility to health care services is divided into physical accessibility, economic accessibility, and acceptability which is social and cultural accessibility. In the second part of the chapter some concealed aspects affecting the health care process are reviewed. These include professional autonomy in health care, labour relationships in health care settings, and ethical issues of utilization.

In Chapter 7 issues of health outcomes and health status are discussed. We propose ways to define the health status of a population and practical means for its measurement. The traditional concepts of death, disease, and disability are discussed from a cross-national perspective and the more modern concepts of positive health and well-being are discussed as indices of outcomes. In addition, the contributions of external influences to the health status of populations, in particular the effects of the environment, life styles, and human biology, are reviewed. In Chapter 8 we concentrate on the relationships of health system outcomes to health outcomes. Here, outcomes relating to the health care system are crystallized. The concepts discussed include effectiveness, efficiency, and quality. Effectiveness is the end result of the health care process. Efficiency is regarded as the relationship between the effects of the process of care and the associated costs of such care. We review four types of efficiency comparatively: allocative, distributive, dynamic, and managerial. Finally, we address the quality of care, and outcome-related quality assurance mechanisms are discussed.

In Chapter 9 are discussed the problems encountered in cross-national comparisons and their limitations. First we consider the methodological perspective. Here we deal with problems arising from ecological fallacy, inconsistency and incomparability in the operational definition of indicators, and the effects of the choice of the measurement method on the final results. Second, we consider the limitations of data collection. Here issues of validity and reliability, feasibility and appropriateness of use are reviewed. Finally, some useful hints are provided to help in finding the delicate balance between correct and inappropriate uses of cross-national or cross-regional data.

Part III concludes the book with four chapters on the application of the modular approach to 'real life' situations. Each chapter provides a distinctive example of such potential applications. On the one hand, we provide in-depth studies of certain phenomena across several countries. On the other hand, we make a comprehensive comparison of fewer countries in broader perspectives. In Chapter 10 we discuss how modules for the *inputs* of health systems affect the modules for processes of care and for health systems *outcomes*. We provide examples of such causal relationships from several different health systems. These examples include comparisons reported in the literature and also some original analyses based on WHO and OECD statistics. In Chapter 11 comprehensive comparisons of health systems using the modular approach are considered. Here the viability of the modular approach is shown by using it for the analysis of a complete national health system. Three health systems are discussed: that of Canada as an example of a fully developed national system; that of Israel as an example of a developed system still facing the problems of a developing nation; and that of Nigeria as an example of a health system of a developing nation.

In Chapter 12 the modular approach is applied to the problem of expanding the number of modules used in international comparisons. The focus is on an attempt by a given country to adopt aspects of health systems from another country. For example, The Netherlands, Israel, and the United Kingdom attempted to adopt aspects of the American competitive model. Such an 'adoption' is often based on an analysis confined to one module only, the organization of health care. Here we show that such a comparative analysis of health care can be improved by the addition of other modules to the analysis. In Chapter 13 we summarize our findings and discuss the future prospects of national and regional cross-comparisons. We raise hopes for improved comparability between health systems, and address some of the difficult problems remaining down the road.

The appendix is useful for linking health systems concepts to their operational terms. First, every concept in this book is listed in order of appearance. Each concept is then provided with an indicator for its measurement. Any special recommendations and/or comments pertinent to the presentation of each topic are also included. The appendix should be helpful to the reader seeking quick solutions to the problem of concept operationalization.

Jerusalem A.Y.E.
December 1991

Acknowledgements

Many people provided the ideas and information necessary in this type of project. I am grateful for discussions held with many individuals and for comments and suggestions made by others: Morris Barer, Ann Crichton, Godwin Eni, Robert Evans, Maureen Law, Annette Stark, Andre Tourigny, and Dean Uyeno in Canada; Stuart Altman, Robert Brook, Marc Chassin, Donald Freeborn, Merwyn Greenlick, Jerrold Michael, Ira Moscovice, and Cyril Rosenman in the USA; Freda Eskin, David Hunter, and Maureen Dixon in the UK; Aad de Roo in the Netherlands. Ideas on the health systems in the Scandinavian countries were contributed by Richard Saltman and Mat Brommels, and information on the African countries was provided by Charles Nagbe and Emmanuel Osnu-Bosni. I am also grateful to many members of EHMA (the European Healthcare Management Association) for useful information on their respective countries.

I am specially indebted to many friends in Israel: David Chinitz who also wrote a chapter in the book (Chapter 12), Zeev Aahronson, Neta Bentor, Marc Cohen, Michael Davies, Rafi Roter. Bruce Rosen, Uzi Salant, Mordechai Shani, Yair Shapira, and Judy Shuval.

Donna Greenberg deserves special mention for her cheerful, patient, and efficient role in the production of the manuscript and Frances R. Warshaw Dadon for her assistance in editing.

Finally, I wish to remember my beloved mother, Shifra. Through the long weeks of her hospital stay at the Sloan Kettering Memorial Center in New York, she encouraged me to carry out this endeavour. In some sense, she forced me to finish it.

Contents

PART I

Concepts

1. Determination of the rules—definitions and concepts

Though it is complicated to investigate a health system, it is even more complicated to investigate and compare among health systems. In the preface, we discussed the importance of comparing health systems. As Victor Sidel (1981) put it, the comparative analysis of health systems is done to improve one's understanding of one's own systems and to learn from experience gained abroad. Such comparisons give us a broad perspective and enable us to pose questions that could not be answered by data from a single region or from a single country. For example, if only one country is examined, there is no way of evaluating the pros and cons of different methods for reimbursing physicians. The methods of several countries should be studied to discern the effects of various economic conditions or the influence of different perceptions of the physician's role. In addition, comparative evaluation allows us to understand the characteristics of the organization of health services, as some variables and their effects can be studied only by comparing different countries or regions. For instance, the so-called benefits of universal health coverage should be carefully evaluated in more than one health system. This is because these benefits probably depend on the particular organizational structures prevailing in each country, as well as on the culture and the economy. What may be considered advantageous in one health system can easily be disadvantageous in another.

Health systems do not only differ from each other; with time they also differ from themselves! This happens because modern societies change rapidly. Before 1948 there were private hospitals and private doctors in England. The enactment of National Health Insurance in 1948 turned this all into a National Health Service. Just a few decades ago, the health system in the US was dominated by private medicine. There were practically no other means for providing medical treatment. Today, social insurance programmes predominate and the central government, once removed from the business of health care, now controls substantial parts of the health care sector.

Having asked 'Why should we compare health systems?' we now ask 'When should we compare health systems?' The straightforward answer is: always. Continuously monitoring changes allows us to detect and identify longitudinal trends within and across systems. This makes comparisons more interesting but far more tedious and complex. In evaluative terminology, comparisons of this kind can be considered as 'Before–After' comparisons with 'control' groups. First, the experimental system is considered, then another system (or more) compared with the experimental system is the 'control' system. A change is introduced into the experimental system, the introduction of a new insurance programme, for example. The time before given changes occur is called the 'before' period; the time after the changes happen is called the 'after' period. Clearly, the change is introduced to the experimental system between the before and the after periods. Both the experimental and control systems are observed in both the before and the after periods. The difference (*D*) in the observed values can be quantitated as follows:

$$D_{BA} = (O_{EA} - O_{EB}) - (O_{CA} - O_{CB})$$

where

D_{BA} The difference in observed value between the control and the experimental groups over the time period BA.

O_{EA} The observed value of a variable for the *'experimental'* system in the after period.

O_{EB} The observed value of that variable for the *'experimental'* system in the before period.

O_{CA} The observed value of that variable for the *'control'* system in the 'after' period.

O_{CB} The observed value of that variable for the *'control'* system in the 'before' period.

Thus D_{BA} is the difference of two differences: the after–before difference in the experimental system minus the after–before difference in the control system. This formula reflects the dual character of the process of comparing health systems. The difference between systems and the difference within systems over time. Though the rationale is simple, there is a fundamental methodological difficulty in comparative health systems' research. It is difficult to find a study design where some variables can be held constant while others can be changed. For example, how does one evaluate the success of a new health insurance programme when several health systems are compared? How can the evaluation be effective when each system is characterized by diverse socio-cultural determinants and by different patterns of financing and reimbursement? Fortunately, some remedies to this problem are available as we shall later see. Before we can continue with our discussion of comparative health research, we must clarify the concepts underlying 'systems' as we shall do in the next section.

The systems approach

One of the major advances in human knowledge in the twentieth century is our increased ability to understand and manipulate the effects of several variables at once. The required skills and methods were first developed in the exact sciences and in engineering. Social scientists and, particularly, management experts were quick to borrow these methods for solving their own operational problems. To explain the interaction of multidimensional parameters in a social network requires that a *system* be well defined. Viewed holistically, a system is a patterned arrangement of activities and values presented in the form of measurable variables and linked by virtue of their contribution to a pre-stated common goal (Ackoff 1971). The systems approach consists, therefore, of the study and analysis of dynamic variables whose values change constantly due to their constant interaction. In this approach the elaboration of the dynamic equilibria between these variables is more important than the study of rigid structures with unchangeable magnitudes. The systems approach provides us with a framework for understanding how the parts making up the system are linked and function together to affect outcomes (Van Gisch 1974).

Social systems, the focus of our attention, are a special category of general systems. According to Miller (1965), social systems are characterized by three elements of 'systems thinking'. First, unlike most physical systems, the boundaries of social systems are flexible. They can be shifted as new social realities are recognized. This is clearly a reflection of the dynamic nature of a social system. Second, Miller claims that a single unidimensional representation cannot explain a social system, but a multidimensional representation is required. He asserts that because reality is so complex no single model can encompass the entirety of social reality. Only a model made up of several variables and their interactions, could explain the complexities of any social system. Third, according to Miller the systems approach assumes that all social systems be open. An open system effects its environment and is affected by it. The open system's outputs affect processes in its environment, and inputs from the environment affect the system's internal processes. Clearly, the openness of a social system stems from its multiple dimensionality and its flexible boundaries. A system with constantly changing boundaries and with many constantly interacting variables needs to be exposed to its external environment in order to remain viable.

Clearly, the systems approach requires the analysis of the system's dynamics as an integral whole. The goal is to build a model and then to measure its 'closeness of fit' to reality. Donabedian identifies the essential components of such a model as shown in Fig. 1.1 (Donabedian 1980). In the figure we see four levels: inputs, processes, outputs, and outcomes. The first step of model building is to identify inputs. Inputs, or 'structure' in Donabedian's terminology, include the characteristics of the providers of goods or services, the tools and resources they have at their disposal and the organizational settings in which they work. More generally, inputs are the human, physical, and financial resources available to the system.

The essence of the process is the transformation of the inputs into services or goods. Donabedian distinguishes between the organization of the

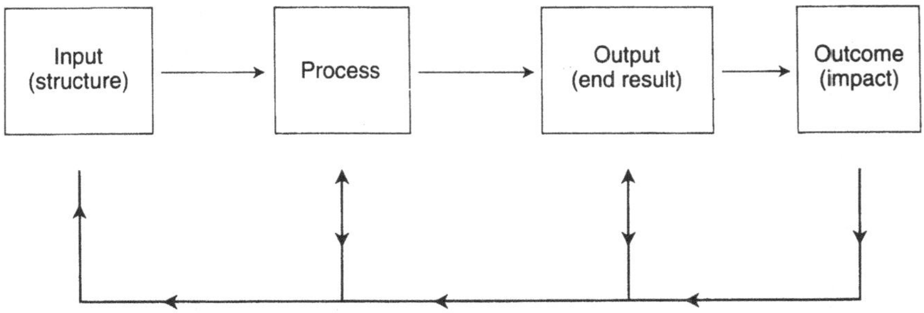

Fig. 1.1 The components of a system. (From Donabedian (1980), Chapter 3, with permission.)

activities of care, which he calls 'configuration' and the performance of these activities which he calls 'content'. Studying of the content may define the activities of the system so that the system's effectiveness in transforming resources into outputs and outcomes may be determined.

Output, or 'end result', and outcome, or 'impact', are distinctively different. Output is the end point of the process; it is the summary of achievement at the moment that the process ends. On the other hand, outcome is results oriented. In the context of health systems, Donabedian defines outcome as a change in a patient's current and future health status which can be attributed to a certain antecedent process of health care (Donabedian 1980). As an illustration of the concepts of output and outcome, consider the modules associated with an immunization programme. *Inputs* to the programme are the funding for running the programme, the manpower for facilitating the programme, and supplies and equipment like vaccines and syringes. The *process* consists of gathering appropriate recipients of the immunization and actually immunizing them. The *output* is the sum of the process, that is, how many recipients actually were immunized. And the *outcome* is the health impact of the programme including, perhaps, some unintended results like illness due to the vaccine itself.

Health systems

As Alan Dever (1980) puts it:

> The medical care systems are one element, or subsystem, within society which seeks to ensure the health of society's members. This subsystem interacts with other subsystems, in carrying out society's goals. In planning for the health system, we must concern ourselves with the interactions both within the system (medical care) and with other systems (lifestyle, environment, biology).

Based on this definition of a health system and its components, we can define a health care system as made up of an internal subsystem of health care and external subsystems. Field (1973) suggests the following conceptual definition: A health care system is:

> . . . a societal mechanism which transforms generalized resources or inputs into specialized outputs in the form of health services aimed at the health problems of the society.

According to Field, generalized resources include intangibles like the political mandate to plan and implement health programmes and health services. They also include tangible assets like professional manpower and physical means. Equally important are the economic resources needed to support programmes and plans.

Clearly, an operational definition for a health system requires a broad vision of society, its values, its resources, and its history. Weinerman (1971) suggested a model to explain the conceptual relationships in a health system. In the model, a stepwise approach is used to determine the influence of

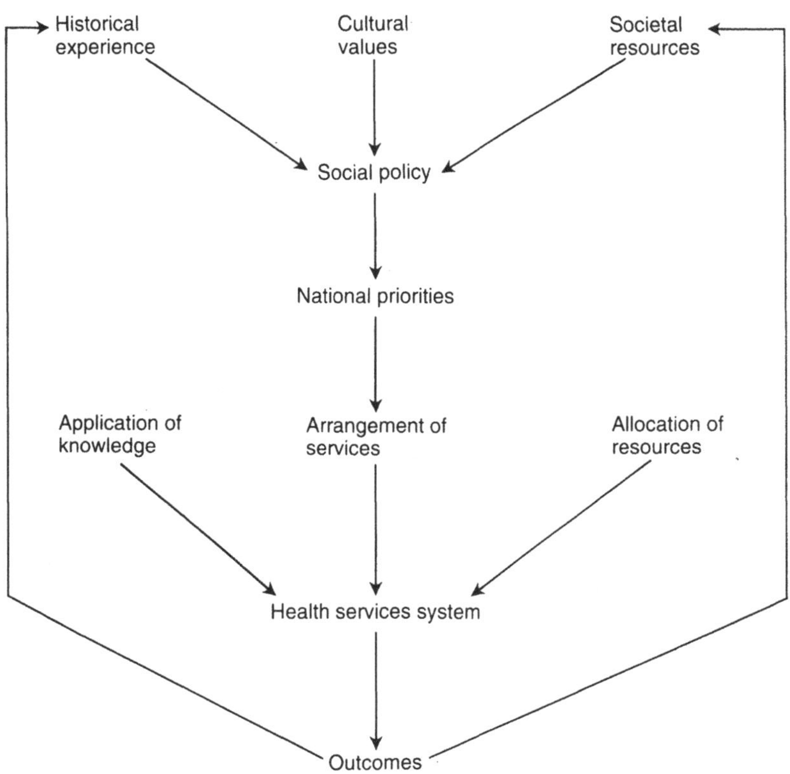

Fig. 1.2 Relationships in development of health services systems. (From Weinerman (1971), with permission.)

the several external factors on the health system. These external factors, which he calls primary factors, are wide societal attributes like historical experience, cultural and moral values, and the resources available to the health system. The interaction among these external factors constitutes a cornerstone in the establishment of a social policy leading to national priorities. In addition, as seen in Fig. 1.2 there are two more components for the production of a health system: professional knowledge and the appropriate allocation of resources.

Although the models cited above provide a conceptual basis for the definition of health systems, we have yet to address the major question relating to the mechanics of operationalizing the health system's conceptual framework. Such operationalization requires a set of measuring instruments which we shall study later. Prior to studying the characteristics of these measurement tools, we still need a broader outlook on health concepts. For example, as we shall discuss in the next section, these concepts often reflect the philosophy of 'where I stand depends on where I sit'. That is, they are seen differently by various health professionals.

The operationalization of health concepts

In this section, we shall concentrate on the problem of the operationalization of health concepts. A major difficulty in operationalizing concepts is the ambiguity of the concepts themselves. As an illustration, let us examine the popular health systems concept 'social medicine'.

During the 'Post-Industrial Revolution', in the second half of the twentieth century, a great number of new groups and organizations have evolved. The tremendous breakthroughs in communication and information systems that also took place have permitted an enormous increase in intergroup communications. Each group has its own benefits in mind, each has its own language. Thus, any definitions of a health concept, including that of social medicine, may depend on which group is defining it and how this group may interact with other groups.

In light of this problem, before we can define social medicine we must ask: Whose 'social medicine'? Politicians and decision-makers will probably answer differently than lay persons; Skilled health professionals would certainly answer differently than economists. Let us examine one of the early WHO definitions of social medicine. As described in Grundy and Mackintosh (1957):

As a comprehensive term, 'social medicine' is used to embrace:

(1) research into social factors which affect health by means of surveys, case studies and statistical investigations;

(2) the reciprocal relations existing between medicine and society (medical

sociology), including the collective responsibility of medicine to society for advising on social problems as they may affect health;

(3) social psychology and social psychiatry;

(4) the agencies of social therapeutics, i.e. social insurance and social aspects of health, medical care and welfare services.

With this definition, or more precisely this mixture of definitions, Grundy and Mackintosh try to satisfy everyone's tastes. Epidemiologists may easily accept article (1). Sociologists and lay persons may accept article (2). Psychologists, psychiatrists, and other behavioural scientists may be pleased by article (3). Finally, decision-makers, politicians, and administrators may welcome article (4).

The difficulty of defining this concept is further seen in several popular textbooks on 'social medicine'. In their *Introduction to Social Medicine*, McKeown and Lowe (1974) deal with contemporary health problems. They consider social medicine as concerned with problems like immunizations, genetic screening, and environmental control. They link social medicine to the action of public agencies in health care systems only as a second priority. On the other hand, Roemer defines 'social medicine' (1976) as exclusively concerned with the role of public agencies in the provision of health care. He complicates the definition even more by dividing agencies involved in 'social medicine' into those providing direct care and those involved in providing care indirectly by reimbursing providers of health care.

As seen from the example of social medicine, it is clear that the operationalization of concepts relating to a health system is a complex process. Keeping this reality in mind, we shall concentrate on this problem in the following chapters. However, any further discussion of an operational perspective requires the understanding of the concept of measurement. Thus, we focus on measurement and its characteristics in the methodological section below.

The concept of measurement

By definition, measurement, is the assignment according to specified rules of numerical values to objects, events or empirical facts. As an example of the measurement of empirical facts, '1' could denote those countries which have nationalized health insurance systems, and '2' could denote those countries without such systems. The definition of measurement requires that one clearly specify the objects to be measured, the range of values to be used, and the rules by which these values may be assigned to the objects being measured. Measurement in comparative health systems' analysis includes five major characteristics: quantification and scale, unidimensionality, reliability, validity, and sensitivity (Veney and Kaluzny 1984). We shall now discuss each of these characteristics in turn.

Quantification and scale

Quantification is the major characteristic of measurement. Three distinct categories of phenomena in health systems may be quantified:

1. Physical states and occurrences: for example, the number of physicians, the number of X-ray machines, or the occurrence of deaths and births. Among these phenomena, physical states are the easiest to quantify and thus to measure.
2. Performance and practice: these include reimbursement of health providers, money spent for financing the health system, and modes of staffing and allocation of authority and responsibility within health organizations. These phenomena are less easily quantified than physical states and occurrences, and thus selecting measurement is more difficult.
3. Attitudes, beliefs, and perceptions: these include the level of physicians' autonomy and attitudes towards health policy issues like the nationalization of health care services or the legalization of abortions. This last group of phenomena poses the most difficult constraints on measurement and require elaborate procedures for the operationalization of their underlying concepts.

There are four measurement scales relevant to our discussion of comparative health analysis:

(1) the *nominal scale*;
(2) the *ordinal scale*;
(3) the *interval scale*;
(4) the *ratio scale*.

A *nominal scale* only permits the distinction between similar and dissimilar. For example, nominal scales are typically used to measure sex, ethnicity, marital status, type of organization, and modes of paying the physician. Real quantification can be achieved only with an *ordinal scale*. Here, unlike the nominal scale, any numerical value used must be greater or less than any other numerical value in the scale. Ordinal scales are commonly used to measure attitudes, beliefs, and perceptions. The Likert Scale is a popular five point ordinal scale often used for measuring attitudes and perceptions. For each particular variable the levels on the Likert Scale are:

(1) strongly agrees
(2) agrees
(3) undecided
(4) disagrees
(5) strongly disagrees.

The Likert Scale is typically used to measure levels of satisfaction with a health service or programme, or attitudes towards a 'hot' health policy issue, like the legal status of abortions.

The two other scales, the *interval scale* and the *ratio scale* are similar in that positions on the scale are equidistant from one another. In addition, on a ratio scale all arithematical operations can be performed including multiplication and division, equivalent to assuming a real zero point in the scale. Among the measurements in comparative health systems' analysis that can be performed on ratio scales, include for example, the number of deaths and births across different regions, the volume of hospital beds, or the number of active physicians in various areas. Several other variables relating to performance and medical practice can also be measured on a ratio scale. For instance, in the comparison of health care organizations it can be used to measure the volume of drug prescription in various areas or the amount of money spent on each specific budget item in a budget of a health care organization.

Unidimensionality

For the sake of simplicity, many researchers attempt to analyse problems unidimensionally. Unidimensionality requires that for any particular phenomenon, only one numerical value to be assigned. In comparative health systems' analysis because health systems themselves are multidimensional many phenomena relating to health cannot be defined unidimensionally. For example, in the macro organization of health services, health systems have often been described as either free market or as social health insurance. But these two models need not be mutually exclusive. In many health systems, including that of the US, both types of models are found. So it is not possible to use a unidimensional scale to assign the numerical value '1' for a 'free market' type of health care system and the numerical value '2' for a 'social insurance' type of health care system. Because of this difficult problem, careful attention is required when operationalizing concepts. We shall discuss these problems in subsequent chapters.

Validity

Simply presented, the validity of a measure is the extent to which it assesses what it purports to measure. With respect to measurement processes, two major categories of validity can be described, *face validity* and *criterion validity*. *Face validity* is whether the measure being used to describe a phenomenon really describes it. In comparative studies, variables such as the per capita rate of physicians in a population or the incidence rate of myocardial infarction are valid measurements of real phenomena because they are easy to agree upon. Because who belongs to the nursing profession is variously interpreted in different countries, and similarly because neurological syndromes are ill-defined, the per capita rates of nurses in a population or the incidence of neurological syndromes are far less valid measurements.

Given a phenomenon for which a certain independent measure has been established as valid, *criterion validity* can be claimed for a second measure sharing a close relationship with the first. For instance, criterion validity can be used to establish the validity of the combination of the three measures of infant and child mortality, maternal mortality, and of age-specific mortality as a single valid index for community health status. Since community health status cannot be directly measured the face validity of each of these three separate measures is used to establish the criterion for the validity of their combination.

Reliability

Reliability or reproducibility is the extent to which multiple measurements of a given phenomenon produce similar results. Some countries have more reliable data than others which makes cross-comparisons difficult. In general, better reliability of data in a given country corresponds to the availability of more accurate sources of data and to the existence of a well organized data collection system. For example, figures on mortality are far more reliable in developed countries where information is gathered routinely, than in most of the developing countries where efficient data collection systems are lacking.

Sensitivity

The sensitivity of a measurement device is the extent to which it changes its value according to actual changes in the real world. If the changes measured are of the same order of magnitude as changes in the real world, then the measurement device is *sensitive*. Measurement devices available for cross-national comparisons are often not sensitive enough for detecting changes in health conditions. For example, mortality is often measured as a proxy for measuring health status. However, a wide range of health concerns are involved in the domains of the mental and social well-being. The use of mortality as a proxy for health status will be insensitive to changes in these domains. Using such a proxy could lead to erroneous conclusions about the actual health status of the population studied because only a few of the many dimensions of health could be highlighted for this population.

From concepts to indicators

Measurement involves measures, not of the concepts but of their properties (Kerlinger 1973). Measuring the properties of a concept requires the use of indicators. Indicators are observable phenomena that are inferred measures of concepts. Indicators can take several forms, these forms are determined by the scale used in a specific measurement. Typical indicators consist of one of the five following types: absolute numbers or values, rates, attributes, perception measures, and composite measures or indices. These five types of indicators will be now reviewed.

Absolute numbers

Very often numbers are used to assign values to indicators simply because numbers are easy to collect and to interpret. For instance, numbers are used to compare the size of the population served, or the number of dollars budgeted or of operations performed in health systems. However, there is a major problem with numbers as such. This problem is related to the problem of relative scales. The process of comparing can be hindered by the use of absolute numbers because numbers alone do not provide a 'common denominator' for comparative examinations. If only the absolute size of the physicians' community is known or if only the health budget in monetary terms is provided, little can be said on the effective and equitable distribution of resources by the system. These problems have lead to the use of *rates* as indicators.

Rates

A rate is the ratio of two measures like the rate of physicians per capita which is the ratio of the number of physicians in an area to its total population. Rates are useful for comparing across a number of countries or across regions of substantially different size, making them valuable for cross-comparisons. Rates used as indicators require that data be made available on interval or ratio scales. When this is not possible, other types of measures are necessary.

Attributes

Attributes used as indicators include such variables as sex, racial composition, and ethnicity. Attributes are generally measured on a nominal scale which can be used to distinguish between categories but not to order them.

Perception measures

In cross-comparisons, attitudes, beliefs, and knowledge are often reflected by perception measures. Perception measures can be used as indicators of several kinds generally defined along ordinal or interval scales. Typically, perception measures are used in needs assessment or in the comparison of political orientations across health systems and within them. A detailed discussion of perception measures can be found, for example, in Miller (1977).

Composite measures

Composite measures, also called indices, may be used to represent several separate indicators grouped by the user in a given predetermined combination usually in the form of an equation. Composite measures are most commonly produced by generating the weighted sum of a given set of measures. For example, the Z-score is a composite measure as shown below:

$$\text{The } Z\text{-Score: } Z = \sum_{i=1}^{k} Z_i$$

$$Z_i = \sum_{j=1}^{n} W_j Z_j$$

where:

Z_i = the index score for the ith case (region or country);

W_j = the weight for the jth variable;

Z_j = a standard score for the jth variable for the ith case (region or country).

A composite measure for mortality may include various variables related to mortality like infant mortality, maternal mortality, and age-specific mortality for several age groups. Such a composite measure is constructed by standardizing each mortality variable*, assigning a weight for its contribution to the measure, and then summing over all variables. Rather than producing a unidimensional measure, it produces a multidimensional measure reflecting several facets of mortality in a region or a country. In the simplest type of composite measure, the weights W_j for each variable j are equal, and the composite measure is the sum of the standard scores. Assigning unequal weights to the variables is necessary when it is clear that some variables contribute more than others to the phenomenon under study. For instance, when studying the effects of poor environmental conditions on mortality, one can increase the sensitivity of the mortality index by assigning more weight to age groups prone to environmental hazards. In such cases substantial weight may be assigned to infant mortality and to the mortality of older groups. Other techniques for constructing composite measures are also available. These will be discussed in relation to specific indices presented in later chapters.

* Standardized variables are evenly distributed around zero, the average value for all standardized variables.

References

Ackoff, R. L. (1971). Towards a system of systems concepts. *Management Science*, **17**, (11), 661–71.

Alan Dever, G. E. (1980). *Community health analysis—a holistic approach*, pp. 41–2. Aspen, Germantown, Maryland.

Donabedian, A. (1980). *Explorations in quality assessment and monitoring*. Chapter 3, Vol. 1, *The definition of quality and approaches to its assessment*. Health Administration Press, Ann Arbor, Michigan.

Field, M. (1973). The concept of 'Health System' at the macrosociological level. *Social Science and Medicine*, **7**, 763–85.

Grundy, F. and Mackintosh, J. M. (1957). The teaching of hygiene and public health in Europe. WHO Monograph No. 34, pp. 55–6. Geneva.

Kerlinger, N. G. (1973). *Foundations of behavioural research*, (2nd edn). Holt, Reinhart, Winston, New York.

McKeown, T. and Lowe, C. R. (1974). *Introduction to social medicine*, (2nd edn). Blackwell, Oxford.

Miller, D. C. (1977). *Handbook of research design and social measurement*, (3rd edn). David McKay, New York.

Miller, J. G. (1965). Living systems: basic concepts. *Behavioural Science*, **10**, (3), 193–237.

Roemer, M. I. (1976). *Health care systems in world perspective*. Health Administration Press, Ann Arbor, Michigan.

Sidel, V. (1981). International comparisons of health services: how? who? why? In *Critical issues in health policy*, (ed. M. Straetz, M. Liberman, and A. Sardell) Lexington Books, Lexington, Massachusetts.

Van Gisch, J. P. (1974). *Applied general systems theory*, p. 2. Harper and Row, New York.

Veney, J. E. and Kaluzny, A. D. (1984). *Evaluation and decision making for health services programs*. Prentice-Hall, Englewood Cliffs, New Jersey.

Weinerman, R. (1971). Research on comparative health service systems, *Medical Care*, **9**, 272–90.

2. Health systems—a critical analysis of existing and suggested models

Health systems are characterized by many complex interactions. The complexity of these interactions permits the creation of innumerable varieties of policies, delivery mechanisms and control mechanisms. Perhaps, the only axiomatic statement that can unify all health systems and their subdivisions would be that they differ from each other. Those differences are not due to chance alone, rather they are rooted in the organization of societies. Societal determinants and attributes which have shaped each system and geared it into its present pattern can be described in several ways as shown in the next section.

The attributes of health systems

In the following section, Roemer's model, perhaps the most basic account on the evolution of health systems, is presented. Roemer's taxonomy (1977) distinguishes between types of health systems by identifying four major attributes: the historical perspective, the political process, the socio-economic environment, and the cultural characteristics.

The historical perspective

First Roemer examines the historical background of the society and shows how it can shape the health system. It is well documented that as far back as Ancient Greece public agencies have been responsible for health care to individuals and groups (Roemer, 1977). However, to understand better the behaviour of contemporary systems, we can start with a discussion of the voluntary guilds of artisans established in the Middle Ages. Among other things, the guild members pooled their funds for the support of their sick and aged, thus sharing the responsibility for individual needs. Though concepts and practices may have changed, this pattern was similar to social insurance systems of our day. Guilds represented individual participation and shared responsibility.

In the Middle Ages charity was another avenue for health support. Often, but not always, charity was inspired by religious motives, and has provided support for health care delivery systems both directly and indirectly throughout the centuries. The direct participation of charitable organizations for the provision of health care in the Middle Ages and later centuries is well known. For many years, charity has been the principal actor in the medical field. Charitable organizations actually operated most hospitals, clinics, and other health institutions. Charity has also substantially contributed to the health field indirectly by assisting it financially and materially. With the industrial revolution, charity became the major financial resource for the emerging modern health system.

In the late nineteenth century a completely different approach was introduced. With the emergence of industrial mass-production Chancellor Otto von Bismarck in Germany adopted the first modern health insurance scheme. Free health care was provided to industrial workers with the aim that medical treatment would return them to work quickly. Economic benefits for employers and for society were implied by this arrangement. In 1911 a similar philosophy encouraged England's mine owners to introduce compulsory health insurance scheme for their mine workers only. In the early 1930s across the Atlantic a similar ideology guided Henry Kaiser to formulate the guidelines of the first social insurance plan in the US since then called the 'Kaiser Permanente' medical organization.

Later on, the philosophy of the welfare state opened new horizons. To quote Wolensky (1980), 'The essence of the Welfare State is government-protected minimum standards of income, nutrition, health, housing and education assured to every citizen as a political right, not as charity'. Then, governments were more motivated by political values than by economic incentives in their pursuit of policies to grant more benefits to the individual citizen. Consider, for example, the introduction of the first social insurance programme of hospital care for the whole population in the Canadian province of Saskatchewan in 1947. Within 14 years this programme was adopted by all of Canada with Quebec entering the system last in 1961. Between 1962 and 1971 the model was extended to include primary care services through the Medical Care Act adopted by all the Canadian Provinces. In practice, to achieve the adoption of this system by all the Provinces required the legislation enabling the central government to contribute over 50 per cent of the total operating costs to any provincial programme meeting certain specified criteria. Thus, provincial governments were encouraged to participate in the plan by financial leverage. In England, the establishment of the National Health Services (NHS) in 1948 threw the country into turmoil. The health services were transformed from a loosely-controlled pluralistic health system into a tightly supervised giant public health organization. As Britons often say, the NHS is the largest organization in Europe outside of the Red Army! This giant organization operates through a network of decentralized structures that include regions and districts. Except for a tiny share of private medicine, the NHS network encompasses practically everybody in the English health business, either directly as NHS employees, like hospital-based doctors and other personnel, or indirectly as NHS contractors, like pharmacists or general practitioners in the community. In contrast to the all-encompassing nature of the NHS, in 1989 the British Government proposed changes in the health system which may remove the hospitals from the NHS network (HMSO 1989). Similarly, the Scandinavian countries have used public funds to institute decentralized health authorities. These are subject to firm control by public representatives. In Sweden, for example, the national Government granted responsibility for the operation of the health system to the 23 county councils, whose members are directly elected. In Finland both primary care and hospital services are the responsibility of the municipalities (Brogren and Brommels 1990).

Across the ocean in the US, trends were remarkably different. The rise of individualism and decentralization in the US can be regarded as a reaction to the tight centralized control held by the British colonialists in the eighteenth century. Thus, for the newly-born health system, decentralization and the sacredness of individual freedoms have caused only minimal involvement of the federal government in the health field for nearly 150 years. The gradual increase of US Government involvement in regulating the market, and later in reimbursing for health services, has changed this traditional pattern. This is particularly true concerning financing mechanisms. However, the system still preserves several facets of a free market: government intervention primarily concerns only the health of the elderly and the underprivileged.

The political process

Roemer's second attribute, the political process, is in harmony with his first attribute, the historical perspective. Since 'today's politics are tomorrow's history', this division into two separate categories is merely a matter of convenience. Politics affect health systems in two ways: it may exert a direct impact on the health field in the formulation of health policies, or it may rather create situations of considerable consequences for the health system. As an example of direct health-oriented policies, let us consider the consequences of the Prospective Payment System (PPS), a programme recently established in the US. The PPS system provides incentives to contain costs for Medicare (for those over 65) and Medicaid (for the socially underpriviledged) patients by requiring fixed and specific rates to cover the acute/high hospital costs for each of the 467 'specific treatment groups', called Diagnosis Related Groups (DRGs), recognized by the plan. Though PPS has been in effect only a short while, lengths of stay have already substantially decreased. As a substitute for long hospital stays, hospitals have developed community-based out-patient services, particularly for diagnostic purposes (Schulz 1985; Feder *et al.* 1987).

The issue of tobacco taxation is a good example of an initially non-health policy affecting health. Between 1965 and 1975 several US local and state jurisdictions increased cigarette taxes by 55 to 130 per cent. It is uncertain whether the primary intent of this legislation was to raise revenues or to control cigarette use. But the effect over that decade was to lower cigarette consumption by 20 per cent (Warner 1977).

The socio-economic environment

Roemer's third attribute in the evolution of a health system is the economy. Generally, economic levels in their operational presentation, like the Gross National Product (GNP) per capita, are clearly related to some macro health indicators, like life expectancy or infant mortality (Maxwell 1981). Economic development can be not only followed directly, by direct macro indicators, but also indirectly using a variety of socio-economic indicators, notably educational or literacy levels, residential density, occupational status, or professional hierarchy. For example, an interesting relationship exists between a direct economic measure (income), an indirect socio-economic level (female literacy), and a health status outcome (infant mortality) as shown in Fig. 2.1.

For each income group in Fig. 2.1, there is a direct correlation between a lower infant mortality rate and a higher literacy rate among women for every country examined (WHO 1985).

Similar kinds of relationships were found at the individual level in more refined studies on the relationship between economic measures and health outcomes. For example, there is an inverse association between unemployment and health. Studies show that mortality, morbidity, and disability all increase with unemployment. These unfavourable health outcomes of unemployment are all extremely costly (Kasl and Cobb 1970; Marshall and

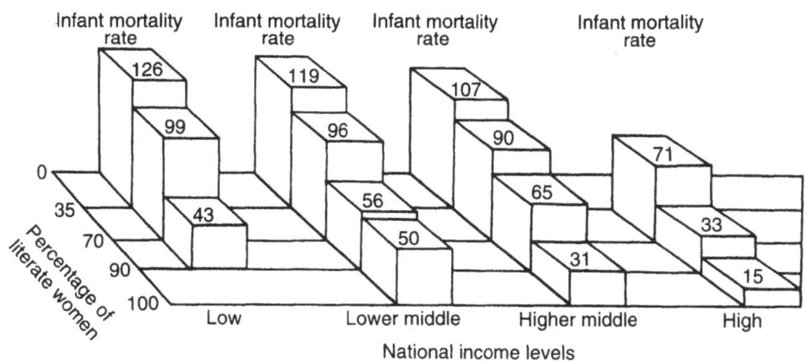

Fig. 2.1 Infant mortality and women's literacy, by broad income-groups. (Data source: WHO (1985).)

Funch 1979). Another example would be the connection between health status and the problem of economic barriers to health care. Among individuals with little or no access to the health system, health status was found to be very poor (Kleinman *et al.* 1981; Dutton 1986). Furthermore, though formally covered by the same medical insurance as everyone else, poor people often get poor service (Newachek 1988). At least in the US, it was suggested that poor women have little chance of receiving perinatal care (Aday, *et al.* 1980). Also, the poor were less likely to receive several preventive health services, including pap-smears, breast examinations, immunization, and dental care (Davis *et al.* 1981; Dutton 1986).

The cultural characteristics

Roemer's fourth attribute is somewhat more ambiguous because it relates to values and beliefs. Values are the inner drives used by society to accomplish its political and economic goals. Thus, it is necessary to understand the values and attitudes governing a society in order to scrutinize the development of its health system. Unfortunately, the multiple facets of societies make this task extremely difficult. Indeed, misinterpretation of societal values by health professionals seems associated with several conflicts that arise in health systems and often accounts for the low acceptability of health care plans by consumer populations. In many if not in all cases there is a mismatch between the structure of the health system and real health needs. Perhaps the most striking presentation of this phenomenon is in the case of the elderly. Elderly populations compose an increasing share of societies in Western countries; in most industrialized countries they average between 10 to 15 per cent nationwide but often amount for a substantially higher percentage of inner-city dwellers. Obviously, age makes the elderly vulnerable to disease and disability. Less obviously, old people often live isolated and alone which adds to their misery. There is a rather frequent transition of their social support networks. From extended families and close-knit supportive communities, self-sufficient elderly people are removed to isolated nuclear families, typically a one-person female household. Acutely ill elderly patients are generally cared for in the sophisticated system of modern hospitals. The need for social support as a substitute for the weakening family ties is rarely satisfied. There is a close association between social isolation, disease and premature death (Anderson and Cowan 1976; Clayton 1974; Helsing *et al.* 1981; Ellencweig and Karger 1983). The problem still continues to bear upon decision-makers at all levels of health systems and probably has been assigned a major priority in every developed health economy.

Another concern affecting society is the desire to achieve equality of access and quality of care. This is a basic need in many societies characterized by an uneven distribution of income and opportunities among socio-economic classes. The search for equality has been the major force in creating and developing national health insurance schemes in virtually all health economies. While the exact classification of these systems will be discussed later, it must be emphasized, at this point, that economic constraints were generally not the primary factors responsible for the development of social insurance plans. Rather these plans emerged as a result of social developments which were based on the concept of mutual assistance. In England, for example, social insurance legislation was enacted in 1911 by a reforming Liberal Government with Lloyd George as its leader. This Government decided that there must be a universal health insurance programme for insured workers. The decision, which later led to comprehensive insurance, namely the National Health Service (NHS) was based on the recognition that social justice can be achieved only if the entire society will support those who are in more immediate need. (USDHEW, United States Department of Health, Education and Welfare 1976).

Comparative analysis of health systems

For a long time, several researchers have been concerned with the striking differences between health systems' structure, modes of operation, and health outcomes. Particularly in the 1960s and the early 1970s, some imagined that the clue for the remedy for the distressing conditions in health systems lies in a better understanding of underlying concepts and their implementation in different environments and locations. The result of these concerns was a flood of several descriptive analyses of health systems, sometimes called comparative. To mention a few of the better descriptive studies, Roemer (1976) systematically reviewed several health systems while Anderson similarly compared the level of equity in three typical systems, in the US, England and Sweden (Anderson 1972). Fry (1970) considered the medical care system in the US, the Soviet Union, and the United Kingdom. Douglas-Wilson and Maclachlan edited an international survey of health systems (1974). Sidel and Sidel (1977) sought to remedy the crisis in the US health system by comparing it with health systems in both Western and Eastern blocks. Fry and Farndale (1972) published an international comparison of the organization of medical care as did Maxwell (1974). More recently, Raffel (1984), using a carefully planned scheme, made a descriptive analysis of 14 countries. Though his analysis is descriptive in nature, comparison between the different health systems is simplified because he used the same framework to analyse each country's health system. Similarly Saltman (1988) posed to his many authors identical questions on how their countries respond to the World Health Organization's 'health for all' strategy. Glaser has written a series of excellent international comparisons focused on different topics, notably physician reimbursement (1970), health insurance (1978) and the hospital system in different countries

(1987). Other authors have made impressive attempts to carry out careful comparisons of several health systems. In most cases, unfortunately, in each of these studies only a few facets of the health system or of health care delivery were examined. Some studies were focused on utilization (Kohn and White 1976) on the financing of health care systems (Abel Smith 1967, 1976) or on analysis of health care expenditure (Maxwell 1981). In a departure from studies based on the general population, Kane focused on the specific population of the elderly (Kane and Kane 1976).

Models for comparative analysis of health systems

There are a few different approaches toward the classification of health systems into categories. Eventually, in any taxonomy used in the literature, there was an attempt to group the 160 or more national health systems into much smaller clusters sharing similar features. While the rationale for such a process is sound, little can be done regarding the considerable variations still remaining within any group. The various taxonomies can be divided into three principal groups. In the following discussion, these groups are labelled:

(1) the health services approach;

(2) the health policy approach;

(3) the epidemiological model.

The health services approach

Roemer is undoubtedly the most outstanding advocate of the health services approach. In his earlier publications (Roemer 1976, 1977) he denotes five types of national health systems: the Free Market, the Welfare State, the Socialist, the Underdeveloped, and the Transition systems.

In a considerable effort to derive a common denominator shared by all national health systems of the same category, Roemer has put together some useful definitions. He views a Free Market System as an open market with minimal intervention of public agencies. 'Supply and demand' are thus determined by market forces only. For example, this was true for the US system until the last decades, before its partial conversion into a social insurance system, in which Government plays a role in ensuring that certain groups of people receive health care.

A Welfare State may be broadly defined as a system in which society assumes responsibility for health care. This results in equal access to the health care system regardless of an individual's ability to pay. The definition allows an extremely wide range of variations. For instance, in the same category are the English NHS on the one hand and the 1100 health insurance organizations (Sick Funds) in Western Germany on the other hand. Obviously there are tremendous differences between these two systems.

To mention a few, the government-owned and financed NHS is a gigantic provider of services to the entire population of England. In Germany, the mostly miniscule funds collect membership fees from their well-defined, limited memberships, but do not provide direct services, rather, these services are purchased from third party providers. In spite of these differences, Roemer's definition is broad enough to contain both these systems, and many others besides.

Roemer's third type, the socialist health systems, embodies the political principles of socialist economies. They are hierarchial and highly centralized systems owned by the Government and well co-ordinated with other public agencies. Naturally, the Soviet health system is the best example of this model. The hierarchy of branches derived from the Soviet Ministry of Health include the intermediate levels of a republic, province, district, counties, and localities, having all health employees on government salaries. The system is structured such that only the higher levels of hierarchy have a say about policies and needs. While information rises up the hierarchic ladder, decisions are made at the top level generally and flow down from top to bottom.

The fourth type in Roemer's health service model is the developing national systems, or, as he puts it, 'underdeveloped' national health systems. The wide variations between systems makes it difficult to define this category thoroughly. Roemer's implicit description of that group may be summarized in his explicit definition: 'a health system typical of the poorest economies, whereas the vast majority of the population is practically denied provision of reasonable modern health care.' (Roemer 1977.) Illustrative examples for this category abound in Africa and South East Asia. For instance, Roemer (Roemer 1985, p. 50) has calculated the percentage distribution of health expenditures for one developing country in Latin America. He showed that only 18 per cent of the population used as much as 70 per cent of the health resources, while only 30 per cent were available for the other 82 per cent. Even taking account of their low per capita GNP, developing countries tend to spend proportionally less on health than do the more affluent countries. This makes the situation even worse for most of the population in these developing countries. The combination of a low per capita income and a tiny share of national resources allocated to health is often disastrous.

Roemer's fifth type, transitional systems, is poorly defined. Into it he groups practically all countries which have some but not all features of the previous categories. In Roemer's taxonomy transitional health systems include national health systems in transition from the state of a developing economy to that of an industrialized economy. Such conditions prevail in Latin America, some Middle-Eastern countries, and in some of the more affluent South East Asian societies. The impression remains that this group is suggested as an escape to group those countries which just don't fit into either categories. Perhaps because of this, it includes bizarre combinations such as China and Brazil.

While Roemer's pioneer classification helps us understand both trends and developments in health systems, it suffers from two major weaknesses. First, the basic definitions of the five groups are not similarly balanced. On the one hand a free market system, a welfare system, and a socialist system all represent a sound philosophy of care which has evolved into a delivery system. On the other hand, the cluster of the developing and transitional types are essentially cross-sectional snapshots of systems not bound by any philosophy or ideology. Second, this classification model does not fit well with the four basic attributes of Roemer's taxonomy. For instance neither socio-cultural nor economic differences play a role in assigning national systems into clusters. To remedy some of the shortcomings of his early model, Roemer and his associate proposed a modified model, the health services system model (Roemer 1985, p. 35–8; Kleczkowski *et al.* 1984). Later on, Roemer suggested the classification of national health systems by economic levels and by health system policies (Roemer 1989). The first modified model retains the three structure-oriented clusters which have somewhat different names: laissez-faire (free market), co-operative (welfare), and socialist (centrally planned) systems. Then it divides each into three sub-categories based on the system's economic strength. These sub-clusters are defined as affluent (industrialized), moderate (developing), and poor (underdeveloped). In all, this classification scheme generates nine groups presented in a matrix form (Table 2.1). The authors emphasized that they would like a further extension into a third dimension, cultural-political, but admit that this is not possible since indicators for political orientations are not available for many countries. In the more recent modification (1989), economic development is classified into four levels determined by the annual

Table 2.1 National health systems: typology based on national economic levels and health system organization

	Degree of health system organization		
National economic level	Modestly organized	Moderately organized	Highly organized
Developed (affluent)	1 USA	2 FRANCE	3 ENGLAND
Developing (transitional)	4 VENEZUELA	5 MEXICO	6 CUBA
Least developed (poor)	7 SUDAN	8 KENYA	9 VIETNAM

Source: Kleczkowski, B.M. *et al.* (1984)

Gross National Product per capita. In addition, a remedy is suggested for the lack of a political component. Roemer develops gradations along a political scale determined as 'entrepreneurial', 'welfare-oriented', 'universal', and 'socialist'. In all, countries are divided into sixteen groups.

A similar approach has been used by Terris (1980) who takes a set of three basic delivery criteria as a guideline for clustering systems. These underlying principles divide groups of national systems into public assistance systems, health insurance models and national health service systems. Field (1980) uses a similar approach in dividing health systems into five types which he calls: anomic, pluralistic, insurance/social security, national health service and socialized. In a more recent classification Field (1989) suggested six characteristics to analyse health systems: the general economic definition of health care, the position of the physician within the system, the role of professional associations, the ownership of facilities, the method of the payment from the recipient of care to the caregiver and the role of government. A health system is then classified into one of five types according to the proportionate levels of these six characteristics.

Abel-Smith (1972) focuses on the physician, the provider of primary care. Here, the basis for the comparison of health systems is the relative independence of the physicians within the system. By 'independence' Abel-Smith means the degree of autonomy of the primary care physician. For example, in the 'American system' the physician has complete responsibility whenever he sees the patient at the hospital or at his office. In the 'Western European' model there are both primary care physicians who retain their private offices out in the community, and also a separate group of salaried, hospital-based doctors who assume hospital care responsibilities. Finally, according to the 'Eastern European' model, physicians are all salaried, public employees and are grouped in a strict hierarchic pyramid. Even in cases of professional disagreement, individual physicians must obey the medical directives of their superiors.

The limitations of the health services approach

The main thrust of the health service model is the identification of various components in a health system. Then the model is engaged in the development of criteria for the classification of each national system into clusters on the basis of a cross-sectional assessment of each component. Two major weaknesses characterize the approach. First, there is an implicit effort to converge the multifaceted profile of a health system into a rather unidimensional presentation. Unfortunately, this is quite impossible if one envisions the many dimensions of health. There are too many effects within the inner system of health care delivery, and those are amplified by several external influences, such as the environment, human biology, and life styles. This simplistic approach can hardly be an accurate classification of the 'real' world. The mere evidence that in most cases there is no perfect 'national' representation of a health system further weakens the validity of the approach for analytical comparisons. For example, the US system is generally considered a free enterprise system; however, welfare programmes such as Medicare and Medicaid lie definitely within the scope of socialized medicine, a model found widely in welfare and even in socialistic economies. Even more homogenous health systems show similar idiosyncrasies, such as the case for private beds (pay beds) in UK NHS hospitals, a demonstration of free enterprise within a classical welfare state pattern (Weller and Manga 1983).

The other deficiency of the health system approach concerns their indifference to time trends. The inability to reflect longitudinal changes in a system, results in a static presentation which often distorts the real processes in health systems. If the model is static and the reality of the health scene is changing, the model is no longer a reflection of reality. A striking example of this incompatibility between model and reality can be seen when examining the recent developments in the Chinese health system. At present this system can hardly be presented as traditional or even as a 'poor' socialist. In a short time, the Chinese people have managed to reform their health system completely. It now consists of a variety of exciting experimental patterns. Indeed, until the economic reform of 1980, especially in rural areas, mere collectivism, with barefoot doctors as its mainstay, reigned in socialist China. After 1980, the health system was abruptly turned into a pluralistic mix including substantial free enterprise. Various health workers now have set up private practices, and they charge patients on a fee-for-service basis and even selling them drugs (Hsiao 1984).

The contrasting case-study approach

A departure from the health services model was suggested by Elling (1974, 1980) and his collaborators (Elling and Kerr 1975). These authors realized that traditional approaches for comparing health services are inadequate for two reasons. First, available data are difficult to use. Secondly, even if data are available and usable, there remains the problem that traditional studies use cross-sectional design and lack procedures for updating. The immediate alternative, to achieve comparability by narrowing the scope of the analysis, does not seem too rosy either, because if a study is to focus on just one aspect, only one facet of a system may be studied. Therefore, Elling has suggested a modified health services approach which is appropriately named 'the contrasting case-study approach'. As defined by Elling and Kerr (1975) it involves: 'identifying countries that contrast in health achievement but are similar in levels of resources and perhaps general political organizations (although this last factor may be so closely linked with variations in health systems that its "control" would be difficult) and selecting in-depth studies of contrasting cases through:

(1) examination of available data and studies; and
(2) field studies designed to obtain data according to a specified framework.'

To establish his model, Elling draws an elaborate scheme (Fig. 2.2). The model identifies economic wealth and education as the two primary factors affecting health systems. Once these factors, called 'context' variables, are controlled for, it is possible to analyse differences between systems that 'contrast in health achievement but are similar in the level of resources and perhaps general political organization' (Elling and Kerr 1975). The model comprises two levels:

(1) inputs to the health care system in the form of the health planning apparatus, and the patterns of the delivery system;
(2) objectives, primary and secondary.

Related to the health status, primary objectives are diverse outcome measures that aim only at reducing mortality, morbidity and disability. Secondary objectives are determined by a wider set of societal attributes. These include environmental pollution and life styles, sophistication about health and health services, that is a greater access to a basis of knowledge, satisfaction with care, appropriate utilization of health care, and a better co-ordination and integration of services. Elling agrees, however, that all the parts of the model can be put together only ideally. In practice, he focuses his analysis on narrowly-selected resources and health information for contrasting countries.

Blanpain *et al.* (1978) take a very similar approach in their study of national health insurance in five European economies. Following an initial presentation of the five systems, the authors delineate their case for comparison. It consists of inter-system comparisons based on national policies regulating and controlling the volume of health resources, the spatial distribution of resources and the system's 'structuring'. This 'structuring' is the degree to which specialized and fragmented resources have been formally structured and integrated to function as a comprehensive delivery system. Though some interesting conclusions as to the relative achievements in specific areas were presented, the authors were not able to satisfy the curiosity of those interested in the ultimate question: was any country doing better?

The limitations of the case-study approach

The case-study approach is easy to apply but severely limited by the simplicity of its preliminary assumptions. In order to compare health systems internationally, the countries in which the health systems are found must be reasonably comparable in their external influences and appropriately

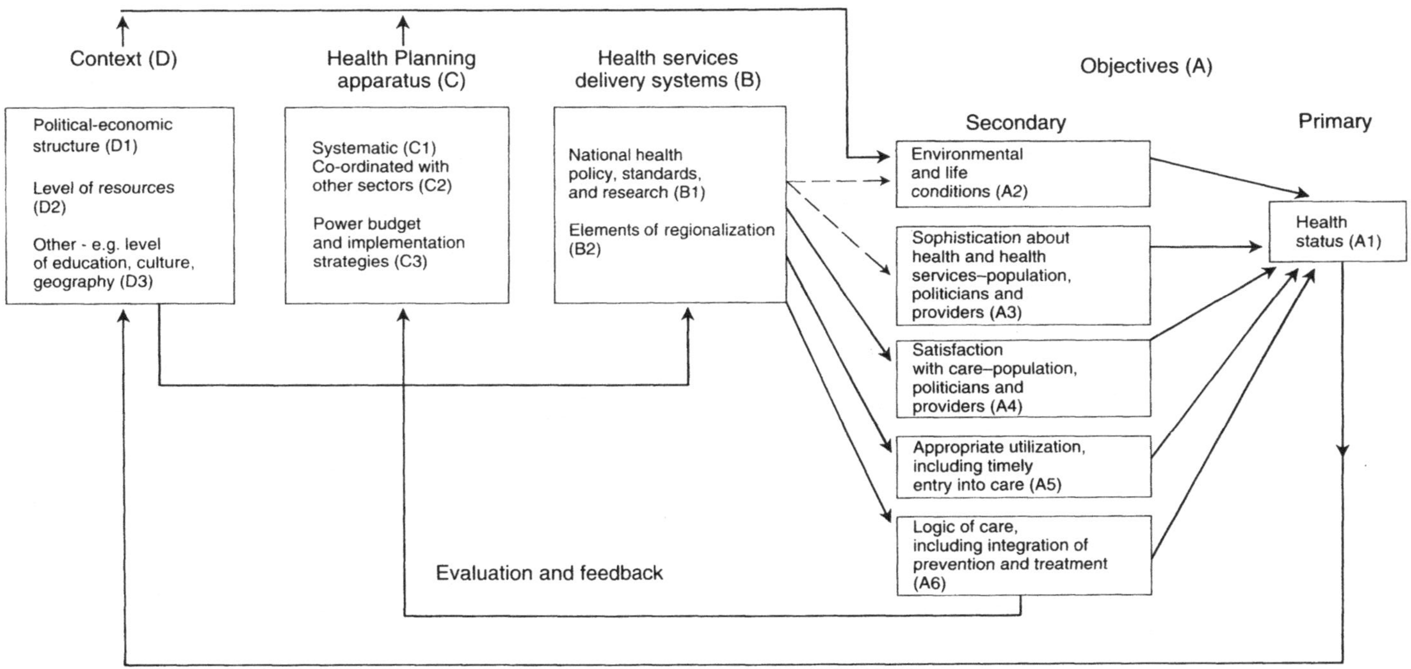

Fig. 2.2 Major blocks of variables and flow of influences in health systems. (From Elling (1980)), with permission.)

chosen. Because they represent external influences, Elling, for example, assumes that economic wealth and education can be used as indicators for country selection. Based on that assumption, he goes on to assume that for countries with similar levels of such external influences, the differences between the health systems can be seen as directly due to intrinsic factors within the health systems themselves.

This simplification masks the real prevailing conditions in health systems. Consider, for example, the United States and Canada, which are very similar with respect to both the educational attainment and the wealth of their populations. The large differences between their health systems, however, can be explained by external influences not included in Ellings' assumptions, like the political climate and differences in historical development.

Furthermore, the case-study approach, while methodologically sound for qualitative comparisons, is far less effective in the quantification of the elements presented for each case. Thus, while good for drawing an overall picture of the developments in a health system it does not permit scrutinizing the details of several systems simultaneously.

The political–economic approach

The political–economic approach is a policy-oriented model which has been adjusted to distinguish between health systems. The classification is goal-oriented and is largely based on the assumption that national health systems really do manifest clear-cut ideologies. Following Rodwin (Rodwin 1984) these ideologies are either conservative, liberal, or radical. The conservative perspective emphasizes the achievement 'equality makes the law'; that is, government intervention is supported only for the maintenance of the law and prevention of coercion. Quite naturally, consumer sovereignty is the guiding principle of this approach (Culyer *et al.* 1980). In the liberal perspective, Government is viewed as a mediating force that aggregates individual preferences into a policy reflecting the interests of large sectors of the population. In doing so, the Government may assume responsibility for the provision of services to the population. This is in sharp contrast to the 'never intervene' philosophy of the conservative approach. The overall goal of policy-setting in a liberal perspective is therefore one of achieving 'equality of opportunities'. The radical perspective aims at targets rather then means; it may justify massive state intervention, whatever its cost, in order to accomplish the ultimate goal, which is 'equality of results'.

For these three perspectives there are many implications in reference to health policy. Under a conservative philosophy planning is critically rejected as an unjust intervention that can endanger the uniqueness of a free market. Therefore, the conservative view would support a free enterprise system in which only two types of actors play: free vendors (the professionals) and free buyers. The interaction between these two groups is shaped by market forces. In its 'purest' representation the free enterprise ideology accommodates a system made up solely of completely independent buyers or vendors, thus precluding any professional organizations at all (Friedman 1962). The model also supports free competition in several professional disciplines so that non-physicians may be encouraged to engage in certain types of medical activities, until then not permitted. Thus, the model provides strong advocacy for the practice of nurse practitioners as a substitute for the physician, and for authorization of chiropractors and paramedics. The free market principle is preserved regarding buyers, but strong co-ordinative mechanisms are set for the supply function. In this way binding mechanisms are set for professional eligibility, price setting, and referral systems. A second option of the conservative model is based on professionalism and advocated the formation of professional groups. This option is fully supported by medical associations, particularly by the powerful American Medical Association (AMA). This model is an accurate reflection of vast sections of the present American health care system. By adopting this option, society accepts professional rather than consumer dominance as the guideline for setting the rules for 'equality under the law.'

As previously stated, the liberal perspective recognizes that the medical market is not a perfect economic system. Society is urged to believe that the establishment of 'equality of opportunities' cannot be left to market force alone but requires some government intervention (Culyer 1973). To achieve this end, the liberal view supports state intervention in order to increase rationality in the resource allocation process, to enhance equity among members of society, and to promote accountability of successes and failures in the health system. The guiding principle of intervention is the improvement of the health of the population at large (Culyer *et al.* 1980). The Welfare State concept is often associated with the liberal perspective. In practical terms it urges the establishment of national health insurance organizations like the British NHS, or of nationally guided insurance agencies like the state controlled voluntary sick funds in West Germany, the Netherlands, and Israel.

The radical perspective presents a classless co-operative society which abolishes exploitation and dominance. In a health scenario this perspective may lead to deprofessionalized medicine as suggested by Illich (1975) who argues for self-care, self-reliance, and full consumer control over the health services. According to his controversial philosophy, only in this way can we remedy the damages to our health which he claims are caused by modern medicine. This damaging intervention by modern medicine to our health he calls 'iatrogenesis'. Obviously, Illich's course can hardly be accepted by any national policy-makers even radical ones. It is not surprising that in practice most radically-oriented ideologists have chosen other avenues for the provision of health care, most often socialized medicine.

Under a system of socialized medicine equity is guaranteed by central planning and by mobilization of all resources by the State. Both the input and the process of health care are thereby strictly controlled to accomplish the end of 'equality of results.' Implementation of a policy based on socialized medicine is not only a matter of ideology. From a practical perspective, models of socialized medicine adopted by some western countries, like England, Sweden, and Finland, do not much differ from those that prevail in communist countries. The most plausible example is a comparison of the NHS in England and the Soviet Health system. Both are centrally planned and regionalized; they both follow a strict hierarchy of command and control. All employees in the Soviet system as well as a vast majority of the NHS are salaried. The several dissimilar dimensions often consist of undercurrents to which the political economic model is insensitive. The manner in which physicians and other health care workers are socialized are very different in the two systems (Anonymous 1987). In England, for example, physicians are trained to have professional autonomy and to exercise freedom of clinical decision-making. In the Soviet Union physicians are more dependent on the professional hierarchy in making their clinical decisions. For example, the volume of surgery and of other clinical procedures in the Soviet Union, are controlled by physicians at a high echelon of command like chief doctors in hospitals (Field 1989).

A critique of the political-economic model

While the analysis of health systems by the health services approach is static, the political-economic approach characterizes systems from a dynamic perspective which encompasses the historical process and the political and economic arena. However, the political-economic approach is too conceptual and lacks tools for comparing elements making up the health system. For example, in its original form, there are no tools for comparing utilization profiles between countries. Some researchers have tried to make the political-economic model more operational by moving from the theoretical level to the more tangible level, the health system itself. Reinhardt (1980), for example, has suggested a political-economic model through which he investigates different health insurance systems from a multidimensional perspective. The model compares the insurance arrangements in Canada, France, and West Germany in terms of their administration of care, the role of private insurance, reimbursement, financing, etc. Though Reinhardt succeeded in making some concepts of the political-economic model operational, its general application to cross-national comparisons remain unwieldy. This is why the model has acquired a relatively high popularity among scholars while use of its underlying concepts in decision-making arenas has been negligible.

The case for an epidemiological perspective

In a health systems context, epidemiologists look for associations between health status, disease, and related factors in a population. The classical epidemiological model embraces a single cause and a single effect and would be appropriate for the analysis of the effects of many infectious diseases. The typical cause for action is that contamination with a causal factor will result in an effect-specific disease caused by a microorganism.

The unidimensional association is not suitable for more intricate scenarios that require, in epidemiological terminology, a multi-causal model. In such circumstances a variety of causes, possibly interrelated, produce a variety of effects each associated with a single or with multiple causes. This situation, by and large, prevails in the typical disease profile of the late twentieth century. Chronic conditions such as coronary arterial disease, cerebral arterial disease, diabetes, angina pectoris, and others, are each caused by many agents. These include hereditary factors, varying ethnic susceptibility, environmental exposure, both physical and social, and lifestyle attributes (e.g. smoking, nutrition etc.). For instance, coronary heart disease (CHD), the major killer of modern society, is associated with four major risk factors contributing to the increased incidence of CHD: cigarette smoking, a diet rich in cholesterol and saturated fats, high blood pressure, and diabetes (Kannel and Gordon 1974). The longitudinal study which established this association suggests also that genetic predisposition plays some role in the development of CHD. It is clear that this type of analysis is useful in establishing the multi-causal factors responsible for a single effect.

Actually, one should also consider the opposite reasoning, that is, a single factor causing multiple effects. The most spectacular argument of this sort is the case against tobacco smoking. Numerous studies showed a direct causal relationship between smoking and the onset of several conditions. For example, relative to non-smokers, 45–65 years old, men who are heavy smokers have a cardiac mortality rate four times higher, as well as a fifteen times higher probability of developing lung cancer (USDHHS, United States Department of Health and Human Services 1982). The risk for developing other types of cancerous malignancies are similarly higher for cigarette smokers compared with the risks among non-smokers or among those who have ceased to smoke. The risk of lung cancer was reduced to that for non-smokers, fifteen years after smokers stopped smoking. A similar reduced risk is observed for cancer at other sites also associated with smoking (USDHHS 1982).

Eventually, one sees that in real situations numerous causal agents contribute to a variety of multiple effects. It is, therefore, the task of the epidemiologist to discern the various effects, to control for confounding influences, and to identify the causal associations between agents and outcomes appropriately. In effect, the modern epidemiologist usually deals with a disease system of the 'modern era', usually a chronic condition, like hypertension or diabetes, or an 'epidemic' of a new type, like road accidents or AIDS. These disease systems are typically open systems affected by a variety of true variables characterized by confounding relationships that make the issue even more complicated.

Do health systems share the basic principles of a disease system? Can health systems be investigated epidemiologically? The answer is unambiguously yes. As Ibrahim states, 'Epidemiology is the investigative science concerned with the search for causes of disease, disability, or death through organized collection and analysis of data about the human population.' (Ibrahim 1985). If so, then a simple rationale will gear it also to 'the estimation of the magnitude of health problems in communities and the planning and evaluation of intervention programmes with the ultimate outcome of improving health status of populations.' (Ibrahim 1985).

A practical approach, however, requires more than a mere conceptual framework. Such an approach requires the operational definitions for causes and effects and the means to carry out an analysis of their interdependence. In the following section of this chapter, previous attempts to operationalize a multiple cause–multiple effect model for use in health services research are described.

The epidemiological perspective

There are a few examples of studies in the literature in which authors used an epidemiological rationale in formulating models for national health systems. It is interesting that researchers did not generally envision their models as 'epidemiological', but rather they applied the terms 'sociological', or 'planning' presumably depending on their professional backgrounds. However, these models are based on definite epidemiological principles. For example Weinerman's model (1971) which we mentioned in Chapter 1, has been further developed by de Miguel (1975). De Miguel divided the health system into four subsystems. These consist of the Individual subsystem, the Institutional subsystem, Society, and 'Larger Systems'. Each subsystem is made up of a variety of causal factors as depicted in Fig. 2.3.

Factors like political structure, socio-cultural patterns, and economic development, in addition to demographic structure, represent the 'society subsystem' while 'institutions' reflect factors like the organization of health services, resources available for health services, and health planning. The 'individual' level comprises psychological factors, biomedical factors and health status. Finally, 'larger systems' refers to the environment. Two interesting features characterize the model: first, it consists of a multi-level analysis of health systems, thus establishing the concept of multidimensionality in the evaluation. This is presumably a step ahead of the unidimensional models which were typically centred in monolithic structures. Secondly, it uses, rather unintentionally, an epidemiological approach, by

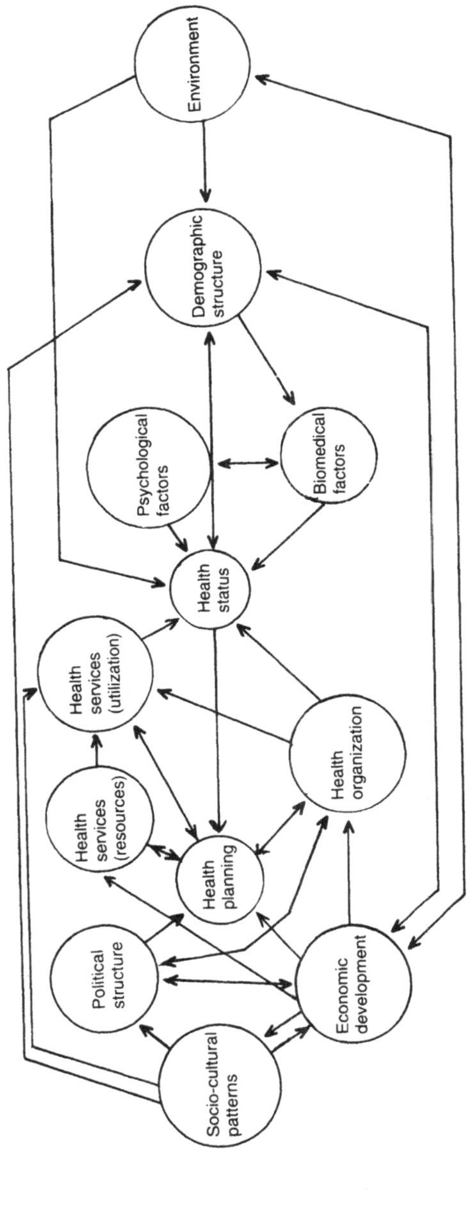

Fig. 2.3 Causal model for health systems. (From de Miguel (1975), with permission.)

assigning causal effects to a variety of factors and by studying the interrelationship between several effects and their causes. For instance, health status is presented in the model as an effect but it truly has a dual character since it also exercises causal influences on other factors, namely the demographic structure and the planning system.

Convergence or divergence

The epidemiological approach hints at possible solutions to problems in cross-comparing national health systems. There is, however, another major problem that has not yet been addressed: do health systems become more similar or do they become less similar with time? That is, do health systems converge or do they diverge? In a hypothetical spectrum of conceptual reasoning, one can find at one end those who support the hypothesis that health systems tend to converge over time. At the other end are those who promote the idea that the evolution of existing health systems will be in the direction of further divergence. Among the strongest advocates of convergence are Marc Field and David Mechanic. Field (1978) perceives the increasing intervention of governments in health systems as an indicator that socialized structures will become more dominant within the health system. Once systems become more socialized, they then tend towards convergence for two reasons:

(1) they have adopted similar philosophies;
(2) there is a gradual structural reorganization such that they become more similar operationally.

On the other hand, Mechanic (1975) conceives that enhanced conversion is caused by developing technology and widespread expectations nourished by the breakthrough in information systems. As Mechanic stated:

> In summary, I have argued that in response to developing technology and knowledge and rising expectations, modern nations are converging in ensuring greater equity in medical care, in organizing services in relation to the needs of defined communities, in integrating the fragmented components of health service, in developing new modes of providing primary medical services, and in attempting to increase the efficiency and effectiveness of the health care system as a whole.
>
> (Mechanic 1975)

Several authors do not believe that this rosy picture is possible. Marxist theorists like Navarro and Elling despair of convergence to an equitable structure. They blame rich capitalist systems for milking the poor and the underprivileged. They argue that the developed economies are oriented to pillage the Third World (Elling 1980, pp. 80–9; Navarro 1986). Thus, within each system, the rich benefit at the expense of the poor, and even between countries, wealthy countries benefit at the expense of poorer ones.

Destabilization of the already weak health systems in developing countries is caused by the migration of their trained physicians to wealthier countries.

Other researchers, believing in divergent trends, have limited their analysis to an empirical level and conclude that there is ample evidence from cross-national comparisons that developmental trends in health systems suggest divergence. For example, Blanpain *et al.* (1978) conclude that for the five European economies that they have studied, the rather similar developmental stages did not yield similarity in the systems' organization:

> Although they have passed through identical stages in health resources development, the countries have not always moved in phase with one another. Each has progressed at its own rhythm, thereby obtaining opportunities to learn and profit from those further ahead in the sequence at any given moment. Germany's system of sickness insurance acted as a model for a number of other European countries. The reaction of organized medicine to the pattern of policy development also indicates a cross-fertilization on positions and tactics among physicians of different countries. By and large, however, none of the countries systematically evaluated neighbouring systems.
> (Blanpain *et al.* 1978, p. 211)

In several publications Roemer (1976, 1977) suggests that systems move on different tracks even though their political economic orientation may be similar. Glaser, in his trichotomy on cross-national hospital systems (1987), on bargaining processes in insurance systems (1978), and on methods to remunerate physicians (1970), also concludes that systems frequently diverge rather than converge.

A rationale for an alternative approach

The conflicting arguments in the literature show that convergence of health systems is not within grasp. Whether convergence theorists might be right in the future or not may be of great concern to ideologists and philosophers but is beyond the rather practical, narrower scope of this book. If the various health systems were to converge, then they would be similar enough to permit their analysis by a simple unidimensional model. However, since *convergence* is not expected in the forseeable future, we are left with a largely unsolved problem. How can we accurately compare systems, or assess different parts of a multisystem in a divergent, multidimensional environment? A distressing comment by Dumbaugh and Neuhauser (1979) summarizes the state of the art: 'Perhaps we are a long way away from the multidimensional modelling that could be the basis for comparative medical systems' analysis. Hopefully that day will come within our lifetime.'

Though there is no immediate remedy for this problem, can we relieve at least some of the agony? A possible alternative is the *modular approach*. A modular model is made up of a number of separate modules which can be grouped together as needed. Symbolically, it shares the characteristics of the popular children's product—the magic 'Lego' bricks. One can use the whole set of 'Lego' to build a dream castle: but for those who are unable to complete an elaborate structure, or for those who do not need the entire set, only a few bricks will suffice. With respect to health systems, the message is unambiguous. Comprehensive cross-comparisons of systems might be desirable but are often beyond reach. The study of longitudinal trends is similarly limited. However, we can still make several comparisons that can be valuable on a narrower perspective, even when only a few modules are available for comparison. The big advantage of the modular approach is that it can be used for solving problems of various sizes. From the many modules making up the system, appropriate modules may be chosen for each problem to be solved.

Obviously, the most restrictive factor in the application of any model is lack of appropriate data. We should only use modules for which comparative data are available. Moreover, even when data are available it is difficult to compare systems when data are not properly standardized or when their validity or reliability are questionable. So, in any given instance, some modules may not be usable for comparison. However, unlike some other models that collapse when data are missing, modular models do not. Modular models are thus more flexible because they are based on comparisons between modules rather than between entire systems.

The modular approach has yet another benefit. One does not have to gather enormous quantities of information if only a handful is needed. For example, those interested in health manpower can simply ignore those modules not concerned with manpower without jeopardizing the possibility for a cross-national comparison. Thus they only need modules containing data about per capita physicians or nurses, but not on the number of available X-ray machines or information about abortion policies.

In the last section of this chapter, we will briefly discuss the modular approach for health systems. The division of the model into modules is based on features already described in the literature that generally had not been formerly separated into clarified units. In subsequent chapters, we shall discuss each module in turn.

Overview of the modular approach

There is an old story about a group of ten blind men in India who were asked to describe an elephant. Since each blind man was located at a different part of the animal's body, they produced ten different descriptions of the elephantine system. Each claimed to have a unique understanding of the system, and an argument ensued.

Many, perhaps too many, health professionals are like the blind men in the story. Familiarity with only portions of the system creates a false and distorted picture of the whole. In this section, we seek a complete model of health systems, which can be used for a comparative analysis of different health systems at a national or at a regional level.

The overall model for health systems is depicted in Fig. 2.4. The figure presents the aggregates of modules contributing to the dynamics of the health system and their causal relationships. Each 'box' in Fig. 2.4 corresponds to a single 'module'. The cornerstone of the model is the principle of producing an outcome by transferring resources through a controlled process. First analysed is the perspective of the consumer, leading to population needs. Then, there are two kinds of modules contributing to inputs which consist of resources and the socio-economic development. Resources include manpower, facilities, commodities, and the financial assets, which are presented in our model as the 'direct effects' of the socio-economic development. On the other hand, the indirect effect on inputs (see Fig. 2.4), is made up of political orientations, the administrative structures of the health system, and the cultural and religious characteristics of the society.

Another set of modules deals with health care delivery. Health care delivery has been further divided into two sections: the organization of health care, or ways resources are deployed, and the actual process of care the way resources are utilized in a health care system.

The next step in the model leads from the process of care to the expected benefits: the outcomes. Outcomes of a health care system can be viewed from various perspectives (Hogarth 1978). One perspective focuses on the

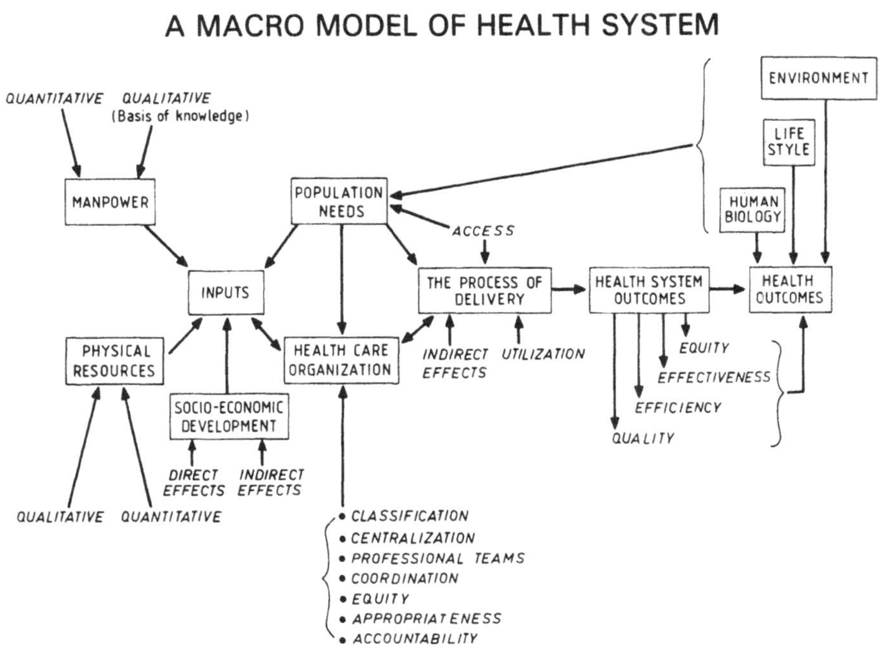

Fig. 2.4 A macro model of a health system.

efficacy of a system. The efficacy is the benefit to the *individual* of the service or control measure applied to his environment. The discussion of efficacy is beyond the scope of this book. A second perspective, effectiveness, emphasized the effect of the service or activities on the *population* at large. A third perspective, efficiency, is the cost-effectiveness in relation to the effort expended in terms of resources. Yet another perspective is equity, the extent to which health care delivery meets the perceived health needs of the population. Finally, quality can be related to all of these, as it is also related to inputs and process, and is a measure of differences between the actual levels of each variable and its desired value.

As shown at the far right of Fig. 2.4, the outcomes of a health system are, unfortunately for our analysis, only part of the general final health outcomes. Environmental, behavioural, and biological influences shape health outcomes in addition to the rather modest effects of the health system itself. Therefore, our model would not be complete were we not to discuss these external influences as we do in the next chapters.

In Part II of the book, each section of the model shown in Fig. 2.4 will be analysed in detail. For each module, we shall review the underlying concepts, and then we shall focus on selecting appropriate indicators for operationalizing these concepts.

References

Abel-Smith, B. (1967). *An international study of health expenditures and its relevance for health planning*, Public Health Paper. No. 32. WHO, Geneva.

Abel-Smith, B. (1972). The history of medical care. In *Comparative developments in social welfare* (ed. E.W. Martin). George Allen & Unwin, London.

Abel-Smith, B. (1976). *Value for money in health services*. Heinemann, London.

Aday, L.A., Andersen, R.M., and Fleming, G. (1980). *Health care in the US: equitable for whom?* Sage, Beverly Hills.

Anderson, O.W. (1972). *Health care: can there be equity? The United States, Sweden and England*. Wiley, New York.

Anderson, F. and Cowan, N.C. (1976). Survival of healthy older people. *British Journal of Preventive and Social Medicine*, **30**, 231–2.

Anonymous (1987). Dawn of a new age. *Health Services Journal*, **96**, 19 November, 1350–3.

Blanpain, J., Delesie, L., and Nys, H. (1978). *National health insurance and health resources: the European experience*. Harvard University Press, Cambridge.

Brogren, P.O. and Brommels, M. (1990). Central and local control in Nordic health care: the public organization spectrum revised. *International Journal of Health Planning and Management*, **5**, 27–39.

Clayton, P.J. (1974). Mortality and morbidity in the first year of widowhood. *Archives of General Psychiatry*, **30**, 747–50.

Culyer, A. (1973). Is medical care different? In *Health economics* (ed. M. Cooper and A. Culyer). Penguin, Middlesex.

Culyer, A.J., Maynard, A., and Williams, A. (1980). Alternative systems of health care provision: an essay on motes and beams. In *A new approach to the economics of health* (ed. M. Olson). American Enterprise for Public Policy Research, Washington, D.C.

Davis, K., Gold, M., and Makuc, D. (1981). Acess to health care for the poor: does the gap remain. *Annual Review of Public Health*, **2**, 159–82.

de Miguel, J.M. (1975). A framework for the study of national health systems. *Inquiry*, **12** (suppl.), 10–24.

Douglas-Wilson, I. and McLachlan, G. (ed.) (1974). *Health services prospects: an international survey*. Nuffield Provincial Hospitals Trust, London.

Dumbaugh, K. and Neuhauser, D. (1979). International comparisons of health services: where are we? *Social Science and Medicine*, **13B**, 221–3.

Dutton, D.B. (1986). Social class health and illness. In *Social science medicine and policy* (ed. L.A. Aiken and D. Mechanic). Rutgers University Press, New Brunswick, New Jersey.

Ellencweig, A.Y. and Karger, H. (1983). Hospital admissions in Israel 1957–1980: a retrospective study. *Israel Journal of Medical Sciences*, **19**, 1082–8.

Elling, R.H. (1974). Case studies of contrasting approaches to organizing for health: an introduction to a framework. *Social Science and Medicine*, **8**, 263–70.

Elling, R.H. (1980). *Cross-national study of health systems—political economics and health care*. Transaction Books, New Brunswick.

Elling, R.H. and Kerr, H. (1975). Selection of contrasting national health systems for in-depth study. *Inquiry*, **12** (suppl.), 25–40.

Feder, J., Hadley, J., and Zuckerman, S. (1987). How did Medicare's prospective payment system affect hospitals? *New England Journal of Medicine*, **317**, 867–73.

Field, M. (1978). *Comparative health systems: differentiation and convergence*, Final Report, Grant No. HS-00272. National Center for Health Services Research, Washington, D.C.

Field, M. (1980). The health system and the polity: a contemporary American dialectic. *Social Science and Medicine*, **14A**, 397–413.

Field, M. (1989). Introduction. In *Success and crisis in national health systems: a comparative approach* (ed. M. Field). Routledge, New York.

Friedman, M. (1962). *Capitalism and freedom*, p. 23. University of Chicago Press, Chicago.

Fry, J. (1970). *Medicine in three societies—comparison of medical care in the USSR, USA and UK*. Elsevier, New York.

Fry, J. and Farndale, W. (1972). *International medical care: a comparison and evaluation of medical care throughout the world*. Washington Square East, Wallingford, Pennsylvania.

Glaser, W.A. (1970). *Paying the doctor: systems of remuneration and their effect*. Johns Hopkins Press, Baltimore.

Glaser, W.A. (1978). *Health insurance bargaining, foreign lessons for Americans*. Gardner Press, Inc., New York.

Glaser, W.A. (1987). *Paying the hospital: the organization, dynamics and effects of differing financial arrangements*. Josey Bass Publishers, San Francisco.

Hsiao, W.C. (1984). Transformation of health care in China. *New England Journal of Medicine*, **310**, (14), 932–6.

Helsing, K.J., Szkalo, M., and Comstock, G.W. (1981). Factors associated with mortality after widowhood. *American Journal of Public Health*, **71**, 802–9.

HMSO (Her Majesty's Stationery Office) (1989). *Working for Patients*. London.

Hogarth, J. (1978). *Glossary of health care terminology*, Public Health in Europe, No. 4. WHO, Regional Office for Europe, Copenhagen.

Ibrahim, M. (1985). *Epidemiology and health policy*, Chapter 4. Aspen, Rockville, Maryland.

Illich, I. (1975). *Medical nemesis: the expropriation of health*. Calder & Boyars, London.

Kane, R. L. and Kane, R. A. (1976). *Long-term care in six countries: implication for the US*. Sage, Beverly Hills.

Kannel, W.B. and Gordon, T. (ed.) (1974). *The Framingham study, an epidemiological investigation of cardiovascular disease*. Section 30, USDHEW (NIH) 74-599. Washington, D.C.

Kasl, S. V. and Cobb, S. (1970). Blood pressure changes in men undergoing job loss: a preliminary report. *Psychosomatic Medicine*, **32**, 19-38.

Kleczkowski, B.M., Roemer, M.I., and van der Werff, A. (1984). *National health systems and their reorientation towards health for all—guidance for policy making*. Public Health Paper No. 77. WHO, Geneva.

Kohn, R. and White, K.L. (1976). *Health care, An international study*. Oxford University Press, Oxford.

Kleinman, J.C., Gold, M., and Makuc, D. (1981). Use of ambulatory medical care by the poor: another look at equity. *Medical Care*, **19**, (10), 1011-29.

Marshall, J.R. and Funch, P.P. (1979). Mental illness and the economy: a critique and partial replication. *Journal of Health and Social Behavior*, **20**, 282-9.

Maxwell, R. (1974). *Health care, the growing dilemma: needs versus resources in western Europe, the US and the USSR*. McKinsey and Co., New York.

Maxwell, R. (1981). *Health and wealth*. D.C. Heath, Lexington.

Mechanic, D. (1975). Ideology, Medical technology and health care organization in modern nations. *American Journal of Public Health*, **65**, 241-7.

Navarro, V. (1986). *Crisis, health and medicine: a social critique*. Tavistock publications, New York.

Newachek, P.W. (1988). Access to ambulatory care for poor persons. *Health Services Research*, **23**, (3), 401-19.

Raffel, M.W. (1984). *Comparative health systems—descriptive analyses of fourteen national health systems*. Pennsylvania State University Press, University Park.

Reinhardt, U.E. (1980). Health insurance and cost containment policies: the experience abroad. In *A new approach to the economics of health care* (ed. M. Olson). American Enterprise Institute for Public Policy Research, Washington.

Rodwin, V.G. (1984). *The health planning predicament, France, Quebec, England and the United States*, Chapter 2. University of California Press, Berkeley.

Roemer, M.I. (1976). *Health care systems in world perspective*. Health Administration Press, Ann Arbor, Michigan.

Roemer, M.I. (1977). *Comparative national policies on health care*, Chapter 1. Dekker, New York.

Roemer, M.I. (1985). *National strategies for health care organization—a world overview*. Chapter 3. Health Administration Press, Ann Arbor, Michigan.

Roemer, M.I. (1989). National health systems as market interventions. *Journal of Public Health Policy*, **10**, 62-77.

Saltman, R.B. (1988). *The international handbook of health care systems*. Greenwood Press, New York.

Schulz, R. (1985) The USA: transitions in health services performance. In *Health services performance, effectiveness, and efficiency* (ed. A.F. Long and S. Harrison). Croom Helm. London.

Sidel, V. and Sidel, R. (1977). *A healthy state: an international perspective on the crisis in United States medical care*. Partheon, New York.

Terris, M. (1980). The three world systems of medical care: trends and prospects. *World Health Forum*, **1**, 78–86.

Thompson, D. (1988). The Griffiths Report in perspective: the place of the NHS management inquiry report. *Journal of Health Administration Education*, **6**, (3), 415–28.

USDHEW (United States Department of Health Education and Welfare) (1976). *The British National Health Service—conversations with Sir George Godber*. USDHEW Publication No. (NIH) 77-1205. US Government Printing Office, Washington, D.C.

USDHHS (United States Department of Health and Human Services) (1982). *Office on Smoking and Health. The health consequence of smoking: cancer*. US Government Printing Office, Washington, D.C.

Warner, K.E. (1977). The effects of the anti-smoking campaign on cigarette consumption. *American Journal of Public Health*, **67**, 645–50.

Weinerman, E.R. (1971). Research on comparative health service systems. *Medical Care*, **9**, 272–90.

Weller, G.R. and Manga, P. (1983). The push for reprivatization of health care services in Canada, Britain and the United States. *Journal of Health Politics, Policy and Law*, **8**, (3), 495–518.

WHO (World Health Organization) (1985). *World Health Statistics Annual*. WHO, Geneva.

Wolinsky, F.D. (1980). *The sociology of health: principles, professions and issues*. Little Brown, Boston.

PART II

The Modular Approach

3. Assessment of needs—population needs and their measurement

To analyse the process of health care requires that we consider the recipients of health care. The needs of these recipients are likely to be presented in the form of health needs. Their needs can then be translated into the demand for health services. Needs can be regarded as the 'difference between observed and ideal levels of health' (Kalimo 1979, p. 64). Need is thus an egalitarian concept because it reflects what is desirable, while demand for health care is a libertarian concept because 'liberty is seldom equally divided' (Boulding 1966).

Individual needs

At the population level, need consists of the sum of individual needs; thus we can consider need at the individual level and then transpose it to an aggregate population level. At the individual level, Kalimo (1979) distinguishes between perceived needs and unperceived needs. As each can take either a medical or social form, Kalimo's typology generates eight groups at any particular point of time.

In Fig. 3.1 the needs of groups represented in boxes A and H are unequivocally clear: they each include individuals with the extreme condition of health or illness. There are various degrees of difficulty in assessing need in the conditions represented in the other boxes. The group described in box B contains persons with social needs but with no medically defined needs. Included are socially isolated individuals: widows, single elderly, or single parent families. In box C are represented all those who are not aware of their medical condition. They may have a hidden or unperceived disease such as a symptomless cancer or unperceived mental disturbances. People for whom such diseases are at a more advanced stage can be categorized in box D. The groups in boxes E and F consist of cases of 'unjustified' need. Typically such persons perceive their own need, but their perception is not supported by professional judgement. The groups in both boxes E and F include persons with psychosomatic symptoms and the degree to which those symptoms alter social function, distinguishes between them. Finally, box G represents a fairly large proportion of the population: though they are restricted by a 'real' medical condition, they are not impeded in their normal role behaviour in the community. In this category are the many people

		MEDICALLY DEFINED NEED			
		NO		YES	
		Socially-determined need		Socially-determined need	
		No	Yes	No	Yes
Perceived need	No	A No need	B Medically unjustified social need without perceived need	C Hidden medically defined need only	D Medical and social need without perceived need
	Yes	E Unjustified perceived need	F Medically unjustified perceived and social need	G Medical and perceived need without behavioural disturbances	H Unanimous need

Fig. 3.1 Typology of a population based on indicators of three concepts of need for health services. (From Kalimo (1979), with permission.)

suffering from chronic diseases or who are physically disabled but continue to live a nearly normal life.

Population needs

Since individual needs are generalizable to a higher population level, the relationship between population needs and the process of care can be determined by the following interrelationship shown in Fig. 3.2 (Blum 1974).

In Fig. 3.2 are emphasized the two basic types of health needs in a community: needs that can be identified and needs that remain unrecognized. Identification of needs is a necessary step, but it is not always sufficient. Some of the identified needs are never met; some others are met by non-

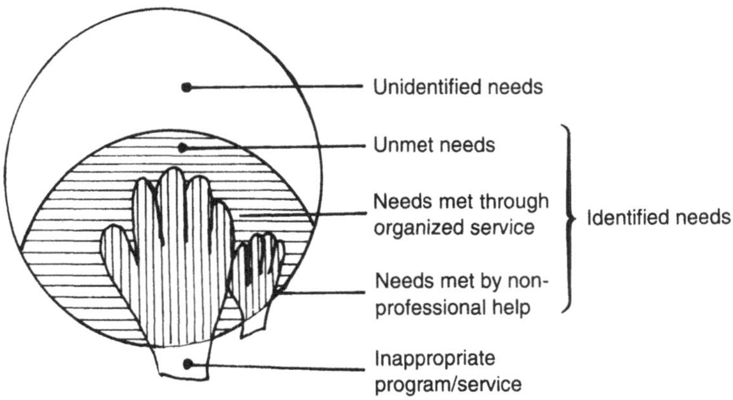

Fig. 3.2 Relationship between needs and service programmes. (From Blum (1974), with permission.)

professional help: only a fraction is met by the organized health care system. Unfortunately, organized health care also includes an additional category of 'deeds' that causes great concern. These are inappropriate services or programmes provided by the system even though there is no need for them. We see this happen when professional 'needs' rather than clients' needs determine the provision of care. For example, consider a region with a surplus of units performing high technology diagnostic imaging. Over-capacity like this may suggest that acquisition policies are determined by competition for clients or a race for prestige rather than the real needs of the population.

The framework for analysis

Now we can turn to determining the framework of our own analysis. Indeed, our analysis is primarily designed to assess service needs and to evaluate the ways in which agencies display their resources for optimal benefits. We shall respond to six questions.

1. What is needs assessment?
2. What are the limitations on shifting the focus of needs assessment from the individual to the community? This question is important because when the emphasis is shifted from the individual to the community, individual needs may not be entirely generalizable or salient at the community level.
3. Are health needs truly assessed in any given health system? What are the appropriate measures for examining the adequacy of the assessment process?
4. Do identified needs affect the process of health care delivery in a system?
5. Should needs assessment at the population level concentrate on identifying new needs or on elucidating the operational meaning of recognized unmet needs. Answering this question can help to orient health planners in establishing health programmes.
6. How do we determine a proper focus for a multi-system comparison? With this last though not least important question the comparative context of needs assessment is considered. Here, we have several options: one can concentrate on the study of discrepancies between 'what has been done' and 'what is needed'. One can also examine strategies for needs assessment in various settings and compare their implementation. Alternatively, a combination of these options can be used.

Let us consider the first question. In needs assessment the relationship between need and demand is studied. When need is translated into care-seeking behaviour, 'demand' is created. Demand is a function of need and of other factors including the availability of services and socio-economic conditions. Needs assessment examines the relationship between needs and demand in determining the degree to which health care services were used by clients in need. In recent years, needs assessment has become a major vehicle in the allocation of services. In the past, resource allocation was based on the simple assumption that the providers of medical services knew better than anyone else what the needs of the population were.

The problem of shifting needs assessment from the individual level to the population level has been described in the literature (Nguyen *et al.* 1981). For instance, typical at the individual level are needs for personal well-being and good health. At the family level these needs are often expressed as concerns about kinship ties and economic stability. At the community level, it has been considered important to preserve political and geographical identities and to secure the social values of the community. Changing the emphasis in this way will require careful analysis in formulating a strategy for needs assessment at the community level. One should always suspect that the aggregation of individual needs may result in a discrepancy between the true needs of an individual and the way that professionals may identify these needs at an aggregate level. A failure to sum up individual needs appropriately will result in the creation of unidentified needs which eventually become 'unmet needs'. In summary, needs must be assessed at all levels of social organization. Thus, assessment at the population level requires a careful integration of the needs identified at individual and family levels.

As an illustration let us consider a practical example. Individual needs are often measured by combining data on health services use with data on individual health status (Andersen 1978; Chen 1979). Unfortunately, simply extrapolating this data to the population level by measuring mean utilization or availability of services is inaccurate. This is so because one cannot ensure that services provided to a community are used by the persons who really need them. In order to solve the problem, several cross-national or cross-regional comparisons should be made and the correlation between indicators of use and indicators of outcome, that is health status, should be measured. Empirical findings suggest that if indicators of utilization and outcome share a common variance of at least 40 per cent, it is tenable that the aggregate represent real trends in the population. (Veney and Kaluzny 1984).

Blum's theoretical delineation of health services needs and health deficiency needs (Blum 1974, 1981) can be used in response to the third question. With his concept of health service needs, he suggests that needs can be translated into service units, so that specific 'service equivalents' are developed for professionally determined health care needs of a community. Thus the problem of needs assessment can be reduced in a professional determination of the minimal quota of services that should be available to the population. The determination of such lists of minimal health services has been addressed by Enthoven (1980, p. 127), and will be discussed further in the section concerning 'The appropriateness of care' in Chapter 5. The amount of service equivalents prevailing in a health system may be determined by listing of all resources available to a community in concordance with accepted standards and norms (e.g. Enthoven 1980). The volume of service equivalents can then determine the extent to which health services needs are met. Satisfying the needs for health services is therefore a plausible response to the average needs of a *general* population. However, responding to needs for health services alone is not a comprehensive response to all health care needs. Blum's concept of health care deficiencies (1981) can be used here. Health care deficiencies represent the components of need stemming from social, economic, and behavioural environments. Having taken the above factors into account, we can concentrate on the particular needs of sub-sections of a general population. A positive response to the specific needs of subpopulations at risk can determine whether the system is capable of modifying patterns of the health care delivery related to specific needs.

Needs brought on by health deficiencies at a health system level can be measured by combining two methods: the Social/Medical Indicators and the Rates Under Treatment (RUTs) (Spiegel and Hyman 1978, Chapter 2) as will be discussed later.

Questions four and five are closely interrelated and concern the preferred 'type' of need assessment at the population level. Setting priorities in needs assessment is always difficult. On the one hand, one must find solutions for known but unmet needs; on the other hand, one wishes to identify unknown needs. One cannot neglect one or the other, so need assessment at the population level includes both identifying new needs and caring for old neglected needs. The principal distinction between the two types of activities is appropriate timing. The first step in needs assessment involves the *recognition of new problems*, that is exploring and identifying areas where there are discrepancies between existing and desired or necessary conditions (Nguyen *et al.* 1981). The second step is the judgement that satisfactory solutions had not been devised for selected problems in the past. In this case one seeks solutions, that is, one attempts to explore the nature of solutions for identified but yet unmet, needs. Finally, the third step is the reallocation of existing resources or the creation of new ones to ensure proper implementation (Nguyen *et al.* 1981).

We now turn to our sixth and last question. We focus our interest on appropriate ways to assess needs in a comparative perspective. Theoretically, one can resort to two interchangeable paths:

(1) compare *the process* of needs assessment in different societies and populations;

(2) consider the *outcomes*. What is the gulf between what is desirable and

what is available across a sample of representative cases in various countries or regions?

In practice, most comparisons are focused on understanding the differences in outcomes. Elucidating the process of needs assessment is much harder because many health systems lack formalized mechanisms for assessing needs. In exceptional cases, the process can be monitored regularly as it is based on a predetermined formula linking health needs to decisions for resource allocation. For instance, in Britain a formula developed by the Resource Allocation Working Party (RAWP) is aimed at responding to variations in needs among geographical regions. These variations are reflected by differences in age, gender, and marital status (Rathwell and Barnard 1985). Using the RAWP formula permits a process-based comparative needs assessment among regions. Needs assessment is then followed by reallocation of resources in accordance with the changing needs of the population. The setting up and use of the RAWP formula thus facilitates the evaluation of the reallocation processes as well.

The evaluation of outcomes is more viable than the evaluation of the process of needs assessment both conceptually and practically. Conceptually, improved outcomes are the ultimate goal of health systems. By comparing outcomes, one can better assess which populations in which regions require the most attention. Practically, procedures for routine data collection are readily available for many outcome variables, simplifying frequent updating of the information and ensuring improved reliability and validity of reports.

Measuring outcomes is often associated with the use of 'health status' indicators; it is tempting to consider outcome indicators used for needs assessment as similar to those used for measuring health status. This is actually not true. As Wolfe and his colleagues note:

> Unmet needs indicators, however, are not health status indicators, and to designate them as such is an error. Assessments of met and unmet needs for health care are not measures of the level of health of an individual or a population, but rather of the social capacity of the society to care for the sick. They measure the extent to which our present state of knowledge is being applied in a given population.
>
> (Wolfe *et al.* 1977.)

In other words, outcome indicators may be used for several purposes and their choice depends on the context of discussion (Mootz 1986). If needs assessment is our present goal, then outcome indicators will serve to distinguish between levels of inequality, distress, or efficiency in health systems. Having set the conceptual framework for our analysis, now we can turn to a more practical direction. In the next section, some useful approaches in comparative needs assessment are presented.

Approaches in comparative needs assessment

Three approaches are presented here:

(1) the single indicator approach which uses a single indicator as a tracer for needs assessment;

(2) the compound approach which concentrates on grouping several separate indicators into a composite index—this is a summary index integrating the many variables measuring need and provides a single index value for each system;

(3) the qualitative approach which deals with the same problem less ambitiously—in it one looks at various need variables separately and then draws qualitative conclusions from differences among the values from different regions or countries.

The single indicator approach

The earliest approach to the study of cross-national or cross-regional differences in needs was the study of differential mortality. Using life expectancy, the conventional indicator of longevity, Matras (1973) noted the great differences in longevity among populations in various countries, regions, and residential groupings within countries, as well as among population strata. When comparing countries, longevity in the Scandinavian countries ranked higher than in the US, where it was in turn higher than in France, eastern and southern Europe. Within the United States, mortality was higher in the South and lower in the West than the mean. Urban mortality was higher than rural mortality, while life expectancy was higher among whites than among non-whites. While these data are interesting, the use of mortality data alone to compare needs is inadequate because of the basic difficulty of conceptualizing health. As we have often mentioned, because health is multidimensional, the use of a single tracer shows only part of the picture, leaving the assessor severely doubting the validity of his comparisons.

Similarly, the use of single indicators other than mortality, such as socio-economic indicators, is inadequate for achieving a full description of the concept of need. A simple illustration of the inherent difficulty of reducing needs assessment to the study of a single indicator is found in a study by Miller and Roby (1970) who focus on income as a single socio-economic measure:

> The connection between family income and basic services is close but incomplete. A fairly well-to-do rural family may have inadequate immediate health care because no health center is nearby while an urban low-income family may have access to an excellent medical teaching center. Or, two families with the same low level of income may live in very different environments—one in an overcrowded area, with few recreational facilities, poor sanitation and garbage control, inadequate police protection, little transportation, the other in a high-density area with outstanding services.

For example in Sweden the poor are better off than in the U.S. because their low incomes are not associated with poor basic services.

The compound method

In the 1960s and 1970s, the health services research community was generally interested in the development of health indices (Berg 1973). The major concern of health researchers focused on the quantification of health states into comprehensive 'health status' indices. Concurrently, composite indices for needs assessment were also proposed. In essence, a single composite index reflects an average state of health for a defined population inhabiting an area or a whole country. If several regions or countries are compared, then the amount of deviation of the index value from the average or 'norm' can serve as a proxy for the population's health needs. Increasing levels of needs correspond to lower levels of the health status and vice versa. For instance, a health status index was calculated for each of the 159 counties in the state of Georgia, US, by selecting six independent variables and then summing up their standardized values (Alan Dever 1980). These variables were: infant mortality; age-adjusted death rates from motor vehicle accidents; age-adjusted death rates from acute myocardial infarction; live birth rates; immature birth rates, and median household buying-power. The calculation of the health status index will be dealt with in greater detail in the section on indicators at the end of this chapter. However, as we have already seen in Chapter 1, the concept of a single health index is associated with numerous pitfalls due to the difficulty in assigning different weights to the contributions of the factors included in the index. In fact, there is no way to assign the weights precisely, diminishing the validity of the index itself. For our current discussion, the immediate consequence is that cross-comparisons based on a single index may not be very valuable for estimating differences in population needs.

Qualitative comparisons

Far more promising and popular among health researchers and planners than the compound method are alternative approaches based on qualitative comparisons of several separate indicators. One of the best known alternatives is the *social indicator approach* (Land and Spilerman 1975). This name is somewhat misleading because indicators other than 'social' indicators are frequently included in the analyses. For example, the social indicator approach may use input variables like demographic and economic characteristics and also health outcome variables like life expectancy at birth. Therefore, in a comprehensive form, the definition of a social indicator is as broad as:

a statistic . . . which facilitates concise, comprehensive and balanced judgements about the condition of major aspects of a society. It is in all cases a direct measure of welfare and it is subject to the interpretation that, if it changes in the "right" direction, while other things remain equal, things have gotten better or people are better off.

(USDHEW 1969)

For a comprehensive discussion of this approach the reader is referred to Smith (1973) and to Land and Spilerman (1975).

Use of the social indicator approach for comparisons is variously described by several authors who called it alternately ecological analysis (Jackson *et al.* 1980) and social area analysis (Piasecki *et al.* 1981). These variations have in common the indirect measurement of need where proxies are used to evaluate needs or problems. Social area analyses are all based on ecological variables. Most often, these variables are descriptive statistics of populations used to compare similar phenomena in several populations. For example, Mustian and See (1973) used small-area analysis to discern empirical correlations between income and high risk for mental disease across several areas.

Another example of a practical application of the social indicator approach in which outcome indicators are used in place of social indicators is found in a 1976 report put together by the British Government team called the Resource Allocation Working Party (RAWP) (DHSS, Department of Health and Social Security 1976) as previously described in this chapter. The RAWP formula takes into account that varying distributions of age groups or male/female ratios in different health regions place different demands on the health system. To reflect those varying needs the allocation process must account for age and sex. The RAWP party also proposed using mortality data instead of utilization variables as a proxy for morbidity because mortality is less affected by the level of the supply of health care resources. In order to examine the variation in mortality between regions according to varying diagnostic conditions, the Standardized Mortality Ratio (SMR) was selected as an indicator. For any given region, SMR compares the actual numbers of registered deaths with the number predicted by the national average modulated by age and sex (Kleinman 1977). In summary, for several in-patient and out-patient services the RAWP party recommends that:

. . . the population weighted for age and sex by national bed utilization for each condition should be adjusted to take into account condition-specific SMRs for each region . . .

(DHSS 1976)

Another example of the qualitative approach was suggested by Kalimo (1979) reporting on an initiative undertaken by Finnish national health and social security surveys. Diseases were divided into 97 categories for each of which a panel of physicians estimated the average requirement for in-patient and out-patient care. Needs in various regions were then assessed according to the incidence and prevalence of each of the 97 disease categories in each region. The requirements for care were adjusted to actual needs and an inter-regional priority list was prepared by the investigators and made available to the Finnish authorities.

The literature on needs assessment deals mostly with developed countries. Estimating health needs in developing countries is particularly problematic because data on social indicators is often scarce and sometimes absent. Chen and Lowenstein (1985) proposed the use of proxy measures as an alternative for needs assessment in developing regions. They found that infant mortality is linearly correlated to the natural logarithm of the ratio of physicians to population. Thus, data on physician availability reflect health services needs.

A departure from the social indicator approach which has particular potential for comparative needs assessment involves its combination with the Rate Under Treatment technique (RUT). RUT is used to estimate needs based on information about the current usage of services. A significant difference between levels of use suggests the presence of a problem. The use of RUT alone is problematic because the technique is not sensitive to variations in the population's socio-economic or demographic composition. This difficulty may be avoided by integrating RUT with social indicators thus controlling for different population mixes. As described by Kohn and White, the model combines data on use with data on social measures in order to assess the perceived needs of a population (Kohn and White 1976, pp. 355–361). The authors present an ecological model for the twelve areas studied in their international comparison of health care in seven countries.

This combined approach is shown in Fig. 3.3. For children aged 0–14 years, sick days—the social indicator—are plotted versus the actual utilization of hospital or ambulatory services, that is physician contacts or hospital days, respectively. Figure 3.4 shows a similar comparison for persons aged 65 years or over. By analysing the two figures it can be seen that for some

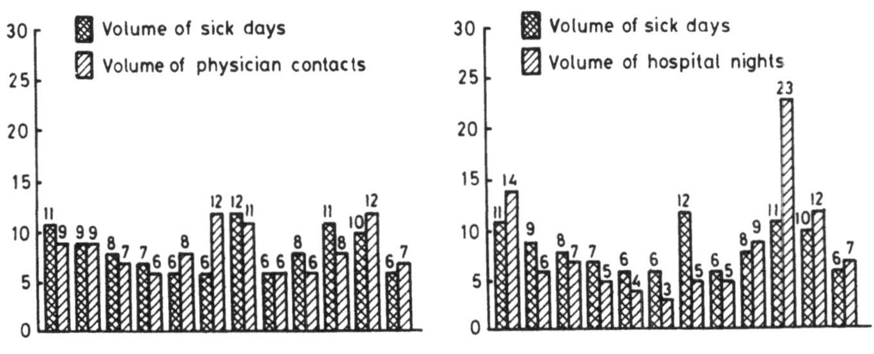

Fig. 3.3 Relative measures of perceived need and use: percentage distributions for children across the study areas. (From Kohn and White (1976), with permission.)

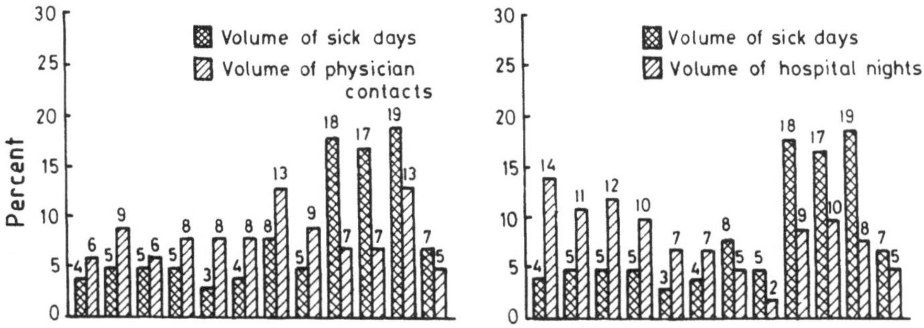

Fig. 3.4 Relative measures of perceived need and use: percentage distribution for adults aged 65 years or older across the study areas. (From Kohn and White (1976), with permission.)

areas there is a poor correlation between the levels of the social indicator and actual utilization. These discrepancies suggest that needs for health services utilization differ between the areas studied as would be expected. In another study, Goodman and Craig (1982) combined RUTs and social area analysis to identify areas where the need for mental health services and actual health service utilization are mismatched. In their study across 31 census tracts within Rockland County, New York, they first identified the several social indicators suitable for assessing the population needs. They used median income, per cent black population, per cent rented housing units and per cent single adult households. Then, they measured utilization. They recommended additional intervention in areas where high levels of social indicators did not result in high levels of utilization.

Indicators of needs

Basic sets of indicators

There are so many social or medical indicators for expressing needs that depending on the conditions, there is always at least one appropriate, valid, and reliable social indicator available for use. A few comments are in order. Concepts can be measured by overlapping indicators. For example, income is related to type and density of residence and often to educational levels and all of these are correlated to ethnicity. Concurrently using several such correlated indicators is not only redundant but also causes statistical problems in analysis like multicollinearity, that is the marked effect of the inclusion of highly correlated independent variables on the findings. It is thus preferable to select only one from any group of highly correlated indicators. This should be the indicator most relevant to the topic of discussion or the one with the most reliable set of data. Alternatively, selection can be by the variable reduction technique, known as factor analysis. By factor analysis a large original set of social indicators can be reduced to fewer artificial constructs, or factors, sharing common features. Health care systems are then compared by comparing the score values of pairs of factors from each system (see for example Gorsuch 1974 and Morrison 1976).

Following is a description relating to the two kinds of comparative approaches mentioned earlier in this chapter: the compound methods and the qualitative comparisons.

Compound methods—indices

The Z-score additive model

The *Z*-score additive model incorporates a series of variables in the form of standard scores (Alan Dever 1980, pp. 204–8). The standard scores reflect a distribution with a mean of zero and a standard deviation of one. If the scores for income and education are not standarized, for example, income would carry more weight than education because monetary values are usually larger than values for years of schooling. Thus, the standardized scores Z_j are defined as follows:

$$Z_j = X_j - \langle X_{av} \rangle / \mathrm{SD} \tag{3.1}$$

where: Z_j = the standard score of a need variable for region (or country) j;
X_j = the original value of a need variable i.e. (unstandardized value) for region j;
$\langle X_{av} \rangle$ = the absolute mean value of a need variable X for all the regions considered;
SD = the standard deviation of a need variable X for all regions.

Once scores are standardized, the sets of weighted or unweighted scores are summed in the *Z*-score additive model as follows:

$$N_j = \sum_{i=1}^{n} W_i Z_{ij} \tag{3.2}$$

where: N_j = the summative need index for country or region j;
Z_{ij} = the standard score for variable i in region j;
W_i = the weight for variable i ($W_i = 1$ for unweighted scores);
n = the number of variables used to determine needs.

Z variables can be either social or medical indicators or utilization variables. An application of this method is illustrated by the following example:

Problem: needs assessment for general health services for the elderly

Suppose that in a hypothetical country there are five regions (A to E) and that we have four need-measuring variables: life expectancy at age 65 (*EX*), proportion of males for those aged 65 and older (*MF*), percentage of people aged 65 and older hospitalized during last year (*HP*), and percentage of people aged 65 or older living alone (*LA*). Table 3.1 shows values for the original values of the indicators:

Table 3.1 Original values of health needs indicators

	Condition			
Region	*EX*	*MF*	*HP*	*LA*
A	15.0	0.46	0.25	0.22
B	13.3	0.47	0.27	0.19
C	17.2	0.50	0.29	0.16
D	16.4	0.42	0.21	0.27
E	15.6	0.44	0.18	0.16
$\langle X_{av} \rangle$ Averages over all regions	15.5	0.46	0.24	0.20
SD	0.55	0.012	0.017	0.018

Suppose that we use unweighted scores, that is $W_i = 1$. Now, longer life expectancy means better health status; also, the rate of health services utilization is higher for females than for males. It follows that higher health needs of the population in a given region may be indicated if in that given region life expectancy is shorter and the male/female ratio is lower than in some other region. Thus we assign a negative sign to both *EX* and *MF* in the following equation for the health needs index (N_j). The positive signs of the two other variables in the equation indicate higher needs if the percentage of people aged 65 or older hospitalized or living alone, increases. Consequently, the standardized scores have the following signs:

$$N_j = \sum_{i=1}^{n} Z_{ij} = Z_{(HP)} + Z_{(LA)} - Z_{(EX)} - Z_{(MF)}$$

where higher levels of N in region j indicate higher needs. According to eqn (3.1), the standardized score for life expectancy in region A would be:

$$Z_{(EX)A} = \frac{15.0 - 15.5}{0.55} = -0.91.$$

and $Z_{(MF)_A}$ would be 0 because:

$$Z_{(MF)_A} = \frac{0.46 - 0.46}{0.012} = 0.00$$

Other scores for standardized values are calculated similarly.

The standardized scores and the summative values of the health index N for all five regions are shown in Table 3.2 below: Table 3.2 demonstrates how the Z-score additive model is useful for distinguishing the five regions with respect to their relative health services needs. The table shows that the summative need index N_j is lowest in region E (−6.70) and is highest in region B (5.14).

Table 3.2 Standardized scores of need variables

	Indicator					
	$Z_{(EX)}$	$Z_{(MF)}$	$Z_{(HP)}$	$Z_{(LA)}$	N	Lower Need
Region						
E	0.18	−0.83	−5.13	−2.22	−6.70	│
C	3.09	2.50	4.27	−2.22	−3.54	│
Country average					0.00	│
D	1.64	−2.50	−2.56	3.89	2.19	│
A	−0.91	0.00	0.85	1.11	2.87	│
B	−4.00	0.83	2.56	−0.55	5.14	↓
						Higher Need

The Socio-economic Status Index (SSI)

The Socio-economic Status Index (SSI), popular in the US, (Alan Dever 1980, pp. 216–17) is a departure from the Z-Score additive model described above. SSI consists of the calculation of standardized scores for three indicators: median education (ED), median income (I), and the ratio of employed workforce to the total workforce (OC). These values are added together and divided by three to obtain the combined SSI as shown below:

$$SSI = \frac{ED + I + OC}{3}$$

The indicators included in the calculation of SSI were selected because they were found to be the most relevant for distinguishing among regions with respect to their health needs.

Multivariate regression

Users of the Z-score additive model wishing to assign weight to indicators must predetermine them according to their best judgement. On the other hand, the multivariate regression method provides a means to calculate the relative weights of each variable quantitatively. The resulting equation is:

$$N_j = \sum_{i=1}^{n} C_i Z_{ij}$$

where: N_j = the index for region j;
Z_{ij} = the standardized Z score for variable Z_i in region j;
C_i = the weight coefficient of the i-th variable.

The uses of the multiple regression method are essentially similar to those of the Z-score additive model. More information on multivariate techniques may be found in statistical textbooks (for example, Morrison 1976).

Qualitative comparisons

Social indicators approach

As shown earlier in this chapter, qualitative comparisons require the use of social indicators. Although information pertaining to social issues is common, it is more difficult to select indicators suitable for cross-comparisons. Such indicators are selected in a stepwise process starting with the analysis of information available for a given population. Then the validity and reliability of each available indicator is examined over time after

Table 3.3 Social indicators for needs assessment

Concept	Indicator
Poverty	Percentage of households beneath the poverty line
Employment	Percentage of workforce unemployed
Racial equality	Ratio of unemployment in minority groups to unemployment in the general population
Mental health	Suicide rate
Health	Infant mortality rates
Traffic safety	Traffic death rate
Air pollution	Air pollution index
Income level	Per capita income
Housing	Cost of housing as percentage of income
Social disintegration	Narcotics addiction rate
Community concern	Per capita contribution to philanthropic organizations
Citizen participation	Voting rates in national elections

which highly redundant indicators are eliminated (Bloom 1981). The Urban Institute in the US has used this procedure to generate the series of social indicators presented in Table 3.3 (Urban Institute 1971).

The indicators listed in Table 3.3 can generally be adjusted for cross-national and cross-regional needs assessment.

The US National Institute of Mental Health uses a similar approach for identifying variables for needs assessment in the field of mental health. Here, too, easy availability has been an important factor in the process of the selection of indicators. Table 3.4 displays the seven categories of indicators chosen by Goldsmith and his colleagues (1975) for this project.

A third initiative of the same kind is based on targets for 'Health for all in the year 2000' of the World Health Organization (WHO). Though the WHO targets were originally designed with the goal of achieving health for all, some of the targets may also be used as indicators for comparative needs assessment. Two sets of indicators are discussed below. The first set, endorsed by the European region of WHO, includes several of the 38 regional targets that we found suitable for needs assessment (WHO 1985).

Table 3.4 Indicators for needs assessment

Concept	Indicators
Social rank	Educational levels (years of schooling) Economic levels (income) Social status (profession, employment)
Life-style	Family status Age Type of residence Residential density
Ethnic status	Ethnic group Ethnic origin
Residential stability	Years in same residence Years in same neighborhood
Female career status	Female professionalism Female employment status Female family status
Social area homogeneity	Ethnic composition Income distribution Distribution of levels of education
High risk populations	Percentage of school drop-outs Percentage of disabled Percentage of narcotic addicts

Source: adapted from Goldsmith (1975)

Table 3.5 Appropriate WHO indicators for comparative needs assessment

Concept	Indicators and their recommended levels	Comments
Elimination of a specific disease	Incidence rate of measles, poliomyelitis, neonatal tetanus, congenital rubella, diphtheria, congenital syphilis, and malaria	Indicator 5 on European list. If needs are met, rate should approach zero.
Life expectancy	Life expectancy at birth should be 75 or more, otherwise needs are not met.	Indicator 6 on European list.
Infant mortality rate (IMR)	IMR should be less than 20 per 1000 live births, otherwise needs are not met.	Indicator 7 on European list.
Low birth-weight (LBW) rate	LBW is a birth-weight of less than 2500 g. Acceptable level is 10% or fewer, LBW births.	For some ethnic groups high LBW rate does not indicate increased needs.
Maternal mortality rate (MMR)	MMR includes deaths during pregnancy or within 42 days of end of pregnancy. MMR should be less than 15 per 100 000 live births, otherwise needs are not met.	Indicator 8 on the European list.
Proportionate mortality from specific disease (PM)	PM is the number of deaths due to a specific disease divided by the number of deaths due to all causes.	Particularly useful in comparisons of needs associated with communicable diseases.
Morbidity-incidence rate	Number of illnesses (spells or persons as applicable) beginning within a specified period of time and related to the average number of persons exposed to risk during that period.	Particularly useful in comparisons of needs associated with acute disease.
Morbidity-point prevalence rate	Number of sick persons existing at a specific point of time related to the number of persons exposed to risk.	Particularly useful in comparisons of needs associated with chronic disease.
Long-term disability prevalence	Number of persons suffering from long-term disability divided by the total population exposed.	In needs assessment, disability is defined as any restriction or lack of ability in performing daily activities.

The second set includes global indicators developed for monitoring the progress towards 'Health for all' (WHO 1981). Table 3.5 lists potential indicators based on 'Health for all' targets and also on the set of indicators for measuring the progress towards 'Health for all'.

Rates under treatment (RUT)

Rates under treatment (RUT) refers to the act of measuring the utilization rates for a given service in order to assess the needs for that service of a given population. There is no internationally accepted set of indicators for measuring RUT. Actually, any available relevant information on utilization can be used and compared cross-regionally or cross-nationally. As shown in a previous section in this chapter, the use of RUTs for needs assessment is seen mostly in the field of mental health which explains why the most frequently used RUTs are associated with the use of mental health services. For example:

(1) Visit rates to community mental health centres: the number of visits per thousand population in a given area per year;
(2) Rate of attendance at community mental health centres: the number of persons attending mental health centres per thousand population in a given area;
(3) Admission rates to in-patient mental services: the total number of patients admitted to mental hospitals per thousand population in a given area;
(4) Mental hospital incidence rate: the number of patients admitted to a mental hospital for the *first* time, per thousand population in a given area;
(5) Rate of drug or alcohol addicts admitted to in-patient mental care: the number of patients suffering addiction and admitted to mental hospitals per thousand population in a given area.

(Wing *et al.* 1967)

Here a note of caution is warranted. The use of RUTs for needs assessment can cause a problem for the identification of trends in utilization. A comparison of RUTs across regions or even countries can reflect differences in utilization levels but cannot reveal actual needs. In other words, smaller RUTs do not necessarily indicate higher needs. Sometimes increased utilization reflects *over-utilization* while decreased utilization reflects an appropriate use of health services. Only experienced observers can properly distinguish between these opposing conditions.

References

Alan Dever, G.E. (1980). *Community health analysis*. Aspen, Germantown, Maryland.

Andersen, R. (1978). Health status indices and access to medical care. *American Journal of Public Health*, **68**, 458–63.

Berg, R.L. (1973). *Health status indexes*, Hospital Research and Educational Trust, Chicago.

Bloom, H.L. (1981). The use of social indicators in the estimation of health needs. In *Assessing health and human services needs* (ed. R.A. Bell, M. Sundel, J.F. Aponte, S.R. Murrell, and E. Lin), Chapter 8, Vol. VIII. Community Psychology Series, Human Sciences Press Inc., New York.

Blum, H.L. (1974). *Planning for health*. pp. 165–86, 213–20, 227. Human Services Press, New York.

Blum, H.L. (1981). *Planning for health—generics for the eighties*, (2nd ed). Human Sciences Press, New York.

Boulding, K.E. (1966). The concept of need for health services. *Milbank Memorial Fund Quaterly*, **44**, 202–23.

Chen, M.K. (1979). Measuring needs for health services: a proposed model. *Medical Care*, **17**, 210–14.

Chen, M.K. and Lowenstein, F. (1985). The physician/population ratio as a proxy measure of the adequacy of health care. *International Journal of Epidemiology*, **14**, (2), 300–303.

DHSS (Department of Health and Social Security) (1976). *Sharing resources for health in England. Report of the Resource Allocation Working Party*. Her Majesty's Stationery Office, London.

Enthoven, A.C. (1980). *Health plan*. Addison Wesley, Reading, Massachusetts.

Goldsmith, H.F., Unger, E.L., Rosen, B.M., Shambaugh, J.P., and Windle, C.D. (1975). *A typological approach to doing social area analysis*. NIMH National Mental Health Statistics Series C, No. 10. United States Public Health Service Publication Office, Washington, DC.

Goodman, A.B. and Craig, T.J. (1982). A needs assessment strategy for an era of limited resources. *American Journal of Epidemiology* **115**, 624–32.

Gorsuch, R.L. (1974) *Factor analysis*. W.B. Saunders, Philadelphia.

Jackson, D.J., Borgotta, E.F., and Goldsmith, H.F. (1980). Data analysis in factorial ecology. In *Aggregate data analysis and interpretation*, (ed. E.F. Borgatta and D.J. Jackson). Sage, Beverly Hills.

Kalimo, E. (1979). Health service needs. In *Measurement of levels of health*, (ed. W.W. Holland, J. Ipsen, and J. Kostrzewski), p. 64. WHO, Copenhagen.

Kleinman, J.C. (1977). *Mortality statistical notes for health planners*. p. 14. National Centre for Health Statistics, Department of Health and Human Services. Washington, DC.

Kohn, R., and White, K. (1976). *Health care. An international study*. Oxford University Press, Oxford.

Land, K., and Spilerman, S. (1975). *Social indicators models*. Russell Sage Foundation, New York.

Matras, J. (1973). *Populations and societies*. Prentice Hall, Englewood Cliffs, New Jersey.

Miller, S.M. and Roby, P.A. (1970). *The future of inequality*, pp. 54–5. Basic Books, New York.
Mootz, M. (1986). Health indicators. *Social Science and Medicine*, **22**, (2), 255–63.
Morrison, D.F. (1976). *Multivariate statistical methods*, (2nd edn). McGraw-Hill, New York.
Mustian, R.D. and See, J.J. (1973). Indicators of mental health needs: an empirical and pragmatic evaluation. *Journal of Health and Social Behavior*, **14**, 23–7.
Norman, G.R. and Streiner, D.L. (1986). *PDQ statistics*, Chapter 15. D.C. Decker Inc., Toronto.
Nguyen, T.D., Attkisson, C.C., and Bottino, M.J. (1981). The definition and identification of human service needs in a community. In *Assessing health and human service needs*. (ed. R.A. Bell, M. Sundel, J.F. Aponte, S.A. Murrell, and E. Lin), Chapter 5, Vol. VIII. Social Psychology Series. Human Sciences Press. Inc., New York.
Piasecki, J.R. and Kamis-Gould, E. (1981). Social Area Analysis in Program Evaluation and Planning. *Evaluation and Program Planning* **4**, 3–14.
Rathwell, T. and Barnard, K. (1985). Health services performance in Great Britain. In: *Health services performance—effectiveness and efficiency*. (ed. A.F. Long, and S. Harrison), Chapter 6. Croom Helm, London.
Smith, D. (1973). *The geography of social well-being in the United States*. McGraw-Hill, New York.
Spiegel, A.D. and Hyman, H.H. (1978). *Basic health planning methods*. Aspen, Germantown. Maryland.
Urban Institute (1971). Measuring the quality of life. *New Human Services Newsletter*, **1**, No. 4.
USDHEW (United States Department of Health, Education and Welfare) (1969). *Toward a social report*. US Government Printing Office. Washington, DC.
Veney, J.E., and Kaluzny, A.D. (1984). *Evaluation and decision making for health services programs*, Prentice Hall Inc., Engelwood Cliffs, New Jersey.
WHO (World Health Organization) (1981). *Progress towards health for all*, WHO, Geneva.
WHO (World Health Organization) (1985). *Targets for health for all*, WHO Regional Office for Europe, Copenhagen.
Wing, L., Wing, J.K., Bahn, A., and Smith, H.E. (1967). The use of psychiatric services in three urban areas: an international case register study. *Social Psychiatry*, **2**, (4), 158–67.
Wolfe, S., Carr, W., Neser, W.B., and Revo, L.T. (1977). Unmet health care needs and health care policy. In: *Health goals and health indicators: policy, planning and evaluation*, (ed. J. Ellinson, A. Mooney, and A.E. Siegmann). AAAS Selected Symposium, No. 2, Westview Press, Boulder, Colorado.

4. Supplying the system—analysis of manpower, physical resources, and socio-economic development

The modular approach is illustrated by the macro-model of health systems as shown in Chapter 2. Those modules of a health system that enable it to operate and that fuel its activities are its inputs. In this chapter we shall examine the content and significance of these input modules which include both resources and the socio-economic environment as discussed at the end of Chapter 2.

Typically, resources are measured in terms of manpower, money, or equipment. Resources are means that the system can use to its own advantage. The system can decide who shall work which jobs, how to allocate its money for different activities, or how to distribute its facilities or equipment geographically. On the other hand, environmental factors are outside the system's control. Examples of environmental influences are economic scarcity, political constraints, or cultural alienation which may support or preclude certain activities of a system. As already shown in Chapter 1, those environmental influences can also directly affect the portion of the model concerned with outcomes. We should distinguish between those direct influences on outcomes and societal influences that affect the system's inputs and whose influence on the outcome is indirectly channelled through the process of health care delivery. In this chapter, we will delineate the essential input components, both internal or external to the system. First we shall discuss them at the conceptual level. Then we shall operationalize these concepts into measurable units.

Resources and the socio-economic development

In their simplest form resources include tangible assets: manpower, and physical resources like facilities and commodities. Intuitively, we tend to evaluate resources quantitatively, by counting the number of physicians and nurses or beds. When considering the resources for industrial production, this quantitative approach is correct. However, when dealing with people involved in a health system, this approach is definitely incorrect. Consider human resources, which we call manpower. Verifying the absolute numbers of doctors, for example, in a given health system is not very informative. Expressing these numbers, as per capita rates somewhat improves the evaluation because a per capita rate can be used as a standard measure for descriptive and comparative analysis. However, a strictly quantitative evaluation is an insufficient basis for decision-making and planning. A qualitative multidimensional analysis of the doctors' professional and even personal attributes, is necessary. These attributes include the basis of knowledge shared by health professionals, professional socialization processes that affected the way in which they acquired their knowledge, skills and ethical codes, their motivation and satisfaction at the workplace, and their interaction with their patients.

As quantitative and qualitative aspects together provide a proper definition of resources, the use of another dichotomy is necessary to define a second focus that makes up inputs: the influences that the general socio-economic development exerts on the system. These influences can be divided into direct effects and indirect effects. The direct effects of socio-economic development consist of finance mechanisms, budgeting, and the costs of the health system, or of health legislation. A typical example of the former is the nationalization of the health system; a sound example of the latter is legalizing abortions. Indirect effects are much wider in scope: they include the economy at large and societal concerns that affect the health system. This voluminous definition contains numerous diverse topics like assessing employment status and income levels, the study of prevailing religious beliefs and their impact on the health system, and the evaluation of the impact of political platforms on the delivery of health care.

Manpower resources

Quantitative aspects

Manpower has long been the most elaborated topic in health systems analysis. As noted in a WHO guideline, 'Manpower is the most precious resource of a country. Whatever other resources are, without trained manpower they can neither be exploited nor properly used'. (Hornby *et al.* 1980.) This great interest in health manpower derives from its crucial role in the intensive and highly professionalized health field. Further interest in health manpower stems from the notorious economic consequences of this labour-intensive field. Some 70–80 per cent of current health expenditures are spent on manpower in virtually all modern health economies. Fortunately, given the relative ease of data collection, indicators measuring several aspects of the volume of health manpower are abundant. However, as we shall see later, those quantitative indicators are still insufficient measures for assessing manpower characteristics.

Absolute figures for manpower are readily transferrable into rates since in most countries census data provides for the population denominator. A wide global account of the absolute number of health professionals and the subsequent rates per population is provided by WHO statistics. The WHO Statistics Annual (for example WHO 1988) is a widely available source that holds a special section on health resources, which is revised every three or four years. It includes rates per population for the major health professions such as physicians. Table 4.1 draws some comparative figures from the report. For example, the rate of physicians per 10 000 population is 32 in France but in the Lao People's Republic it is only 2.8. Even among developed countries, there are great variations: though the United Kingdom and France have similar populations, the United Kingdom has only half the absolute number of physicians that France has. These figures are unreliable, however, because of standard definitions for health professionals are severely lacking.

Another valuable source for the member countries of the Organization for Economic Co-operation and Development (OECD) is the series of social policy studies; these include interesting cross-national comparisons on physicians' supply (OECD 1985). Numerous other publications are available for nationwide and areawide comparisons. For example, the US Department of Health and Human Services produces an annual report showing trends in health manpower with reference to US geographical zones. (USDHHS 1983). In Canada, data on physician manpower can be drawn from federal publications (*Canada, Health and Welfare Canada* 1984, for example). This source gives numbers of active civilian physicians and populations per physician for each province since 1970. Data for other health personnel are also available.

On a more analytical basis, geographical variations in manpower staffing have been compared between countries. For example, Morgan *et al.* (1985, Chapter 6) show that regional variations in the number of physicians per 1000 population in England were much smaller than in France, Germany, or the Netherlands. Quantitative determination of supplies may also involve exploration of longitudinal trends. For instance, Barer and Evans (1986) used the multi-annual distribution of physicians in Canadian provinces to discern a gradual increase in the availability of physicians across the provinces.

Measuring the rates of health personnel to population can facilitate the determination of shortages or oversupplies in health manpower. This is extremely important in planning and has clear relevance for comparative research. In this respect, Sorkin (1977) has suggested three methods to estimate shortage as follows:

1. Normative standards based on comparisons of existing manpower ratios to standards determined by professional experts: with this method, quantitative volume indicators are used directly. While easy to apply, the

Table 4.1 Personnel in major health professions: latest available year; selected countries

Country/area	Absolute number	Rate per 10 000 population
Australia, 1986		
Physicians	36 610	22.9
Medical assistants	–	–
Professional nursing/midwifery personnel	139 434	93.4
China, 1986		
Physicians	926 603[a]	9.1
Medical assistants	1 784 425	16.9
Professional nursing/midwifery personnel	759 485	7.2
Hong Kong, 1986		
Physicians	5 147	9.3
Medical assistants	–	–
Professional nursing/midwifery personnel	22 982	41.5
Japan, 1984		
Physicians	181 101	15.1
Medical assistants	–	–
Professional nursing/midwifery personnel	651 660	54.1
USSR, 1985		
Physicians and dentists	1 170 000	42.1
Medical assistants	315 900	11.4
Pharmacists/chemists	91 000	3.3
Pharmaceutical assistants	180 300	6.5
United Kingdom, 1981		
Physicians	92 172	16.4
Dentists	17 472	3.1
Pharmacists/chemists	17 589	3.1
Professional nurses	182 897	32.5
Lao People's Democratic Republic, 1985		
Physicians	551	2.8
Medical assistants	2 088	5.8
Professional nursing/midwifery personnel	6 753	18.7
Canada, 1984		
Physicians	48 860	19.6
Nurses	–	–
Nursing auxiliaries	85 539	34.3
Dentists	12 271	4.9
Pharmacists	15 337	6.2
Nutritionists	4 304	1.7

Table 4.1 *continued*

Country/area	Absolute number	Rate per 10 000 population
Brazil, 1984		
Physicians	122 818	9.3
Nurses	25 889	2.0
Nursing auxiliaries	84 163	6.4
Dentists	16 696	1.3
Pharmacists	4 630	0.4
Nutritionists	1 930	0.1
United States of America, 1984		
Physicians	501 200	21.4
Nurses	1 943 700	83.0
Nursing auxiliaries	1 269 000	54.2
Dentists	137 950	5.9
Pharmacists	158 000	6.7
Nutritionists	71 000	3.0
Uruguay, 1984		
Physicians	5 756	19.3
Nurses	1 000	5.0
Nursing auxiliaries	1 500	5.0
Dentists	2 300	7.7
Venezuela, 1984		
Physicians	24 038	14.3
Nurses	8 914	5.3
Nursing auxiliaries	6 300	3.7
Dentists	4 342	2.6
France, 1986		
Physicians (Ordre des Medecins)	173 116	31.9
Dentists/dental surgeons	38 980	7.2
Pharmacists/chemists	50 296	9.3
Germany, Federal Republic of, 1984		
Physicians	153 895	25.6
Dentists/dental surgeons	34 415	5.7
Pharmacists/chemists	30 865	5.1
Professional midwives	5 366	0.9
Professional nurses	200 997	33.4
Greece, 1984		
Physicians	28 212	28.5
Dentists/dental surgeons	8 379	8.5
Professional midwives	1 831	1.9
Professional nurses	19 980	20.2

Table 4.1 *continued*

Country/area	Absolute number	Rate per 10 000 population
Hungary, 1985		
Physicians and dentists	34 758	31.9
Pharmacists/chemists	4 548	4.2
Professional midwives	2 569	2.4
Nurses and infant nurses	58 853	54.1
Israel, 1983		
Physicians	11 895	29.0
Dentists including therapists	2 900	7.1
Pharmacists/chemists	2 540	6.2
Midwives and nurses	12 110	29.5
Professional nurses	14 785	36.0
Netherlands, 1985		
Physicians	32 193	22.4
Dentists/dental surgeons	7 118	4.9
Pharmacists/chemists	1 900	1.3
Professional midwives	971	0.7
Poland, 1985		
Physicians	73 199	19.5
Dentists/dental surgeons	17 440	4.6
Pharmacists/chemists	16 064	4.3
Professional midwives	19 850	5.3
Professional nurses	171 364	45.6
Romania, 1985		
Physicians	40 050	17.3
Pharmacists/chemists	6 558	2.8
Spain, 1984		
Physicians	121 362	31.3
Dentists/dental surgeons	4 682	1.2
Pharmacists/chemists	28 748	7.4
Professional midwives	5 770	1.5
Professional nurses	142 542	36.8
Sweden, 1985		
Physicians	21 596	26.4
Dentists/dental surgeons	9 000	11.0
Professional nurses	69 261	84.6

[a] Includes doctors of traditional Chinese medicine
Source: World Health Annual Statistics (1988)

method suffers from lack of standard definitions for several health professions.

2. Demand/supply differential: this is a strict economic definition of shortage or oversupply which may be directly measured only in free-market conditions. In health systems where most people carry health insurance, demand/supply are not affected by direct economic forces. In such cases, non-market measures can be used as tracers for demand/supply measurement. The common measures are:
   (a) unavailability of service (for example, a physician refuses to see new patients);
   (b) long waiting queues;
   (c) a short and inadequate process of care.
3. Relative income: may be used in free-market systems or in systems where physicians are paid on a fee for service basis as in Canada. This criterion has been used to demonstrate differences in physicians' income and activity levels across the Canadian provinces (Barer and Evans 1986).

Qualitative aspects

While the quantitative evaluation of health manpower is relatively simple, the dimension of quality in evaluating health manpower is much more complicated and raises great concerns. In an input-related context, quality is the way in which resources are managed so as to achieve the best balance between health benefits and risk. However, caution is recommended before attempting to operationalize it. First, unlike the quantitative measures, quality cannot be extracted in a univariate presentation, but must be assessed with respect to several attributes. Second, assessment of manpower as a resource addresses only a few features of quality. There are several other quality characteristics relating to the process and to the outcomes of the health system which will be discussed later. The present evaluation, restricted to quality issues of manpower, may be divided into two main classes: personal attributes and professional characteristics.

Personal attributes

Personal attributes have been extensively studied in the literature, particularly for physicians (Eisenberg 1986). Factors such as age, gender and cultural background influence physicians' decisions about the level and patterns of their activity. In several studies, age is significantly correlated to physicians' activity levels: younger physicians are more active then older ones (Freeborn *et al.* 1972; Eisenberg and Nicklin 1981). Similarly, female physicians are less active than male physicians in the same age bracket

(Eisenberg and Nicklin 1981). Culture and socialization also play a role in physician behaviour, though the findings, for physicians who practice in the US are controversial. For example, in comparing domestic with foreign medical graduates. Eisenberg and Nicklin found more laboratory tests used by foreign medical graduates, while Danzon (1982) found an opposite trend.

Professional attributes

Among the professional attributes, professional socialization warrants special attention. There is ample evidence that diverse patterns of medical practice are strongly correlated to the length and intensity of the training programme, to the place of training and to general ethical and societal values. Where there are substantial immigrant populations, these may hint at wide variations in medical practice. In Israel, for example, a considerable proportion of primary care physicians are immigrants trained elsewhere and who possibly still hold features of their original socialization. On the other hand, Israeli hospital-based specialists are almost entirely graduates of local medical schools. This contributes to stereotyping general practice as unprestigious (Ellencweig 1983).

Even in more homogenous physician populations, professional socialization tends to vary. Numerous studies have explored the differences between activity patterns of specialists and generalists. Studies have revealed that specialists take more time with their patients, counsel more, apply a more elaborate mix of resources (Rosenblatt *et al.* 1982) and use more diagnostic testing than generalists (Eisenberg and Nicklin 1981; Noren *et al.* 1980).

Professional background also consists of the type of medical school attended. Epstein showed greater diagnostic—test use by specialists (internists) trained in more academically-oriented settings compared with those trained in less academically-oriented medical schools. Similarly, public school graduates in the US used laboratory tests more extensively than graduates of private medical schools (Epstein *et al.* 1984).

In addition to the personal characteristics, physicians are motivated by the style of medicine they desire to practice, and the lifestyle they seek outside of their practice. The many inevitable gaps between their desires and their actual styles of practice create stressful situations which affect both their motivation and satisfaction (Friedson 1970).

Yet another influence is due to group norms. The pressure to conform to group standards may influence patterns of practice for physicians working in large groups as in hospitals (Eisenberg 1979) or in organized community settings (Dorsey 1983). Some authors argue that in the long-run the accumulating effect of professional regulation in organized groups of collaborating physicians is more important than the professional socialization that occurs during medical training (Pineault 1976).

Quality assurance for health manpower

In most countries the quality of health manpower is regulated by the authorization of only those meeting required standards of education and experience. When a government authorizes persons to engage in any given profession or occupation it is called licensure. When a professional agency authorizes a person to practice it is called certification or registration.

Usually, as in the cases of state governments in the US, the Government grants primary, or basic, licensure. Often, a variety of non-governmental agencies are involved in certification beyond primary licensure. To quote the American Nurses' Association (1975),

> Although registered nurse licensure represents a minimal level of safe and effective practice, it cannot be construed to imply a level of quality above the minimum. Consequently, quality assurance as it relates to structure, specifically the qualification of nurses, cannot rely solely on state licensure.

Licensure and certification can each be viewed from two different perspectives:

(1) the comprehensiveness of the process;

(2) the specificity of the requirements.

The comprehensiveness of the process is the extent to which there are regulatory mechanisms for professional practices in a system. In some health systems several disciplines must be regulated. For instance, there are seven different health professions registered in all the Australian states, and twenty different professions registered in at least one of the Australian states (Roemer and Roemer 1981). Even within a single discipline, there are wide variations among countries. Responses to an International Council of Nurses questionnaire from 60 member countries showed that 32 countries reported having registered nurses, assistant nurses, and aides, 9 countries had only registered and assistant nurses, and 16 countries had only registered nurses and aides (Hall and Mejia 1978).

Licensure requirements specify the criteria for licensure and their definitions. These licensure requirements will affect which of these criteria are developed for various health disciplines. For example, one may ask, what are the specific requirements for the board certification of physicians in each of several health systems? In Sweden and West Germany academic institutions are free to determine the eligibility of physicians to practice. In Britain and in most states in the US, physicians must pass medical examinations before registering (Roemer 1976; Vuori 1982). Presently, in Israel, while locally trained physicians are exempt, immigrant physicians must pass special compulsory examinations.

Indicators of manpower

Research on input characteristics of medical manpower suggests several indicators potentially useful in cross-national or cross-regional comparisons:

Age

The implication of age distribution for planning of future supplies and for scheduling of retirement is evident. Retirement, rate of premature death, and migration are all associated with age distribution; therefore, age is an essential element in manpower evaluation. For a more elaborate discussion on this specific topic the reader may consult a manual on health manpower planning (for example, Sorkin 1977).

Gender

Gender, much like age, may affect retirement, since women are generally required to retire earlier than men. Temporary or final cessation of work among female professionals is also linked to child-bearing and child-rearing. Gender also tends to affect the choice of specialities. For example, proportionately more women than men have entered the fields of paediatrics and psychiatry than orthopaedics and surgery. Women, as physicians, are also likely to select a primary care setting to reduce the conflict between the traditional woman's role and the exigencies of the professional life (Lopate 1968).

Family and dependents

Family may influence health professionals in two distinct patterns: first, the size and age-structure of the family relate immediately to personal decisions like the search for more profitable positions, the desire to attain a less demanding work environment, and the choice of part-time jobs in addition to or instead of a full-time job. In addition to those 'universal' choices, specific dilemmas arise in the health system due to the nature of the medical professions. The heavy burden of shiftwork or 'around the clock' duties, the exhausting confrontation with the dying and the severely disabled, all cause inevitable conflicts between professional responsibilities and the care of the health worker's own family (Brown 1975). This is particularly true for members of the primarily women's professions like nurses, paramedics, laboratory workers, or those who practice health-related social sciences.

Second, the informal support that can be provided by the family is a great asset for the health professional. The structure of a health worker's family may provide indirect information about the nature of this support. Measurement of familial status is relatively easy since it is commonly reported to employers and to management.

Culture and socialization

Culture and socialization may be subdivided into two classes, each deserving a separate category of indicators. First, there are the general socialization processes that exist in society at large. For example, such general processes account for the differences in the attitudes and behaviour between American 'WASPS' (White Anglo-Saxon Protestants) and American Blacks from an urban 'ghetto'. These differences are found even when both manage to gain admission to the same medical school. These general indices can be found for comparative studies by considering ethnic distribution, birthplace, and years of immigration to a new country (if any) for health professionals.

Professional socialization follows the general socialization process and has often a more pronounced effect on the practice of care than general socialization alone. It is not surprising that the two concepts are closely related. Consider again the suburban WASP and the black ghetto-dweller in terms of their likelihood of admission to a given medical school. A failure of the black to pass admission criteria to a 'highly prestigious' institution would not be surprising. In other words, the gap already present in the general socialization process triggers a gap in professional socialization: The ghetto dweller will probably find his alternative in a far less prestigious school than the one he has initially selected. As Miller and Miller summarize it:

> Sixty per cent of medical students (in the US) come from only 100 of the most elite undergraduate colleges, and this has changed little since 1960. Consequently, the poor high school and college training of most lower-class and minority students make it unlikely that they will significantly increase their share of admissions vis a vis achievement oriented middle class students in the near future.
>
> (Miller and Miller 1981, pp. 144–5)

A useful source for international comparisons of culture and socialization is presented in the final report of a WHO study on migratory flows in which some 40 countries were randomly selected for analysis (Mejia *et al.* 1979). The study concludes that in the mid-seventies some 6 per cent of the world's physicians work neither in their own countries nor in the country where they were trained. Though the wealthiest countries always received many physicians trained elsewhere, not all the recipient countries were rich and industrialized. Several developing countries, particularly in Africa, admitted graduates from other developing countries in Asia and Africa.

Professional socialization can be measured using a variety of indicators. Notable examples include: place and year of graduation, place and year of postgraduate education, level and type of specialization, and the characteristics of their training institutions (e.g. academic affiliation, size).

The study of health manpower is related to several other features of professional socialization, including the type of practice, the mode of practice, and remuneration, which may affect its supply and behaviour. Because these factors are primarily determined by the system's organizational setting, we will discuss them separately in the section on the configuration of the health system.

Quality assurance indicators of manpower

Licensure may be viewed from several different perspectives for which we can suggest the following indicators.

Comprehensiveness

This indicator measures the extent to which health professions require licensure in a given country if at all. Then, comprehensiveness expresses the balance between *mandatory licensure*, or certification, and *voluntary certification*, or registration.

Depth of licensure/certification

This indicator reflects the extent to which there are either solid explicit criteria (gold standards) or normative criteria for licensure or certification. This indicator is used mainly to focus on physicians because though physicians are licensed in all countries, the extent of the licensure procedures varies considerably. In this respect we wish to note a variety of sub-indicators that can be used in cross-national comparisons:

(1) basic statutes for licensure of locally-trained physicians;
(2) basic statutes for licensure of foreign-trained physicians;
(3) re-licensure;
(4) requirements for specialization and subspecialization;
(5) special requirements in addition to licensure for independent medical practice.

Physical resources

Quantitative aspects

Like data on manpower, information on physical resources and equipment is easy to obtain since the number, size, and geographical disposition of health institutions are the cornerstones of any description of a health service. Most countries publish hospital statistics regularly, and also issue data on community settings. These data can be used to obtain crude estimates on disparities in physical resources between countries and regions. For example, disparities can be evaluated by comparing uneven distribution of hospital beds, health centres and other health institutions in different geographical regions or different social segments of the population.

Comparative health statistics for hospital beds is available in WHO publications, particularly in the *WHO Statistics Annual* (for instance, WHO 1984). The OECD also provides comparative data for selected countries (OECD 1985). At the national level, regional bed-availability is regularly reported by numerous countries. Consider the example of the US where figures on distributions of hospital beds are provided on a statewide basis by the American Hospital Association (AHA publications). Similar information is available for Canadian provinces (Statistics Canada publications). Data on the regional distribution of hospital beds in Europe is provided in Eurohealth (1985).

Qualitative aspects

While quantitative data are readily available, the mere distributional consequences of 'quantities' of resources are not generally sufficient for achieving a complete assessment of physical inputs. Rather, the qualitative component should also be evaluated. Consider the following argument as an illustration. Let us assume that input can be described in terms of 'quality' equivalents. The concept of quality equivalents applies, for example, to levels of expertise and 'professionalism' of skilled manpower, to levels of sophistication in modern technology, and to degrees of modernization in physical facilities. While quality equivalents may seldom be defined operationally, they are particularly relevant to comparative studies. This relevance may be examined by linking quality to the cost of resources. The cost of resources consists of two principal components: the cost of personnel and cost of facilities and equipment. Personnel is the major item on the current budget while facilities or equipment represent, for most purposes, capital investment. The argument is illustrated in Fig. 4.1, adapted from a Rand publication (Brook *et al.* 1979).

Figure 4.1 shows how the cost of the acquisition of resources into the system is related to quality. Limiting our discussion to capital investment only, the figure shows that in Region I there is a linear relationship between each unit of cost invested and a hypothetical 'unit of quality' generated. For each unit of cost a full equivalent of the hypothetical 'unit of quality' is produced. This is the condition prevailing in some developing nations. For example, building a hospital from scratch in a previously unserved area results in an absolute improvement of the quality of care from nothing up to a certain level of acceptable modern health care. Effecting this improvement requires only moderate professional expertise and very basic instrumentation, mostly manual aids to health professionals like stethoscopes. Now, suppose the poorly-equipped hospital is further supplied with diagnostic (e.g. X-ray) or surgical equipment (e.g. operating rooms). The

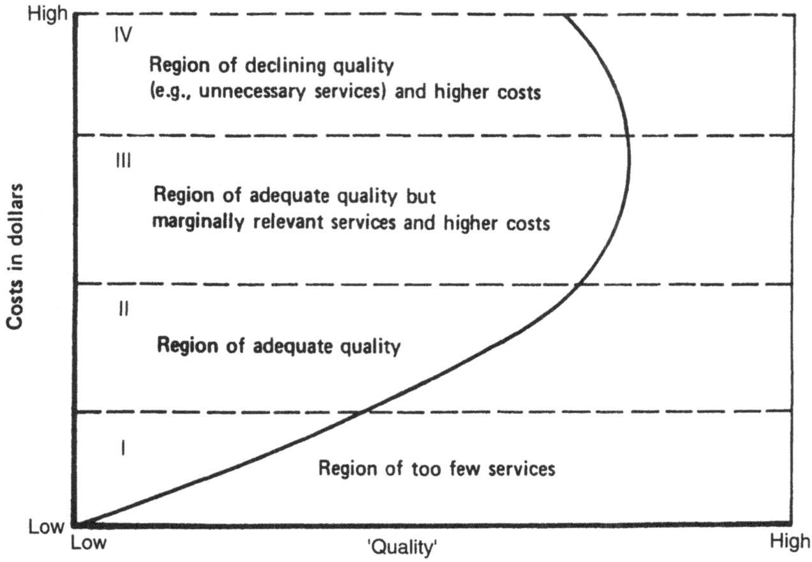

Fig. 4.1 Conceptual cost/quality trade-off curve. (Adapted from Brook *et al.* (1976).)

addition of such an advanced technological dimension to the facility, moves our analysis to Region II. Since new technologies replace human expertise alone, the relationship remains positive: that is, every new technology adds to the previously implemented technology. However, the slope of the graph is more moderate than that of Region I: that is, there is less than a full equivalent of 'quality units' for each full unit of cost.

In Region III, the curve is almost vertical, showing that the marginal improvement in quality decreases to almost nothing with each additional unit of cost invested in the system. This may occur when a hospital management replaces old machines by newer models. Moreover, even the introduction of new technology may fail to cause an improvement in cost-effectiveness ratios, as when an X-ray machine is replaced by a new CT-scanner for exploring suspected pathologies. There are benefits—in improved diagnostic quality—but the marginal value of slightly better quality *vis-à-vis* costs, decreases. Region IV shows that further investment has a deleterious effect on the quality provided by the health system. This happens in our example when the hospital management decides to open certain 'high tech' facilities like departments of thoracic surgery. If sufficient units are already active within the same catchment area, it is likely that opening additional units will only reduce the volume of surgical procedures per unit. This could diminish the volume of activities to a level which is well below the recommended standards—in the US, 400 procedures per unit per year (Alan Dever 1980 pp. 252–3). Inevitably, such a trend dangerously degrades the quality of care, at a higher level of cost per unit of service.

Another measure of the quality of physical resources is credentiality. Credentiality, of utmost importance in upgrading the quality of resources in the health care system, often takes the form of accreditation. Accreditation is the process by which a government, or other authorized agency, evaluates and recognizes institutions and programmes. Though regulatory processes of accreditation across countries are not standardized, accreditation still has a good potential for use in cross-comparisons.

There are two major prevailing approaches to accreditation. In North America many health professionals have long advocated accreditation as a means to improve quality. In the US, accreditation includes a wide array of activities varying from the examination of buildings and equipment to staff training and assessment. Hospitals may be evaluated for accreditation by a prestigious non-government voluntary organization, the Joint Commission on Accreditation of Hospitals (JCAH). The JCAH gained its authority from several medical organizations as well as from public (e.g. Medicare) and private funding agencies. These organizations and agencies require the JCAH's evaluation in order to be eligible for hospital reimbursement (Meisenheimer 1985, pp. 51–3). A special feature of the American accreditation system is that it is subject to periodic examination by the JCAH, thus increasing awareness and concern on the part of the evaluated agency. In Europe, where the other approach prevails, accreditation is project-oriented. Especially regarding the approval of building construction and of new activities or institutions, project-oriented accreditation is confined to a rather narrow scope of conditions. Particularly with respect to major changes or extensions, criteria for accreditation are rarely reviewed (Roemer and Roemer 1981, pp. 400–1).

Indicators of physical resources

General level of resources

One can attempt to measure the qualitative aspects of physical resources by using the RAND model (Brook *et al.* 1979). This can be achieved by using an index including the four categories in Fig. 4.1. Each country or region is than assigned to an appropriate category. For example, in countries where basic resources are not yet available to the great majority of the population, the index scores I (the lowest level). Such conditions may be encountered in several African countries. In countries with basic minimal care, that is universal coverage, but a relatively low level of physical resources, the index scores II. This situation occurs in several South American countries. Levels III and IV are typical of developed nations.

Differentiating between the levels III and IV is difficult when an entire health system is considered. However, it can be concluded from case-studies that some health systems are closer to level IV than other health systems. Typical examples are the US and Britain. Costly physical resources are far more available in the US than in Britain. For instance, there are far more CT-scanners per capita in the US and far more tertiary care beds per capita, such as beds in neurosurgery or in thoracic surgery (Banta and Kemp 1982). Therefore, the US is more likely to represent level IV of the model and Britain level III.

Indicators of accreditation and affiliation

Whenever agencies or organizations in a health system evaluate and recognize an institution or a programme as meeting certain predetermined criteria, the accrediting agency, the criteria and standards, and the scope of the accrediting processes may be evaluated and compared. Two indicators may be studied:

Comprehensiveness

This indicator is used to specify the types of institutions that are subject to accreditation and certification. These may include acute care hospitals, mental hospitals, extended care hospitals, polyclinics, and laboratories. The indicator is also used to measure the balance between *mandatory* and *voluntary* processes. This may be useful for a first approximation in cross-national comparisons.

Depth of accreditation/certification

This indicator is used to measure the extent or the depth to which accreditation/certification is performed in a health system. Specific topics to be examined and compared across countries are:

(1) the time-frame for evaluation, either concurrent (ongoing processes of quality assurance) or retrospective processes;
(2) the areas subject to structural evaluation (e.g. equipment, staffing, training, organizational arrangement, financial mechanisms);
(3) the kind of criteria used in the evaluation, either explicit (predetermined standards) or implicit (value judgements and norms).

Evaluating these indicators for several health systems may provide a better insight into the structural components of quality in different health systems.

Control of capital investment

A companion indicator of quality measures the ways to control for hospital construction and to some extent, other capital investment. If new construction is subject to regulation, and hospital standards are developed centrally, this tracer indicator for quality of inputs scores high, otherwise it scores low. Examples of countries in which standards for investment in physical resources are available are Britain, Netherlands, France, and Canada (Roemer 1976). In the US, standards vary between states, while efforts to establish national criteria have failed (Miller and Miller 1981).

Socio-economic development—the direct influences

Socio-economic development covers a wide range of variables and their relationships. A thorough examination of inputs representing social development requires separate consideration of two types of influences: direct economic characteristics and indirect socio-economic effects. As already mentioned, direct influences are far easier to identify and measure. They would typically include presentations of financial resources available in a system or cross-systems comparisons of those resources. There are several sources available for cross national comparison (Freeland and Schendler 1983; Maxwell 1981; OECD 1985, 1989; Schieber 1990). These sources provide comparative data on the basic macro-economic indicators, in particular the Gross National Product (GNP) and its derivatives like the National Expenditure on Health. Similarly, some countries provide data suitable for cross-regional comparisons. For instance, *Health United States-1987* (USDHHS 1988, pp. 150–151) reports the per capita expenditures on personal health care and the annual percentage changes for selected years. All the information is provided both nationally and at the state level. For example, in 1982, in the wealthy state of California, the annual per capita health expenditure was $1450; in South Carolina it was only $875, a significant 70 per cent less.

We shall now consider specific indicators most frequently used in the operational measurement of direct economic effects.

Indicators for direct economic effects

Size of health expenditure

The health expenditure as a percentage of the Gross Domestic Product (GDP)* or of the Gross National Product (GNP) is probably the most popular indicator for measuring and comparing health expenditures. It is also readily available from national governments' statistics. WHO has set an operational standard for this variable with the recommendation that at least

* GDP, the gross domestic product, is the gross national product minus net transfers. It is considered more suitable than GNP for measurement since it reflects health expenditure as a percentage of the net national product.

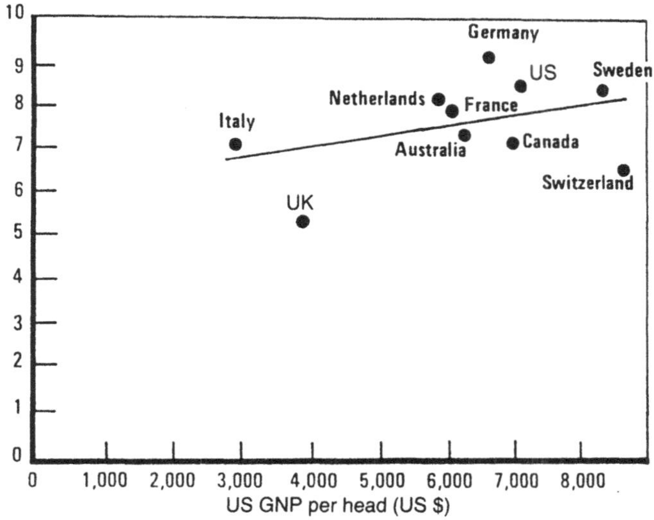

Correlation:	R = 0.446	
Regression coefficients		Significance
Slope:	0.00027	P < 0.1
Intercept:	5.9	P < 0.001

Fig. 4.2 Total health-care expenditure as percentage of GNP. (From Maxwell (1981), with permission.)

5 per cent of the GDP (or sometimes GNP) should be spent on health (WHO 1981). Figure 4.2 illustrates the total health care expenditure as percentages of the GNP in 10 developed countries (Maxwell 1981).

Per capita expenditure on health

Fixed currency terms are usually used in the determination of the per capita expenditure on health. By far the most popular measurement unit is the US dollar. As an indicator, the US dollar provides a direct means to compare actual health expenditures, though it is confounded by the relative wealth of nations as well as by variations in exchange rates between currencies. By suggesting universal purchasing power as the basis for calculations, purchasing-power parity rates (PPP)** provide some remedy to the too-high volatility of the exchange rate. Table 4.2 provides international comparisons for per capita expenditure on medical care, based on these two methods of

** The purchasing-power parity rate (PPP rate) reflects real price levels and the acquisitive power of populations in each country.

Table 4.2 1982 per capita expenditure on medical care ($US 1982)

Country	Per capita expenditure	
	Measured at current exchange rates	Measured at current GDP purchasing-power parity rates
Germany	874	883
Australia	828	796
Austria	644	684
Belgium	534	636
Canada	989	1058
Denmark	746	736
Spain	302	417
United States	1388	1388
Finland	692	629
France	931	996
Greece	187	256
Ireland	436	532
Iceland	865	832
Italy	441	607
Japan	602	673
Luxembourg	601	719
Norway	930	822
New Zealand	440	481
Netherlands	836	851
Portugal	132	248
United Kingdom	508	539
Sweden	1168	1239
Switzerland	1158	990

Notes: The second column reflects a broad order of magnitude of the resources allocated to medical care expressed in a common numerary. The approach is still experimental and subject to caveats. Small inter-country differences (e.g. Belgium and Finland, or Greece and Portugal) can be neglected.

Source: OECD (1985)

calculation. The table shows that the slight differences between the two methods do not affect the demonstration of the basic distinction between countries of different economic wealth.

Structure of expenditures

The next direct indicator measures the structure of expenditures for medical goods and services. In national health accounts, several broad categories of health expenditure are usually distinguished: hospitalization, ambulatory

Table 4.3 Health care expenditure by service; percentages of total expenditure for selected countries 1963 and 1983

Country	Institutional care			Ambulatory care			Drugs		
	1963	1983	% change	1963	1983	% change	1963	1983	% change
Australia	n.a.	54.0	–	n.a.	16.1	–	n.a.	9.4	–
Belgium	n.a.	39.2	–	39.2	45.4	15.8	26.8	18.6	−30.6
Canada	47.1	55.1	17.0	23.9	21.8	−8.8	11.7	9.4	−19.6
Finland	47.3	48.8	3.1	33.2	29.7	−11.7	17.2	10.4	−39.5
France	34.9	46.2	32.3	32.1	25.8	−19.6	30.5	15.7	−48.3
W. Germany	n.a.	38.6	–	n.a.	26.6	–	n.a.	20.3	–
Japan	28.5	32.8	15.1	39.4	35.5	−9.9	n.a.	n.a.	–
Switzerland	44.6	46.4	4.0	n.a.	44.7	–	n.a.	14.0	–
UK*	55.0	58.5	6.4	12.9	10.8	−16.3	5.5	10.0	81.8
US	37.6	49.5	31.6	30.1	27.8	−7.6	12.6	6.7	−46.8

*public expenditure only
n.a. not available
Source: OECD (1985)

services, long-term care, preventive medicine, drugs, and other expenditures. Included in this last category will typically be expenditures for administration and for research. The absolute and proportionate expenditures for each category can be compared between nations and regions, or cross-sectionally, or over time. A comparative overview of health care expenditures by service is shown in Table 4.3.

Income of health professionals

Since the health sector is a labour-intensive industry, the income of health professionals, especially physicians, warrants special attention. The gross income of physicians and other personnel may be compared with the average gross income in the economy, and then cross-sectionally or longitudinally in several health sectors across nations. This would permit us to assess developments in relation to identifying problems in the labour market. Unfortunately, data are not available for most countries. Whenever there is data, comparisons are possible, as for example, physician income in the US and Canada (Barer and Evans 1986, p. 100).

Socio-economic development—indirect effects

The study of the indirect effects upon the health system poses some difficult questions. On the one hand, indirect effects are important because they reflect the many facets of society at large. On the other hand, their study is cumbersome, time consuming, and often made impossible by data scarcity and partiality. Furthermore, several socio-economic variables show strong inter-class interactions and so are subject to multicollinearity. This is why tremendous efforts invested in data collection may result in little additional information relevant to planners and decision-makers. A more thoughtful approach requires concentrating on variables that are both less prone to ambiguous definitions and readily available. Here we shall consider four interpretative frameworks for the examination of indirect effects. Then we shall propose specific indicators for measuring the contents of each of these frameworks. The four suggested frameworks are: the demographic structure, the socio-political process, the economic environment, and levels of individual achievement.

The demographic structure

Demographic structures have attracted the attention of many health systems analysts. For example, the increased percentage of individuals reaching advanced age presents new problems affecting society in general and the health system in particular (Shanas *et al.* 1968). Though future patterns of ageing are controversial (Barer *et al.* 1987), it is generally accepted that the highest utilization ratios for health services are found for the aged population. For example, Gibson (1979) reports that in the US, some 27 per cent of the national health expenditure is spent on the 11 per cent of population over 65 years of age. At the other end of the spectrum, the second largest health expenditure per capita is spent on the youngest population, those one year old or less. The actual expenditure by this second group is considerably magnified if one also considers costs incurred by women in their child-bearing periods. Needless to say, the care of infants and toddlers constitutes a particularly heavy burden for countries with high fertility rates.

Another demographic issue is internal migration. This phenomenon, most frequently described as urban growth, is often associated with the creation of poverty belts in and around large metropolitan areas. The population in these neighbourhoods often consist of low income, unskilled workers with large families, or of those living in nuclear families lacking close-knit supportive communities (Miller and Miller 1981).

Along with internal migration, external migration presents also a major challenge for health service analysts. Before continuing, we must distinguish between 'migration' and 'ethnicity' (Colledge and Svensson 1986). 'Ethnicity' generally refers to conditions affecting particular ethnic groups, like sickle cell anaemia among people of Afro-Caribbean ancestry or Tay Sachs disease among Ashkenhazi Jews. 'Migration', the subject of our current interest, refers to the interaction points between cultures, particularly to the differing ways that various groups perceive social and health reality. Migration is an important problem for the health services in typical immigrant societies like that of Israel. In such societies cross-cultural differences have long affected attitudes, perception, and consequently the demand for, and utilization of, health services (Shuval *et al.* 1970). It is also of utmost importance in Europe where some fifteen million or so immigrants, mostly 'guest workers' from southern Europe and North Africa, are now living in the affluent Northwestern part of the continent (Colledge and Svensson 1986).

The socio-political process

Another cornerstone of the indirect effects of inputs on a health system is the socio-political process. Kohn and White (1976) characterized it as a process consisting of three principal components: health as a societal value; a political balance between collectivism and individualism; and the amount of distributional responsibility.

The way societies may value health forms a continuum from society's assuming minimal to full responsibility for financing and organizing the provision of health services to individuals. In a given health system, a society may assume responsibility for organization, or finance, or both. The British National Health Service is a good example of the society having a full discretionary power for both organizing health care in a hierarchic pyramid and for funding the system from general taxation. In the US, health care for the aged is mostly funded by society, with Medicare as its principal vehicle. Yet, organizational responsibility for the general provision of health services is fragmented. Israel is an example of society's being responsible for the organization of care. This is mainly achieved by strongly advocating membership in publicly-owned, non-profit making sick funds. Yet, societal responsibility for funding the health system is only partial, and Israeli sick funds depend on individual membership fees or other contributions to balance their budgets.

The balance between collectivism and individualism may range from maximum collectivism to maximum individualism. In maximum collectivism, the system is almost entirely concerned with providing benefits to the society as a whole, leaving little or no choice to the individual. In the state of maximum individualism, ill health and its care are viewed as problems of the individual only, unless, as in the case of epidemic disease, they pose a direct threat to society. Collectivism at its best, is probably seen in traditionally socialist societies like the USSR. Here society determines individual choice in almost every respect. Even professional autonomy in medicine is governed by the administrative hierarchy. At the other end of the spectrum, the US health system, particularly in its 'free market' components, idealizes the individual and individual free choices.

Distributional responsibility is a measure of the extent to which society assumes responsibility for the distribution of its health resources. Distributional responsibility scores high when society guarantees standards of service like equity of access. It scores low, when society assumes little responsibility for the distribution of resources and services, or when planned intervention is limited to selected purposes. For advocates of the 'Welfare State', distributional responsibility is the utmost goal. Distributional responsibility is mostly found in decentralized systems with similar established equitable standards in their various social clusters and geographical areas as in Sweden and Finland. On the other end of the spectrum are several African and South American nations whose health systems are distinguished by lack of planning accompanied by striking maldistribution of resources.

The economic environment

The general economic environment is known simply as 'the economy' in well accepted socio-political jargon. Even though the 'economy' is closely related to other determinants of the health system, particularly to 'direct' economic affects, it still merits a separate discussion. There are two main reasons justifying the consideration of the 'economy' as a separate component in our model. First, an analysis of international data reported by Maxwell (1981) and others (for example, Cochrane *et al.* 1978) shows that there is a nearly linear relationship between some major health outcome variables like life expectancy and infant mortality with general economic measures like the GNP. This is a clear inverse linear relationship: infant mortality rates increase as the GNP decreases. Secondly, it is important to note that a nation's wealth is reflected not only by absolute measures of affluence like the GNP or the presentation of the average values of economic indicators like the average per capita income, but also by general internal patterns of economic distribution among population deciles (a decile is any of the nine values that divide the range of a probability distribution into ten equal parts of equal probability). With respect to these internal distribution patterns, it has been shown that the poorest nations have the most major health problems. Therefore, any analysis of health systems would be more comprehensive and sensitive if measures of income distribution were included (Roemer 1985).

Individual achievements

The fourth component in the study of the indirect socio-economic effects is the level of individual achievements. Individual achievements are defined as social determinants affecting the status of an individual in his society. The most dominant factors are education, housing, and work conditions (Dutton 1986). In most national settings these factors are readily available. However, users are advised to withstand the temptation to use all the available factors because they tend to show collinear associations. For example the level of education is closely related to both housing conditions and to levels of income. A sound alternative is either to select carefully the most meaningful variables from a broader list, or to use statistical techniques for data reduction. Principal component analysis with or without factor analysis is frequently the most successful method for this type of analysis (see for example, Lawley and Maxwell 1981).

Indicators for indirect effects

As discussed above, the four categories of indicators for indirect effects are:

(1) demographic patterns;

(2) socio-political;

(3) general economic;

(4) individual achievement.

The following variables may be used as indicators for the measurement of these indirect effects:

Variables measuring demographic patterns

Birth rates during a given calender year

Life expectancy at a given age For a worldwide evaluation of these variables see the *United Nations Demographic Yearbook* (UN publications).

Age/sex distribution within a population

Death rates These can be crude rates, adjusted rates, age-specific rates, or cause-specific rates for a given calendar year. Crude death rates are obtained by dividing the actual number of deaths, by the total population at the end of a given period. Adjusted death rates account for differences in age/sex composition of a studied population. Adjusted rates are always preferable to crude rates for cross-comparisons. Direct or indirect adjustment techniques are available in several textbooks (see for example, Fleiss 1981). Cause-specific death rates refer only to deaths due to a specific cause. Age-specific death rates refer to a specific age group. The advantage of using age-specific death rates or adjustment techniques in cross-comparisons is that confounding effects due to differences in age compositions across populations are eliminated. Age- and cause-specific death rates are reported in the *WHO Statistics Annual* (WHO publications).

General infant mortality This is an annual measure of the deaths of children less than one year old. It is most frequently presented as a rate of deaths (age 0–1 year) per one thousand births. General infant mortality can be divided into two sub categories:

(1) Neonatal mortality rates, which refer to infant deaths in the first 28 days of life;

(2) post-neonatal mortality rates, which refer to infant deaths in the remainder of the first year.

- Cause-specific infant mortality rates are constructed similarly to general cause-specific mortality rates.
- Maternal mortality rates refer to maternal deaths from puerperal causes.

Type of residence This is mostly expressed in terms of urban/rural ratios. The size of the rural population is inversely proportional to the health status of the population and/or to poorer accessibility to the health care delivery system (Dutton 1986). Data are available from the *United Nations Demograhic Yearbook* (UN publications).

Migration Migration is usually measured as the percentage increase or decrease in populations during a given period. For a whole country, external migration reflects trends in immigration and emigration. For a region, internal migration reflects changes of populations within national/regional borders. Though universal sources for information of migration are generally unavailable, data for cross-comparisons can be extracted and compiled from national sources. National census data are particularly useful for this purpose.

Dependency ratio This is an index reflecting both demographic and socio-economic features. It denotes the ratio between 'dependent' persons (i.e. those under 15 years and over 65 years of age) per 'active' persons (aged 15–64 years) as follows:

$$\text{Dependency ratio} = \frac{\text{Number of persons aged } \{(0\text{–}14) + (65+)\}\text{years}}{\text{Number of persons aged } (15\text{–}64) \text{ years}}$$

This index is particularly suitable for cross-regional comparisons and thus is seldom used for national populations. The dependency ratio is a particularly useful index for industrialized societies, where it has a potential for identifying areas in greatest need. However, industrial societies are often troubled by unemployment or partial employment whose measures are confounding variables severely limiting the usefulness of the dependency ratio.

Before turning to the next section, notice that the use in cross-comparisons of all indicators on demographic patterns consists of measuring the value of each indicator for each case and then studying the variations among several cases. Using the indicator for age distribution, for example, consists of measuring age means and their standard deviations for a particular population of a nation or region. After making similar measurements for other regions, the statistics for those several populations are compared. The study of the percentage changes over time for the individual variables can add a longitudinal dimension to the analysis.

Indicators for socio-political variables

Percentage expenditures on health from public sources The indicator is probably the best proxy for measuring the societal values placed on health. There is a strong association between the extent of public participation in the improvement of health status, and the responsibility assumed by the State for health issues. A useful source for this indicator is the World Bank *World Development Report* series (World Bank publications).

Health sector structure This is a plausible indicator for studying the balance between individualism and collectivism. One may construct a nominal scale based on any one of the several typologies suggested in Chapter 2 like Roemer's (1977) or Terris's (1980). Using these typologies is legitimate so long as the user remembers that, in the vast domain of a health system, the typology determines only one or two modules of the health system and not the entire set. For example, Table 2.1 shows nine categories into which national health systems fall. Types 1, 4, and 7 are individualistic, while types 3, 6, and 9 are collective (Kleczkowski *et al.* 1984).

General economic variables

GNP per capita GNP per capita is a general indicator which is relatively easily obtained, and has been shown to be valid for cross-national comparisons (Maxwell 1981). Its reliability, however, is suspect in countries where data sources for national accounting are dubious as in the developing countries. Information on per capita GNP can be found in the World Bank *World Development Report* series (World Bank publications).

Distribution of income (Gini Index) This indicator combines economic and socio-economic perspectives. Technically, a Gini coefficient is used for calculating the degree of inequality of income among various percentiles of the population. The Gini coefficient is zero in a state of perfect equality when members of each percentile earn exactly their proportional share. In a hypothetical setting that is fully inequitable, where one tenth of the population earns all the country's income, the Gini coefficient would be 1.0. Thus, the Gini coefficient increases with an increase in maldistribution of wealth. Obviously, the assessment of distributional trends is subject to several measurement errors and is infrequently calculated, limiting its usefulness. Values for income distribution are largely available from the series of World Bank *World Development Reports* (World Bank publications).

Indicators of individual achievement

Levels of education Education consistently appears as a significant correlate of good health (Fuchs 1979). For several countries, a choice of several indicators is provided by national statistics or international agencies. Included are average years of schooling, percentages of those who completed various levels of education (mostly suitable for developed regions), adult literacy ratios, percentage of educated children (mostly suitable for developing regions). International data are reported in World Bank publications.

Employment and professional achievement Labour force statistics provide information on the size of the working force and on several other labour-related dimensions. Data are presented by type of industry, occupation, sex, and employment status. Routine international statistics are available from the International Labour Office *Yearbook of Labour Statistics* (ILO publications). Some data are also available from the World Bank *World Development Report* series (World Bank publications).

Unemployment rates/levels This indicator is specially relevant to health systems since a cause–effect relationship between unemployment and health has been shown (Brenner 1973, 1977). However, unemployment status has varied definitions, and the condition is often seasonal and changing with time. Furthermore, partial employment is under-represented in unemployment statistics. Because of these several drawbacks, the validity of the indicator and its reliability are questionable. Longitudinal data on unemployment as well as stratification by industry and occupation can be found in ILO year-books (ILO publications).

Research on indicators of individual achievement show that they are strongly associated. For example, education is a confounding variable in measuring levels of employment (Fuchs 1983, pp. 166–7). Moreover, indicators of individual achievement are also correlated with certain economic indicators like income. For this reason, for most purposes, only one indicator of the individual achievement class should be selected for analysis. This selection can be based on the relevance for health systems' analysis and on the ease of data collection.

References

Alan Dever, G.E. (1980). *Community health analysis*, Aspen, Germantown, Maryland.

American Hospital Association *Hospital Statistics*, Chicago, Illinois. (Various years.)

American Nurses Association (1975). *A plan for implementation of the standards of nursing practice*, ANA, Kansas City, Missouri.

Banta, H.D. and Kemp, K.B. (1982). *The management of health care technologies in nine countries*. Springer, New York.

Barer, M.L. and Evans, R.G. (1986). Riding north on a south bound horse. In *Medicare at maturity, achievements, lessons and challenges*, (ed. R.G. Evans and G.L. Stoddart). The Banff Centre, School of Management, Banff, Alberta.

Barer, M.L., Evans, R.G., Hertzman C., and Lomas J. (1987). Aging and health care utilization: new evidence on old fallacies. *Social Science and Medicine*, **24**, (10), 851–62.

Brenner, M.H. (1973). Fetal, infant and maternal mortality during periods of economic instability. *International Journal of Health Services*, **3**, (2), 145–59.

Brenner, M.H. (1977). Health costs and benefits of economic policy. *International Journal of Health Services*, **7**, (4), 581–623.

Brook, R.H., Williams, K.N., and Avery, A.D. (1976). Quality assurance today and tommorrow: forecast for the future. *Annals of Internal Medicine*, **85**, 809–17.

Brook, R.H., Davies, A.R., and Kamberg, C.J. (1979). *Selected reflections on quality of medical care; evaluation in the 1980s*, A Rand Note N-1308-HEW. Rand, Santa Monica, California.

Brown, C.A. (1975). Women workers in the health service industry. *International Journal of Health Services*, **5**, 173–84.

Canada, Health and Welfare Canada (1984). *Canada Health Manpower Inventory 1983*. Policy Planning and Information Branch, Health Information Division, Ottawa.

Cochrane, A.L., St Leger, A.S., and Moore, F. (1978). Health service 'input' and mortality 'output' in developed countries. *Journal of Epidemiology and Community Health*, **32**, 200–5.

Colledge, M. and Svensson, P.G. (1986). Introduction. In *Migration and health*, (ed. M. Colledge, H.A. Van Geuns, and P.G. Svensson). WHO, Regional office for Europe, Copenhagen.

Danzon, P.M. (1982). *Economic factors in the use of laboratory tests by office based physicians*, (R-2525-1-HCFA). Rand Corporation, Santa Monica, California.

Dorsey, J.L. (1983). The use of diagnostic resources in health maintenance organizations and fee for service practice settings. *Archives of Internal Medicine*, **143**, 1863–65.

Dutton, D.B. (1986). Social class, health and illness. In *Applications of social science to clinical medicine and health policy*, (ed. L.H. Aiken, and D. Mechanic). Rutgers University Press, New Brunswick.

Eisenberg, J.M. (1979). Sociological influences on decision-making by clinicians. *Annals of Internal Medicine*, **90**, 957–64.

Eisenberg, J.M. (1986). *Doctors' decisions and the cost of medical care*. Health Administration Press Perspectives, Ann Arbor, Michigan.

Eisenberg, J.M. and Nicklin, D. (1981). Use of diagnostic services by physicians in community practice. *Medical Care*, **19**, (3), 297–309.

Ellencweig, A. Y. (1983). The new Israeli health care reform: an analysis of a national need. *Journal of Health Politics, Policy and Law*, **8**, 366–86.

Epstein, A. M., Begg, C. M., and McNeil, B. J. (1984). The effects of physicians' training and personality on test ordering for ambulatory patients. *American Journal of Public Health*, **74**, 1271–73.

Eurohealth (1985). *Eurohealth handbook*. Robert S. First, New York.

Fleiss, J. L. (1981). *Statistical methods for rates and proportions*, (2nd edn). Wiley, New York.

Freeborn, D. K., Baer, D., Greenlick, M. R., and Bailey, J. W. (1972). Determinants of medical care utilization: physicians' use of laboratory services. *American Journal of Public Health*, **62**, 846–53.

Freeland, M. and Schendler, C. (1983). National health expenditure growth in the 1980s: an aging population, new technologies and increasing competition. *Health Care Management Review*. **4**, (3), 7.

Friedson, E. (1970). *The profession of medicine: A study of the sociology of applied knowledge*. Dodd, Mead & Co., New York.

Fuchs, V. R. (1979). Economics, health and post industrial society. *Milbank Memorial Fund Quarterly*, **57**, 153–82.

Fuchs, V. R. (1983). *How we live*. Harvard University Press, Cambridge, Massachusetts.

Gibson, R. M. (1979). National health expenditures. *Health Care Financing Review*, **1**, 1–36.

Hall, T. L. and Mejia, A. (1978). *Health manpower planning*. WHO, Geneva.

Hornby, P., Ray, D. K., Shipp, P. J., and Hall, T. L. (1980). *Guidelines for health manpower planning*. WHO, Geneva.

ILO (International Labour Office) *Year-book of labour statistics*. ILO, Geneva. (Various years.)

Kleczkowski, B. M., Roemer, M. I., and van der Werff, A. (1984). *National health systems and their reorientation towards health for all*, Public Health Papers, No. 77. WHO, Geneva.

Kohn, R. and White, K. L. (1976). *Health care: an international study*. Oxford Medical Publications, London.

Lawley, D. N. and Maxwell, A. E. (1981). *Factor analysis as a statistical method*. Butterworth, London.

Lopate, C. (1968). *Women in Medicine*. John Hopkins Press, Baltimore, Maryland.

Maxwell, R. (1981). *Health and wealth*. Lexington Books, Lexington, Massachusetts.

Meisenheimer, C. G. (1985). *Quality Assurance*. Aspen, Rockville, Maryland.

Mejia, A., Pizurki, H., and Royston, E. (1979). *Physician and nurse migration*: analysis and policy implications. WHO, Geneva.

Miller, A. E. and Miller, M. G. (1981). *Options for health and health care. The coming of post-clinical medicine*. Wiley, New York.

Morgan, M., Calnan, M., and Manning, N. (1985). *Sociological approaches to health and medicine*. Croom Helm, London.

Noren, J., Prazier, T., Altman, I., and Delozier, J. (1980). Ambulatory medical care—comparison of internists and family-general practitioners. *New England Journal of Medicine*, **302**, 11–16.

OECD (Organization of Economic Co-operation and Development) (1985). *Measuring health care 1960*–1983, Social Policy Study, No. 2. Paris.

OECD (Organization of Economic Co-operation and Development) Secretariat (1989). Compendium, health care expenditure and other data. *Health Care Financing Review*, Annual Supplement, pp. 11–194.

Pineault, R. (1976). The effect of prepaid group practice on physicians' utilization behavior. *Medical Care*, **14**, 121-26.

Roemer, M.I. (1976). *Health care systems in world perspective*, Health Administration Press, Ann Arbor, Michigan.

Roemer, M.I. (1985). *National strategies for health care organization—a world overview*. Health Administration Press, Ann Arbor, Michigan.

Roemer, M.I. and Roemer, R.J. (1981). *Health care systems and comparative manpower policies*, chapter 9. Marcel Dekker, New York.

Rosenblatt, R., Cherwin, D., Schneeweiss, R. et al. (1982). The structure and content of family practice: current status and future trends. *The Journal of Family Practice*, **15**, 681-722.

Shanas, E., Townsend, P., Wedderburn, D., Friis, H.J., Milhoj, P., and Stehouwer J. (1968). *Old people in three industrial societies*. Atherton, New York.

Schieber, G.J. (1990). Health expenditures in major industrialized countries 1960-1987. *Health Care Financing Review*, **11**, (4), 159-67.

Shuval, J.T., Antonovsky, A., and Davies, A.M. (1970). *Social functions of medical practice*. Jossey-Bass, San Francisco.

Sorkin, A.L. (1977). *Health manpower*. Lexington Books, Lexington, Massachusetts.

Statistics Canada. *Canada year-book*. Ottawa. (Various years.)

Terris, M. (1980). The three world systems of medical care: trends and prospects. *World Health Forum*, **1**, 78-86.

UN (United Nations). *United Nations demographic year-book*. UN, New York. (Various years.)

USDHHS (US Department of Health and Human Services) (1983, 1988). *Health United States, 1982, 1987*. US Government Printing Office, Hyattsville, Maryland.

Vuori, H.V. (1982). *Quality assurance of health services*, Public Health in Europe, No. 16. WHO Regional Office for Europe, Copenhagen.

WHO (World Health Organization). *World Health Statistics Annual*. WHO, Geneva. (Various years.)

WHO (World Health Organization) (1981). *Guiding principles for its application in the managerial process for national health development*, Health for All Series, No. 6. Geneva.

World Bank. *World Development Report*. Oxford University Press, New York. (Various years.)

5. Preparation for the process—analysis of health care organization

The organization of health care systems is a crucial element in our analysis. Unfortunately, studying complex organizational patterns is also complex, often cumbersome, and sometimes ambiguous. Because of this complexity, the analysis requires a step-by-step consideration of several organizational dimensions. Following are seven dimensions which we have chosen for the comparative study of health care systems:

(1) the organizational classification;

(2) the centralization/decentralization paradigm;

(3) the co-ordination in a health system;

(4) the configuration of professional teams;

(5) organizing for equity;

(6) the appropriateness of care;

(7) the accountability of the system.

Dimensions 1 and 2 are macro dimensions and refer to the broad view or macro perspective of the health system. Dimension 3 refers to the co-ordination between the several components of the health system. Dimension 4 is a typical micro dimension used in organizational studies, and deals with the particular configuration of the personnel in medical and health teams. Finally, dimensions 5, 6, and 7 refer to the three major quality attributes of the health system's configuration: equity, appropriateness, and accountability. Starting with the macro dimensions and moving sequentially to the micro dimensions of the organizational complex, we hope to shed light on each dimension in turn.

Dimension 1: The organizational classification

As stated in Chapters 1 and 2, socio-economic input variables may determine the organizational classification of a health system either implicitly or explicitly. Because these input variables strongly influence the structure of the health system, there is a wide range of possible organizational classifications for the system. At one extreme it could be a government-owned and government-operated system, in which nearly all health personnel are government employees. At the other extreme, it could be an essentially private system in which most health care is provided by private individuals or group entrepreneurs. However, the analytical problem is not in classifying the health care system into well-defined organizational categories, but rather the multitude of such classes and categories that are regularly found within a single health care system.

How can we avoid being bogged down by so many classes and categories? First we could distinguish between principal and marginal organizational classes within a health system, and then for a crude analysis, we could ignore the minor classes. For example, in Britain, a minor though still measurable amount of the expenditure on health care (about 6 per cent) goes to the private market. However, for simplicity's sake, we can ignore this minor contribution of the private market, and categorize the British health system as a system operated by the National Health Service—a government-owned, health service provider.

Unfortunately, not every health care system can be simplified so easily. When a system is composed of several nearly equal parts, with no 'minor contribution,' it is more difficult to ignore any of the parts. This makes it more difficult to label the system as a whole. For instance, can the American health system be defined as a health insurance market supervised by public agencies as suggested by the view of Health Maintenance Organizations (HMOs) and even of the non-profit third party insurers? Or is it, perhaps, a system of social benefits funded by the Government as manifested by Medicare and Medicaid? Is it a local government-operated public system as suggested by the presence of inner city public services? Could it simply be a free-enterprise system consisting of buyers and sellers of health services? Could it be something else again? Well, the answer seems to be a little of everything. Even for this complex case there is some hope: one should simply consider the American system as one having a variety of subsystems sharing some common aspects (Torrens 1984).

Having noted the methodological difficulties in classifying systems into appropriate 'boxes', we turn now to identifying those 'boxes'. Now we shall discuss three perspectives of organizational classifications: administrative structure, decision-making and planning styles, and financial arrangements.

Perspective I The administrative structure

The term 'administrative structure' encompasses two aspects: the extent of government involvement in the health sector, and the levels of pluralism within the system. The first aspect is the way that governments are involved in the activities of the health system. This involvement ranges from full governmental control to exclusively private initiatives. At one end of the scale one can envisage an arrangement where the Government is very powerful, leaving very little room for private enterprise. This pattern occurs in the state-owned, nationalized systems of socialist countries like the USSR and, until recently, other Eastern European countries. At the other end of the scale, private hospitals and medical services are robust and flourishing while governmental health programmes are weak and marginal. This case is nicely illustrated by the US system, particularly during the nineteenth and early twentieth centuries. It is not surprising that high levels of public ownership and control as in Britain or Sweden, are associated with high levels of public funding as seen in Figure 5.1 (Maxwell 1981).

There is also a broad range to the second aspect, levels of pluralism. Health systems may range from a pluralism to a monopoly. The multi-faceted system of the US perfectly exemplifies pluralism. It consists of: profit and non-profit health insurers (HMOs), commercial insurers, private and public providers, Government, charitable organizations and so on. Britain, with its gigantic health provider, the National Health Service, reflects a considerably more unified network because almost all the activities carried out in the health system are performed by just one provider.

At first glance, one would expect a monopoly to correspond to massive government involvement, and pluralism to correspond to a decreasing level of government involvement. With this in mind, Kleczkowski and his co-workers (1984*a*, *b*), proposed to use a single aggregate variable called

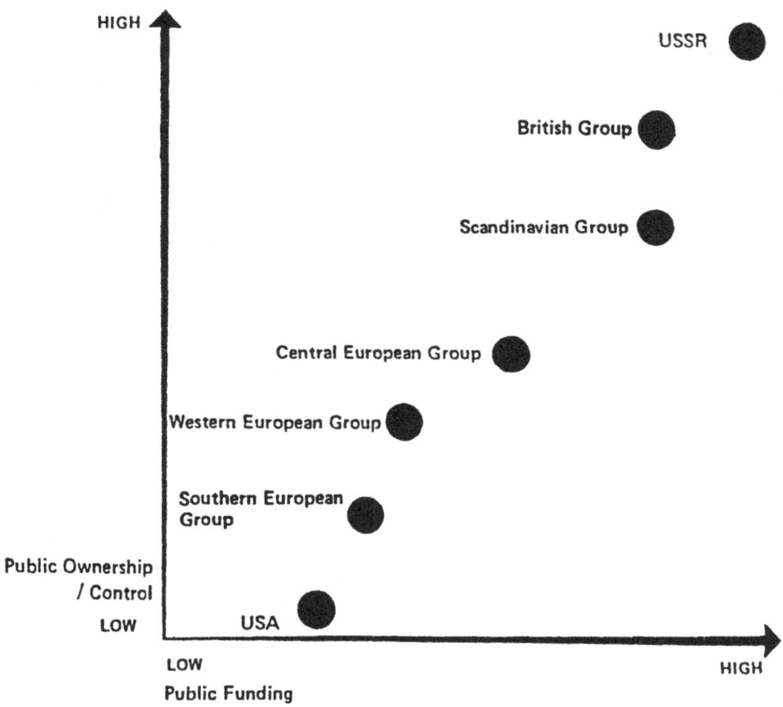

Fig. 5.1 The organization spectrum. (From Maxwell (1981), with permission.)

'level of organization' as a descriptive measure for administrative structures. In a later paper (Roemer 1989) this single variable was labeled 'health system policies.' However, the use of such a single measure is inadvisable because there are 'near' monopolies with relatively little government involvement. In Israel, for example, while the gigantic General Sick Fund controls the majority of health services, the Government exerts very little influence on it (Ellencweig 1983).

Perspective II Decision-making and planning styles

The second perspective of organizational classification consists of the frame of reference within which the decision-making and planning processes take place. Planning is related to decision-making in that planning is the process of 'decision-making for the future'. Planning and decision-making represent the two sides of the same coin and can be studied simultaneously. Hyman (1976) identified four basic planning types, and designated them as systems' planning, partnership planning, alliances planning, and individual actions. Frequently found in Eastern European nations, systems' planning provides full control over resources, and the span of control lies within a single hierarchy of command. The Central Authority issues general plans for various time periods, like a Three Year Plan, or a Five Year Plan, for example. The central plans are then used as a basis for regional and local planning. Approved plans become legally binding for the central and peripheral units. In the USSR, it takes the form of ministerial 'orders' that govern activities throughout the health system (Davis 1988). A more moderate form of control, called partnership planning is found, for example, in Sweden, the UK, and Israel. Authority is divided among agencies or between different levels of government. Particularly for budget allocations or collective wage agreements for the health professionals, decision-making is carried out through bargaining and negotiations: in the UK, for example, responsibility is shared by the NHS, independent providers like general practitioners and pharmacists, local authorities, and other government agencies. In Israel, there is a partnership between the Ministry of Health representing the Government, and the largest provider of health care, the Kupat Holim (General Sick Fund).

Central to the third type of planning, alliances planning, are voluntary agreements or alliances. Compulsory measures, in the form of legal action, are seldom undertaken and agreement is reached through compromises. This type of planning prevails in the US where those representing the consumer (e.g. employers) agree with potential providers on the development of health care delivery services. Finally, the fourth type of planning style, individual actions, is commonly found in African and other developing countries. In 'no planning', individual action prevails. On the one hand, the central governments of these developing nations suffer from a weak decision-making process. On the other hand, there are no organized health care providers with whom to establish partnerships or alliances. In these cases, micro systems of health care develop, where individuals, like those covered by their employer's health policy, can 'plan' their own health care delivery processes. Those who cannot enter such 'micro' systems have hardly any access to health care.

Resource allocation is also germane to planning styles. Blum (1974, p. 400) suggests an interesting model addressing the allocation of resources for planning. In the model are identified four essential components of the planning process:

(1) organizational structure (or system structures);
(2) purposes (or system goals and objectives);
(3) the roles of participants in the planning process (in a macro context, roles are essentially institutional or agency rather than individual);
(4) functions (functions represent the necessary means for achieving the desired outcomes).

Figure 5.2 illustrates the three possible patterns of the sequential relationships between the four components. While the model is valuable for both macro and micro scales, we are most interested in translating the model into a system's perspective. From this standpoint, the model clearly demonstrates why structural hierarchies generally fail to create adequate means for planning (Pattern I). Pre-imposed structures tend to shape purposes and roles resulting in inappropriate functioning of the entire system. The 'centralized planning process' in socialist economies is a typical Pattern I system. Due to inadequate sequential order, the system focuses on the build-up of hierarchical structures whose survival becomes the health system's major function. This emphasis is obviously at the expense of the problems associated with the health needs of the population.

Pattern II is an example of another departure from an optimal sequence. Roles and functions are of prime importance in the planning process. This can lead to an inadequate structure and to an imbalanced setting of priorities. This pattern is typical of power struggles in the health systems of several Western societies. Power lobbies may exercise pressure on decision-makers in shaping the health sector to meet their needs. Alternatively, these lobbies may formulate their institutional (or agency) policy regardless of the interests of other players or the needs of the rest of the population. Pattern II behaviour was seen in the massive opposition to Certificate of Need (CON) regulation in the US. The regulation attempted to control the growth of hospital expenditures by limiting investment to those services assessed as needed by regulatory agencies. However, pressures from industry representatives and state governments who shared concerns for loss of their roles and functions, yielded to the practical elimination

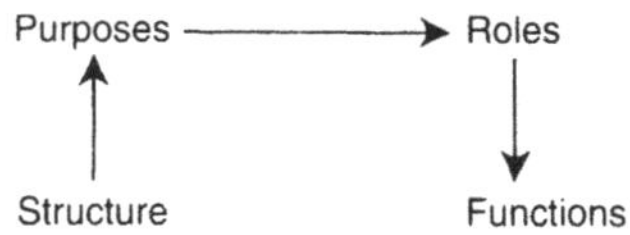

PATTERN I
Structure has commonly been set up as the first step in creating a new institution such as comprehensive health planning. Structure tends to shape Purposes, which are then seen as calling for certain Roles. This pattern seems to be the result of 'needing' the security of an edifice before defining its utility.

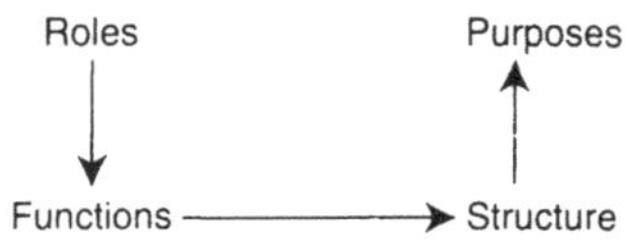

PATTERN II
Others see Roles and Functions as the starting point and proceed to Structure. Purposes tend to be rationalized from this set of structured and functional influences and are likely to remain unclear. As a result, the choice of Roles and Functions may be illogical or inconsistent and the Structure inadequate to do more than the initial comprehension called for.

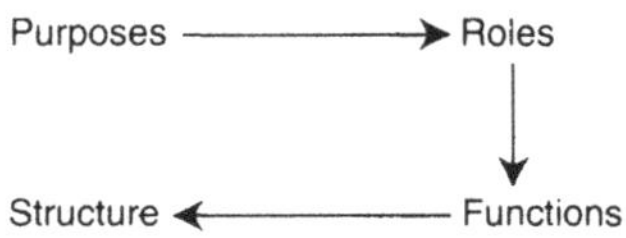

PATTERN III
Purposes visualized as the starting point are then seen as the determiners of Roles. Roles require that certain Functions be performed. Functions, then, place demands on the Structure of the planning body. This is the logic of setting up a planning body to which we subscribe. Once a Structure is conceived in this way, the probabilities will be performed. This in turn should contribute to Role success and lead to the fulfilment of the Purposes which gave rise to the planning body in the first place.

Fig. 5.2 Sequential relationships between Purposes, Roles, Function and Structure. (Modified from Cyril Roseman, *Planning, structure, roles and relationships*, delivered at Advanced Comprehensive Health Planning Seminar, Yakima, Washington, 30 March 1970.)

of the programme and to reinstituting a Pattern II cycle (Heidenheimer *et al.* 1983).

Pattern III reflects the preferred logic for setting up a health system. Purposes and objectives are formulated first and then roles and their functions are appropriately defined. Only then is the system structured along these lines. The British NHS is perhaps the best example of Pattern III planning. Created in 1948, the NHS has been twice restructured, once in 1974 and once in 1982, and another reorganization is planned for 1991. In the reorganization of 1974 the roles of professionals in the system were redefined when the 'voice of the expert' was given greater and more formal powers in the institutional structure (Klein 1983, p. 95). However, the increase in the powers of the professionals was accompanied by the establishment of overly complex organizational structures. The attempt was to achieve a variety of policy aims and in promoting managerial competence and satisfying the professionals (Klein 1983, p. 99). The reorganization of

1982 was similarly designed to achieve the purposes of greater efficiency in the system. Managerial roles were redefined and strengthened and team management was abolished. The responsibility for the operation of health services was given to a single executive manager within each geographical area. For the sake of a simpler bureaucratic structure, one level of hierarchy, the health authority, was abolished.

Perspective III Financial processes

The financial processes of a health system may shape it in several ways. They may affect the availability of resources, access to them, and, consequently, their utilization. They may also influence distributional equity and the quality of the process of care. Finally, the financial processes may determine the system's impact on health outcomes. The following discussion will address only the effects of financial processes on organizational patterns. Other financial influences have already been discussed in Chapter 4.

There are three possible financial funding processes:

(1) direct reimbursement of health professionals;

(2) funding of institutional providers (e.g. hospitals);

(3) financing of health insurers.

Clearly, the financing of insurers can only be relevant for countries where the social insurance systems are separate from the Government. Naturally, health professionals and institutional providers must be paid everywhere. The process of payment, however, varies substantially in different organizational settings.

Reimbursement of individual health professionals

Due to the immense influence of physicians on the performance of health systems, the reimbursement of physicians has naturally attracted considerable interests of decision-makers, planners and researchers. Salary, capitation, and fee-for-service are the three major options widely used for physicians' compensation. In a salaried system, payment is based on the amount of time the physician works. In a capitation system, payment is based on the number of patients for whom the physician is responsible. In Fee-For-Service (FFS) systems, remuneration is based on the physician's activity level, usually measured in terms of the number of visits and/or the number of procedures performed.

Reimbursement based on FFS is generally more expensive than either capitation or salary arrangements because under FFS the physician has a financial incentive to increase his professional activities. However, salary and capitation also contain cost-enhancing components not found in FFS systems. For example, while physicians working in FFS systems have an incentive to process patients quickly and efficiently, salaried physicians, and especially those on capitation, have no such financial incentive. Empirical studies in the US have shown that even though overall costs have been lower for salaried physicians practising in an HMO, the main savings resulted from reducing the rate of hospitalization and not from cost-containment in the ambulatory setting (Luft 1981).

Fee-for-service systems tend to be relatively expensive in terms of billing costs, though this depends in part on the degree of disaggregation of the fee schedule. In the absence of control mechanisms, it is relatively simple for a physician to overcharge the insurer by categorizing simple procedures into more lucrative billing codes. At the same time, the FFS billing system generates a great deal of information about the content of medical care, its distribution, and the efficiency of its provision. This has been shown particularly in Canada, where availability of detailed utilization data prompted extensive research on the functioning of the health system (Roos *et al.* 1987).

Salary systems are the easiest to administer. Reporting costs are low, and because the system imposes few reporting requirements on the individual physician, opportunities for misinformation are limited. The information from the payment system itself, however, is minimal.

Between FFS and salary models, capitation models have intermediate benefits. Physicians must generally submit reports on the size of their patient rosters, but preparing and processing such reports involves far less effort than processing the detailed claims required in the FFS system. The billing system under capitation generates little information about the content of care. Further, under capitation, physicians generally work in their own offices, so there are few opportunities for developing standard methods for data collection.

Reimbursement of institutional providers of health care

Institutional financing and reimbursement is even more complicated and problematic than individual provider reimbursement. Quite a number of recent books and review articles include very detailed classifications and analyses of the hospital reimbursement systems found in developed countries (see, for example: Glaser 1987; Evans 1984). Many of the analyses consider the advantages and disadvantages of each method, taking into account differences in institutional settings and national traditions.

In analysing systems for institutional reimbursement, we ask three basic questions:

1. What is the reimbursement method?

2. Who pays the institution or institutional system?
3. How is the money distributed?

1. There are several methods for institutional reimbursement. Reimbursement can be based on a global hospital budget, which is fixed annually, as in Canada (Evans 1984). It may consist of a standard daily charge averaged over the costs of caring for all patients. In Israel for example, the daily charge can be all-inclusive for all the costs incurred during a hospital stay (Ellencweig and Rosen 1989). Alternatively, with the exception of physicians' fees, it can consist of reimbursement for clinical services only, as is frequently found in the Netherlands (Glaser 1987, p. 16). Another method for institutional reimbursement is itemized billing with charge lists of separate fees for each item of care. This method, often labelled Fee-For-Service (FFS), is also widespread in the United States. The most recent specification for a unit of service is called case payments; a system of predetermined hospital rates. In the United States, these widely accepted units of service are based on diagnoses in the form of Diagnosis Related Groups (DRGs) (Glaser 1987). In this case, reimbursement is not directly linked to the cost of an individual treatment but rather to an average cost for each given diagnostic group.

2. Paying the institutional providers of health care can be achieved via four different means. The first is Government at its various levels: national, regional, and local. In most nationalized health systems, as in the USSR or England, and in most systems of social insurance, as in Canada, Germany, and Israel, institutional providers are reimbursed by the Government. The second means is via the recipient of care himself. Naturally, personal payments are the main vehicle in reimbursing providers under free-market conditions. In social insurance systems, the recipient of care frequently shares this responsibility with the Government. This is done by introducing into the system, prepaid insurance premiums and co-payments or deductibles for services actually rendered to the recipients of care. (Glaser 1987).

The third means is via employers' contribution to the cost of health care given to their employees. In some countries, like the US, this is an enormous contribution, as the cost of care for a substantial proportion of the active workforce is carried by employers (Glaser 1987). This instrument has been widely used in other countries, too. In Israel, for example, about one third of the national expenditure on health is indirectly covered by employers (Ellencweig and Rosen, 1989).

The fourth means is through philanthropic contributions. Though philanthropic organizations exist everywhere, their major impact as a source of reimbursement lies in the developing countries (World Bank 1980).

3. There are also several methods for the distribution of funds received by the institution. Consider three models for the organization of the hospital

system: it can be composed of several individual hospitals, of a system of regional networks of hospitals, or of a multi-hospital system. The first model, prevailing in the US, Germany, and France, is the classical organization for a hospital system. Reimbursements for services are transferred directly to the hospital management (Roemer 1977). The second model prevails in large national health systems where public ownership allocates funds to the regionalized structures, which in turn fund the individual hospitals. Good examples of this process of allocation are the NHS in England or the network of interorganizational relationships of hospitals as found in the Netherlands (Breemer ter Stege 1980).

The multi-hospital system model consists of the formation of hospital conglomerates. Here the system can take advantage of the economic benefits of large scale operations. The parent corporation, rather than the individual hospital, is reimbursed for services rendered to recipients of care. In the US, this fast-spreading model can be seen to be replacing the classical organization for a hospital system. It has been popularly predicted that within two decades, corporations will dominate all health care delivery in the US (Iglehart 1986).

Studying intra-organizational differences is another way to distinguish between reimbursement processes at the institutional receiving end. There are two models for examining differences in organizational structure. In the classical model, two separate groups, management and workers, create the active organization. Here, workers are not involved in the process of institutional reimbursement because hospital workers are salaried employees. This is typical of the health systems in Britain, Scandinavia, and Israel. In the second model, some professional groups in the hospital are in a more independent position. For instance, even when their activities are performed within the hospital complex, physicians in the US or in Canada are reimbursed on a separate payment scheme. Physicians' reimbursement can either be at an individual rate or at a group rate like those paid to physicians practicing in HMO-owned hospitals in the US (Luft 1981).

In conclusion, the three perspectives of the organizational classification:

I the administrative structure;
II decision-making and planning styles;
III financial processes;

reflect the substantial variation among health systems. The reader should not be discouraged by these variations, because they are easily articulated and measured. In the next section, we shall consider the use of indicators for the measurement of characteristics of the organizational classification.

Indicators of organizational classification

The indicators of the organizational classification can be divided into five categories which are:

(1) an examination of control and governance in the system;
(2) indicators for planning and evaluation;
(3) financial controls;
(4) reimbursements to individuals;
(5) reimbursements to institutions.

Perspective I The administrative structure

Government involvement

Control and governance This is an indicator reflecting the extent of the *structural* involvement of the government (national, regional or local) in the design and organization of a health care system. We suggest an ordinal scale to measure the extent of government control in a health system. The levels of the scale are as follows:

(1) complete ownership by the State as in the USSR;
(2) partial ownership by the State plus state-controlled insurance plans as in Britain, Israel, and the Scandinavian countries;
(3) no direct ownership by the State, but state-controlled insurance plans as in France and Germany;
(4) partial ownership by the State with no further intervention in the health care system as in Kenya and many other African countries;
(5) no ownership by the State or state intervention except for special groups like the elderly in the US (Medicare) or for special health domains like environmental health;
(6) no state control at all: free enterprise as was found in the US in the past.

Perspective II Planning and evaluation

Resource allocation

We suggest three indicators for measuring resource allocation processes in health systems.

Type of resource allocation This indicator is based on the typology suggested in Fig. 5.2. Countries can be divided into the three following categories:

(1) Pattern I

(2) Pattern II

(3) Pattern III

The examples from our discussion of Perspective II—decision-making and planning styles (p. 99), are helpful for categorizing health systems into their appropriate pattern.

Autonomy of health planners

The autonomy of health planners is often restricted by intervention by prominent 'outsiders'; in many countries for example, the Ministry of Finance (or other agencies of central government) intervenes in planning decisions. (Marmor and Bridges 1980). The extent of intervention in allocating resources by the Treasury or by other agencies of central government can be used as tracer for the autonomy of health planners. There are two possible levels:

(1) restricted authority, as in Israel and Germany where the Ministers of Finance have a final veto power over the health planning process, or in Norway and Finland where national governments strongly influence plans of local planners;

(2) lightly-restricted authority, as in the Canadian provinces or the regions of the NHS in England, where lack of outside intervention by central government's bureaucracy affords health planners more flexibility.

Centralized/decentralized resource allocation

This indicator measures the extent to which regional and local levels of government may make choices and plans. We suggest two broad categories:

(1) a centralized system where there is almost no power to allocate resources at a regional level, as in Israel and in most socialist countries;

(2) a decentralized system, where regional authorities can allocate resources within budget ceilings; among other places this arrangement is found in Scotland, Finland, and Canada.

Strategic planning

The following indicators measure the extent of strategic planning applied within a system.

Type of planning

Types of planning can be divided into four categories:

(1) systems planning;

(2) partnership planning;
(3) alliances planning;
(4) individual activities.

In the introductory section of this chapter we explained how to categorize countries into each group (see Perspective II – planning and evaluation).

The extent of implementation

This indicator measures the extent to which planning agencies can exert pressure on the implementation of health care programmes. Because the determination of the extent of this leverage is difficult, we suggest only two levels of the indicator. The indicator has a high value when planning agencies have strong administrative or legal leverage over the health care implementors, as seen in the NHS in England or in the Ministry of Health in the USSR. The indicator scores low when this leverage is absent, as in the national systems in the US and in Japan.

Perspective III Financial processes

Levels of financial control

In the analysis of the characteristics of a health system, yet another indicator of control must accompany the indicator of 'control and governance'. This second indicator is a measure of the extent of government control over the health system's financial arrangements. For the analysis of the extent of government leverage achieved through the control of financial sources, we suggest the following levels for the indicator:

1. *A fully-supported system* Though it can take many forms (e.g. subsidy, budgeting, or rebates) this arrangement reflects complete governmental financial control over the system as in Britain and the USSR.
2. *Partially supported system including government control over the resource allocation process* This method shares financial control between government and other agencies (e.g. local authorities), yet it permits nearly complete governmental control as in the Scandinavian countries.
3. *Partially supported systems with no governmental control over resource allocation* (as in France, Germany, and Israel) In addition to support from the Government, financial support is derived from membership fees in health insurance organizations, employers' contributions, and clients' co-payments for health services rendered to users.
4. *Government support only for specific programmes or populations* These would include health programmes for the elderly and the indigent, or financial coverage of environmental health programmes, as in the US.

5. *Minimal governmental or public support* This is very typical of developing countries, where employers' contributions or out of pocket payments constitute the major mode of financing health care services.

Types of reimbursement—individual providers

The following arrangements prevail in health systems:

1. *Salary* Health professionals on salary are mostly non-physicians. They also include physicians employed by institutional providers in some countries. This category includes physicians in Sweden, Israel, and hospital-based physicians in England.
2. *Fee-for-service* Fees may be negotiated at the time of service delivery as is done by private practitioners in several countries, or global fees may be set by agreement with professional associations, as in Canada.
3. *Active capitation* Capitation fees are paid to health professionals for only those clients who were actually seen during a reference period.
4. *Passive capitation* Capitation fees are paid for every client on physician rosters—as for GPs in England. Since, with the exception of physicians, most health workers are predominantly salaried, this mode of reimbursement is generally applicable only to physicians.

   In any given system, a further distinction can be made between primary care and hospital-based physicians for whom there are often different reimbursement schemes. For example, in England, hospital-based doctors are salaried while general practitioners are reimbursed by passive capitation.

Types of reimbursement—institutional providers

Institutional providers are frequently hospitals or hospital networks. Often institutional providers consist of large health insurers and other forms of health care organizations (e.g. HMOs, Sick Funds). The major reimbursement formulas are as follows:

1. *Negotiated budgets* Budgets are based on a forecast of future expenditures, sometimes according to a 'cost plus' formula which accounts for previous costs, inflation, and profits. An alternative option is a fixed formula which takes into account needs for health services, the general health of a population, etc. as found for the reimbursement of regions and districts in England and for the reimbursement of sick funds in Israel.
2. *Payment by unit of service or a fee for service scheme* In this mode, the cost of each given service is accounted for and fully reimbursed. This is the regular reimbursement system in the US.
3. *Payment on a per diem basis* The unit of payment is a hospital day and may or may not be according to the type of wards. For example in West

Germany's public hospitals it is averaged across all clinical services in the hospital.

4. *Payment by episode of care* For each episode there is a predetermined rate based on a severity index. A typical example is the Diagnosis Related Groups system (DRG) in the US which applies for elderly patients (under Medicare).
5. *Payment by capitation* Reimbursement is based on a per capita cost projection for the population of a catchment area.

Dimension 2 Centralization or decentralization?

The second dimension in the study of the organization of health systems addresses the question: to what extent has the system been decentralized? Arguments for either centralization or decentralization are usually based on three major components of organizations: power, authority, and responsibility. In the fifteenth century, Machiavelli wrote in *The Prince*:

> When states [are] newly acquired . . . there are three ways to hold them securely: first, by devastating them, next, by going and living in person (i.e. **centralization**). Thirdly, by letting them keep their own laws, exacting tribute, and setting up an oligarchy which will keep the state friendly to you (i.e. **decentralization**)
>
> (1988 edn; author's italics, AE.)

In the continuation of this discussion, Machiavelli strongly recommends the third approach, that is, when properly managed, decentralization is preferred.

Like Machiavelli, many health professionals today also recommend decentralization. In health systems, power—the first characteristic of decentralization—can be delegated into professional and administrative spheres. Given the notorious autonomy of professionals—particularly clinicians—in making health and clinical decisions, decentralization rules in the professional sphere. Concerning the administrative sphere, the picture is more ambiguous. On the one hand, the needs of a particular population are best served by decentralization because a decentralized system has the potential for dealing with local problems in small areas (Smith 1973). On the other hand, as often happens, formal decentralization does not delegate authority and responsibility. If formal delegation of authority is lacking, decentralized processes are ineffective. This problem can be illustrated by the health system in the USSR. Though formally it has a highly decentralized structure, the central bureaucracy in Moscow made regional planning efforts irrelevant, because authority remained in the headquarters (Ryan 1978). Some other decentralized systems like the Canadian (Taylor 1978) or the Australian health systems (Roemer and Roemer 1981) have been more successful in delegating power and authority regionally. For instance, the Canadian provinces and the Australian states have full jurisdiction over the provision of health care. This jurisdiction includes almost every segment of the population except for some specific groups like the armed forces and prisoners who are cared for by the federal government.

These examples imply that the use of structural indicators alone cannot predict the actual delegation of power, authority and responsibility in regionalized systems. Since indicators for delegation of either power or authority are not generally available, the use of proxies is recommended. Specific proxies are presented in the forthcoming section on indicators.

Indicators of centralization versus decentralization

Here we suggest two indicators: the first is purely structural and measures the extent of formal geographical decentralization in the system. The second, the index of democratization, was developed by political scientists (e.g. Vanhanen 1979) as an empirical measure for estimating the degree of political competition and electoral participation. The index of democratization may be used as a proxy measuring the delegation of power and authority to decentralized organizational structures. It is generally believed that in democratic societies authority and power are delegated to a large number of individual decision-makers: local governments, other agencies and citizens who are making their decisions on the basis of their individual preferences. At the other extreme, in non-democratic systems, a governing group like a political party makes all the decisions on behalf of the population (Berliner 1988).

Decentralization Index (DI)

The following alternative formal structures prevail:

1. *A fully decentralized system* Health care delivery is carried out in regional structures; the central government assumes responsibility for special activities like research or health education campaigns as in Britain, Sweden, Canada, and the USSR.
2. *A mostly decentralized system* Delivery of health care is decentralized, but central authorities assume jurisdiction over certain types of service; in the US system, for example, Medicare is under federal jurisdiction.
3. *A partially decentralized system* Some functions only, are decentralized; in Israel most preventive and some curative services are decentralized and provided on a geographical basis, while hospital services are mostly centralized.
4. *A fully centralized system* Central authorities assume all the responsibility and authority for the provision of health care; this model prevails in smaller countries as in Malta or Singapore.

The Index of Democratization (ID)

The index is a combination of two empirical variables, competition and participation. Competition is measured by calculating the share of the smaller parties in parliamentary or presidential elections. Participation is measured by estimating the percentage of the total population that actually voted in those same elections. The ID is calculated by multiplying the percentages of the two variables and by dividing the result by 100. A list of IDs for 119 countries can be found in Kurian's *Book of World Rankings* (1984).

A thorough examination of the issue of centralization versus decentralization must include the use of both indicators, the Decentralization Index (DI) and the Index of Democratization (ID). Using the DI alone can cause an incorrect interpretation. For example, from a purely structural and geographical perspective as reflected by the DI, the health care system in the USSR is fully decentralized (see above). However, because the ID is much lower in the USSR than in Western countries, the amount of actual decentralization is lower there than in most democratic countries.

Dimension 3 Levels of co-ordination and continuity

By levels of co-ordination, we mean the extent of collaboration within a health system, between institutions at the same or at different organizational levels. Collaboration at the same organizational level is called 'horizontal co-ordination'. For example, this co-ordination can be seen in the relationship between two separate agencies providing two interacting kinds of ambulatory care, like community mental health care services and social welfare services. 'Vertical co-ordination', on the other hand, which may also be viewed as decentralization, regularly involves delegation of authority and responsibility, because it requires the establishment of control mechanisms between different hierarchic levels in the system. In the case of horizontal co-ordination, health care workers at the same level of responsibility have no authority over each other. If conflicts in the organization prevent successful horizontal co-ordination, problems at any given level must be solved by some higher authority in the management. If such an authority is not willing or not able to exert power, then the lack of vertical co-ordination in a health system reflects an absence of central responsibility. One of the most striking examples of impotence of this sort is seen in the health system in the US. One of its better-known planning efforts, the Hill Burton programme, attempted to achieve better co-ordination between central authority and providers of care by using the leverage of a grant mechanism to supervise hospital construction. These efforts were unsuccessful due to relative lack of funds and mostly because alternative funding sources helped providers in bypassing the control desired (Gottlieb 1974).

In a later experiment in the 70s, Health System Agencies (HSAs) were assigned the task of producing plans and co-ordinating the allocation of resources for their respective service areas. Because this legislation required the HSAs to exercise greater authority over the organization and financing of health care than had earlier planning efforts, there was opposition from both state authorities and professional associations. This opposition caused the HSAs minimal achievement in planning and co-ordination. Things became even worse under the Reagan administration, which was idealogically resistant to intervening in institutional business. Planning efforts were eroded, and the HSAs became a skeleton agency with very limited responsibilities (Roemer 1986). It was finally abolished in 1987 (Sofaer 1988).

The lack of success of co-ordinating efforts in the American health system leaves an important question unanswered: how can successful collaboration in health systems be achieved and measured? Since determinations of success depend on adequate measurements, we will focus on how to measure co-ordination. For example, it has been suggested that levels of co-ordination in health systems be categorized according to the extent of the interdependency between organizations. There is continuum of levels of co-ordination ranging from contrasting parties, with a form of weak agreement between them, through coalescing parties with partial coalitions, up to a complete merger between parties (Thompson 1967; Starkweather and Cook 1988). In operational terms, a more practical approach is presented by Van de Ven and Ferry (1980) who suggest three basic co-ordination modes: impersonal, personal, and group. As presented in Table 5.1 they delineate several specific mechanisms for achieving co-ordination within each mode.

From Table 5.1 it is evident that it is worthwhile to study in cross-national

Table 5.1 Alternative co-ordination modes in health systems

	Impersonal	Personal	Group
High	*• Computerized information systems	• Co-ordination departments	*• Use of Task forces *• Use of standing committees
Medium	• Manual reports of plans and schedules	• Staff co-ordinators	• Use of *ad hoc* group meetings
Low	• Rules • Policies • Procedures	• Simple line hierarchy	• Simple direct contact

* Relevance to cross-national comparisons.
Adapted from Van de Ven and Ferry (1980, p. 248.)

perspective only those mechanisms that have scored 'high' in terms of the amount of communication they produce. In the course of practical evaluation, it is advisable to use indicators reflecting qualities of such 'high' co-ordination mechanisms. For example, the establishment of widespread management information systems, the extent and variety of standing committees, and the frequency of the use of 'task forces' in a health system.

Indicators of co-ordination of services

We suggest two approaches: the first is merely the study of structural co-ordination, vertical and horizontal within a system. The second approach focuses on the assessment of co-ordinative arrangements like use of information systems or committee work in a health system.

Horizontal co-ordination: co-ordination of curative and preventive networks

This indicator can be operationalized by creating an ordinal scale for potential levels which include:

1. *A fully co-ordinated system* Curative and preventive services are provided concurrently by a single agency; this is typical of the USSR.
2. *A partially co-ordinated system* Curative and preventive services may be provided by different agencies. Co-ordination is maintained among them by the exchange of information about the client's health status. In Israel, for instance, the Government provides preventive care while sick funds provide curative care. Some information exchange is present.
3. *Separate systems of curative and preventive medicine* Except for occasional flows of information, the systems are not co-ordinated. Such systems, for instance in the Mexican health care system, are often found in Latin America. Preventive care is under the responsibility of the Government or private practitioners, curative care is fragmented among several agencies.
4. *No system co-ordination* Curative care is provided mostly by individual practitioners. Preventive care is only partial and wherever it is found it is provided by volunteers or by international agencies. This is commonly found among African countries.

Vertical co-ordination: co-ordination of ambulatory and in-patient services

This indicator is very similar to the indicator of horizontal co-ordination, and a similar ordinal scale can be created to include the following:

1. *A fully co-ordinated system* A unified system for hospital and ambulatory care. Such fully co-ordinated systems are typically found in

socialist countries like the integrated health services in the USSR for example.

2. *Professional but not administrative co-ordination* Health professionals, in particular physicians, have privileges in hospitals. Co-ordination at the level of the care for individual patients is achieved by these physicians. On the other hand, there is no administrative linkage between community and in-patient services. This method is generally found in the US and Canada.
3. *Hierarchic administrative co-ordination* There is administrative co-ordination for planning and for resource allocation, for example, but there is no integration among health professionals in the ambulatory and hospital settings. Hierarchic administrative co-ordination is found in the NHS in England. At the professional level, there is no formal relationship between hospital and ambulatory services. The process of resource allocation for both these services is carried out by a single regional authority.
4. *Partial administrative co-ordination* That is, administration of health care is co-ordinated for only certain population groups. There is administrative vertical co-ordination for certain segments of the population covered by a specific health care plan as for members of Kaiser-Permanente plan (the largest HMO in the US). These health plans own and autonomously operate a network of ambulatory and in-patient services.
5. *No vertical integration* There is no vertical integration at either the professional or administrative levels. This condition is most frequently found in countries having weak managerial structures and lacking enough professional health care workers, as in many African countries.

Use of information systems

With respect to effective co-ordination, the necessary information consists of population profiles in the form of needs, utilization data, and medical, social, and psychological outcomes. In several health systems, routine data collection on these elements consists of the compilation of information originating at the *ecological*, or *population* level. Such data only reflects central tendencies and distributional trends but does not provide specific information to health agencies like hospitals, clinics, etc. Unfortunately, a higher degree of co-ordination among such health agencies can be achieved only if information is available not only at the *population* level but also at the *individual* or *epidemiological* level. The specific indicator here is the 'level of data aggregation'. This indicator can score high, moderate, or low. A health system with a high level of data aggregation is one in which there is a good assessment of its population's needs, utilization and health outcomes at the *individual* level. A typical example is the well co-ordinated

Finnish system where there is a constant flow of information on individual patients between health agencies. Other systems such as the US can be classified as moderately co-ordinated. If there is no or little data at the individual level, as in most African countries, systems can be classified as having a low level of co-ordination.

Use of group co-ordination

Group co-ordination is a measure of the extent that a group of people from several backgrounds or organizations can work together in planning and decision-making. Though the indicator is conceptually sound, it is difficult to assess what exactly is to be measured. One might want to measure team or committee activities; but such activities can only be evaluated subjectively, and some bias due to value judgement cannot be escaped. It is, however, possible to measure objectively the *extent* and *frequency* of the *establishment* of committees or project teams in a health system as a proxy for assessing co-ordinative efforts. The ordinal variable on 'use of group co-ordination' scores 'high' for health systems that openly endorse committee work as a basic component of managerial decision-making, as in Britain. It scores 'medium' for the US or Canada where inter-agency committees have more of an *ad hoc* character. It scores low for many developing countries in Africa for example, that have not yet established co-ordination networks between health agencies.

Dimension 4 The configuration of professional teams

Among different nations, there are very different structures of professional teams and different layouts between them. For instance, in the US; office-based solo practitioners dominate the scene; in the USSR, organized work in clinics; in Sweden, ambulatory functions provided by the hospital staff in out-patient clinics are frequently found. For practical purposes, one can separate the professional configurations of health care providers into two classes: those providing primary care, and those providing care in hospital or other institutional settings. Primary care is delivered either by physicians in solo practice, or by physicians working in organized health centres. Sweden and Finland have based their primary care services on such centres, called clinics, each having a team of general practitioners and nurses with specific responsibilities, (Weiner 1987). There are very similar arrangements in Israel also, where the largest health insurer—The General Sick Fund—operates several hundred clinics (Ellencweig 1983).

Clearly, in institutional settings there is no substitute for teamwork. There are, however, different ways to organize professional teams in hospitals or in other institutions. The conventional organizational model emphasizes functional design; this kind of structure is found when labour is divided into specialized departments according to function. Historically, hospitals were an excellent example of functional design because each department included a permanent staff with a fixed hierarchy. More recently, the appropriateness of traditional organizational function has been questioned, and hospitals have moved towards designs that allow better co-ordination and interaction between units. For example, in a matrix design, multidisciplinary teams comprising health professionals from different units, develop or conduct special programmes or plans. Matrix organizations are gaining in popularity in health settings particularly because many functions of modern hospitals require interdisciplinary collaboration (Neuhauser 1972; Crampton *et al.* 1978, Webber and Peters 1983).

Examination of the employment status of people in organizations may clarify yet another perspective of professional configuration. Clearly, health professionals are often employed by health organizations. This is true for most paramedical and nursing staffs in many health systems. It is also true for physicians in several nations like the USSR and Sweden, and in the hospital sector in Britain and West Germany. In another arrangement, some health professionals, particularly physicians, remain independent, but they are linked to a monopolistic buyer. This is the arrangement between general practitioners and the NHS in Britain, and between physicians and provincial insurance plans in Canada. Sometimes independent physicians may contract more than just one insurer, as seen in the sick funds in West Germany or in the insurance associations in France. Finally, although health professionals may maintain some loose arrangements with insurance organizations, their role as private practitioners remains mainly entrepreneurial. This is typical for most physicians in the US and for dentists in most Westernized societies.

In the next section we shall use appropriate indicators to determine operationally various arrangements for the establishment of professional teams.

Indicators on the configuration of professional teams

The different typologies of professional configuration may be presented divided into groups, each one relating to a particular type of health setting, primary (or ambulatory) care and institutional care.

Indicators for work teams in primary care

Percentage distribution of physicians in a health system in different modes of practice They may be categorized as follows:

(1) solo practitioners;
(2) physicians in group practices;
(3) physicians based in other clinical settings like hospital-based clinics, and so on.

The ratio between the number of physicians in primary care and the number of independent non-physicians in primary care In several countries, where physician manpower is either scarce or expensive, non-physician health care workers have filled the gap for providing primary health care. These include nurse practitioners, medical or physician assistants, physician extenders, and so on. The ratio between physicians and non-physician health care workers providing primary health care can be used as an indicator. The indicator can be further subdivided to reflect the number of workers in preventive and curative care. Thus, two ratios are produced, each reflecting a different dimension of the issue.

Indicators for work teams in institutional care

Distribution of the various types of institutional arrangements The indicator provides information on the arrangements in the hospital sector. They are expressed as percentages as follows:

(1) institutional networks or multi-hospital systems; this type is characterized by for-profit or not for-profit ownership in a competitive market as in hospital networks in the US;
(2) single private institutions;
(3) independent public institutions, these are autonomous entities each having a separate board of directors—typical of Canada;
(4) public institutions owned by the central government, corresponding to a 'government network';
(5) public institutions owned by local government;
(6) other types of public ownerships.

Intra-institutional configuration This indicator is also expressed as an estimate of a percentage distribution. Categories include:

1. Percentage of institutions still operating in classical modes. In the classical model, there is a central management team, often made up of an administrator, a physician, and a nurse. Alternatively, it can consist of single-handed management by a physician. This management is typical of community hospitals as in the US, Japan etc.
2. Percentage of institutions in decentralized configurations which enable more autonomy for peripheral units. This is seen in hospitals where there is a formalized departmental structure, and management teams are functional.
3. Percentage of institutions sharing a multi-disciplinary configuration in matrix form. A direct evaluation of the extent of matrix structures within a system is often unavailable. A reliable proxy are tertiary academic

centres, because the complex operation of tertiary centres requires collaboration between various departments or units. Such collaboration can only be achieved in a matrix configuration. Thus the proportion of beds in tertiary centres in a country will roughly correspond to the volume of matrix structures in the system.

Employment status Employment status is defined as a percentage distribution of each of the employment statuses in a system.
Following are examples of frequently encountered employment types:

(1) full-time employees;

(2) part-time employees;

(3) contracting independent health professionals;

(4) non-contracting independent health professionals.

Often, a single health worker can be categorized by more than one employment type. For example, in Britain and in Israel, top hospital-based specialists—called consultants in the UK—also carry out a fully entrepreneurial practice as non-contracting independents. These physicians maintain full-time employee status as salaried senior members of their hospitals, and thus must be categorized both as 'non-contracting independents' and also as 'full-time employees.'

Dimension 5 Organizing for equity

Organizing for equity requires the clarification of the concept of equity, often discussed together with equality. Though the two terms are easily distinguishable, many health professionals tend to use 'equity' and 'equality' interchangeably. Intuitively, 'equality' is an objective term indicating that similar quantities of health care, of equal quality, are provided to each individual or group under similar conditions. Further examination reveals, however, that there is little meaning to the provision of equal quantities of health care to different individuals (Ellencweig and Grafstein 1986), because needs as well as interpersonal, social, and behavioural factors are so highly variable. The more realistic term, 'equity' reflects an egalitarian approach based on the different needs of individuals in homogenous groups and their aspirations, and on the general environmental and social conditions pertinent to the health care system (Fein 1972).

Unfortunately, equitable health care goals are rarely met. The inequities in the provision of health care facilities, personnel and procedures have been discussed by various authors (Alan Dever 1980; Ellencweig 1983; Shuval 1987; Wyszewianski and Donabedian 1981). Research has shown that the interaction of care-seekers with the system varies among groups (Shuval 1979). A demonstration of an integrated approach including both structural and attitudinal perspectives is the Black Committee Report (Townsend and Davidson 1982). It details the manifestation of patterns of inequality in access to care in the British health care system. Considering the differences in trends of utilization and in health outcomes within the context of poverty and class structure. The Black Committee Report shows that there is a positive correlation between utilization and social class: the higher the social class, the more frequent the utilization. Similarily, wealthier people generally have better health outcomes.

Even with this evidence of harsh reality in mind, one can opt for an operational definition of equity. This is certainly not easy because the concept of equity embodies subjective as well as objective measures. However, in a pioneer study on this topic Aday and colleagues suggest a plausible solution. They argue that 'the greatest "equity" of access is said to exist when need, rather than structural factors (for example, availability of physicians), or individual factors (for example, family income) determine who gains entry to the health care system' (Aday *et al.* 1980, p. 26; see also Andersen *et al.* 1975, pp. 10–11). In other words, access is equitable if utilization, as operationally defined, is related to health status in an optimal way.

According to this argument, in order to evaluate the extent that conditions are equitable, one should first assess needs and then correlate them to the actual utilization process. We considered this process in our discussion on needs assessment. However, the measurement of equity requires far more than the mere assessment of the gulf between needs and actual utilization of health services. As Sloan and Bentkover (1979) put it:

> Specifically, variations in certain potential access variables, especially process variables, can have equity implications even if they do not show up as important on the Aday and Andersen* criterion, that is, by reference to their effects on utilization rates. Time spent in a waiting room, or out-of-pocket health-care expenditures, if they vary with income group (corrected for health status), are differentially burdensome even if utilization rates (or use per need rates) are not affected. More generally, someone may argue that some inequalities in potential access variables between subgroups raise equity questions even if they do not affect the outcomes of health-care-seeking behavior, as measured by utilization rates. They still affect other outcomes—for example, what else someone has the chance to do with his time or money.

A plausible solution for these problems is to add, beyond utilization, new dimensions to the measurement of equity. These new dimensions focus on process measures like the quality of service rendered to the patient, or on outcome measures like patient satisfaction. A detailed discussion of those measures is given in Chapters 6, 7, and 8.

* Aday and Andersen 1974.

Indicators of equity

As shown in the previous section, issues of equity are closely related to both the process and to the outcome of health care. Therefore, considerations of equity should by no means be restricted to the study of distributional equity, that is equity from an organizational perspective. While further measures of equity, related to outcome, will be discussed in Chapter 8, here we shall elaborate on measures related to the organization of health care. Such equity measures can be approached either descriptively or analytically.

Descriptive evaluation of equity measures

A descriptive evaluation of equity consists of comparisons of the availability of health-related resources among smaller areas within a country or among different nations. For example, equity may be assessed through the geographical distribution of:

- manpower (physicians, nurses, etc.);
- hospital beds;
- dwellings with running water (in developing countries);
- dwellings with sewage disposal (in developing countries).

Though these simple ecological indices are easy to obtain, they provide only a crude picture of equity because ecological information does not reflect individual needs. More sensitive indicators are required for the examination of individual differences in equity. A promising approach is to compare output measures, like levels of vaccination coverage which can be used as a universal 'tracer' of coverage and of effectiveness in health systems.

The analytical examination of equity (Lorenz curve approach)

In Chapter 4, we discussed the use of the Gini coefficient as a measure of distributional allocation. The Gini coefficient can also be used to measure equity. Similar to the use of the Gini coefficient is the qualitative comparison among various countries or regions of the shape of Lorenz curves for selected indicators.

For example, Fig. 5.3 provides information on the Peruvian health system (Musgrove 1986). Two indicators are considered simultaneously, the per capita government expenditure on health (*E*) and the per capita geographical distribution of physicians (*O*). The diagonal represents a state of full equity. The lower Lorenz curve reflects the relation between cumulated population to the cumulated percentage of the number of physicians per capita. The upper Lorenz curve reflects the relation between the cumulated population to the cumulated percentage of per capita expenditure on health.

If one wishes a quantitative value for each indicator its Gini coefficient can be calculated by measuring the area between each Lorenz curve and the diagonal. From Fig. 5.3 it is easily seen that inequity in per capita government expenditure is smaller than the inequity in physician distribution. Thus, the indicator (O) overestimates inequity.

The ability to distinguish between inequity and inequality is another interesting feature of the analytical approach. Consider again Fig. 5.3; the lower diagonal A represents the estimated level of per capita government expenditure on health if adequate medical care could have been given to needy patients. That is, if duplication or unnecessary treatment were eliminated and efficient use of services were guaranteed, the cumulative per capita expenditure would have amounted to only 85 per cent of its actual value. The hatched area in the graph represents real inequity, and the dotted area represents inequality.

In conclusion, the use of the Lorenz curve approach in cross-national or cross-regional comparisons requires the completion of the following sequence of steps:

1. Selecting one or multiple adequate indicator(s) (see Fig. 5.3).
2. Drawing a Lorenz curve for each indicator for the first country or region.

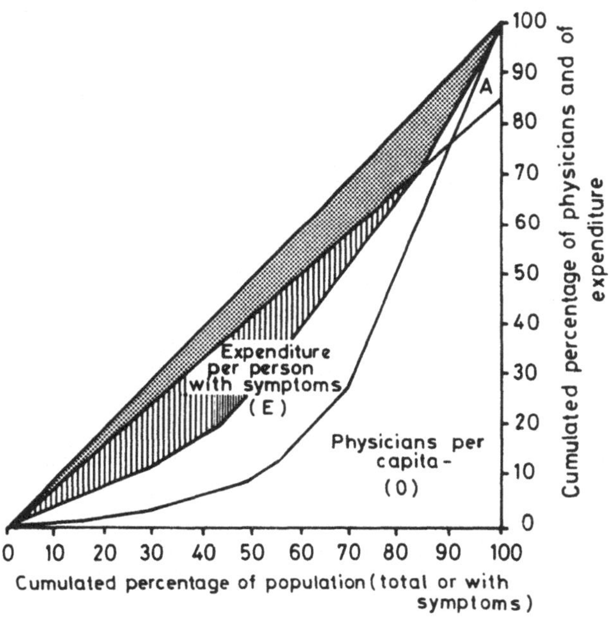

Fig. 5.3 Lorenz Curves of inequality of the distribution of physicians relative to population (by department) and of Ministry of Health patient-related expenditure relative to population with symptoms (by health region), Peru; 1982. (From Musgrove (1986), with permission.)

3. Optional: Calculating the Gini coefficient for the first country or region.
4. Repeating steps 2 and 3 for the other countries and regions to be examined.
5. Comparing these regions and countries for inequity by using a qualitative method (Lorenz curve) or a quantitative method (Gini coefficient).

Dimension 6 The appropriateness of care

Closely related to equity is the appropriateness, or adequacy, of care. In an organizational context, appropriateness relates to levels of available resources with respect to population needs, or to the 'extent to which needed or indicated services are sufficient' (Lane and Kelman 1975). These levels of appropriateness can be determined with reference to quantity and quality. Indeed, there was an intense effort in the literature to determine the extent of 'sufficient care' through definition of a decent basic minimum of care. One interpretation is suggested by Fried (1976) who argues that the decent minimum health care should reflect values generally accepted or tolerable to society as a societal commitment, like mother and child health care. The problem with Fried's approach is that it does not allow for an operational definition of what is 'tolerable' or 'acceptable' and therefore just extends the difficulty from the definition of appropriateness, *per se*, to that of other concepts. Alternatively, Enthoven (1980) suggests that the concept may be interpreted in two ways:

(1) by reference to a criterion indicating whether services have reached the minimum accepted by society;
(2) by listing services which are essential for appropriate care.

The translation of the concept of a decent basic minimum of care to an operational definition, which Enthoven labels 'basic health services approach', requires a set of minimal standards and criteria. He delineates the essential components of this minimal list of health services as follows:

> . . . a qualified plan would be required to cover, at a minimum, the list of services called 'basic health services' in the Health Maintenance Organization (HMO) Act of 1973 (as amended). This list includes physician services, inpatient and outpatient hospital service, emergency health service, short term outpatient mental health service (up to twenty visits), treatment and referral for drug and alcohol abuse, laboratory and X-ray, home health services, and certain preventive health services.
> (Enthoven 1980, p. 128.)

Further clarification of such a minimal list would require breaking general health care services into operational blocks of care and then defining a minimal list for each one. One such useful classification divides health services into primary, secondary, and tertiary levels of care. The primary level comprises curative and preventive services rendered to the community; the secondary level includes in-patient care and out-patient specialist care at the hospital or the extended care unit. Tertiary care consists of subspeciality in-patient functions like thoracic or plastic surgery, burns units, intensive care units and rehabilitation facilities (Numerof 1982, p. 67).

The appropriateness of health care systems can also be measured in the relationship of the competence of health care personnel to the responsibility and authority which they have assumed (Donabedian 1980; Mechanic 1986). The role of nurses, for example, is judged differently in different countries. In the US, it is appropriate for nurse practitioners to see patients, prescribe drugs, and to refer the patient to a physician for further care when necessary (Bacon and Kotkin 1983). Such independence on the part of a nurse, even a highly qualified one, is not tolerated in most European countries. There, according to the classical model of the physician–nurse relationship, nurses lack the training and authority to make simple clinical decisions necessary for the safety and comfort of patients (Stein 1967).

Indicators for the appropriateness of care

A series of indicators for appropriateness of care can be developed according to the conceptual outline described above. These indicators should address the balance between primary, secondary, and tertiary services in various geographical areas or population groups. The indicators should also relate to the distribution of health professionals for these service areas and populations. Closely related to the previously described group of indicators measuring equity, indicators for the appropriateness of care can be exemplified as follows:

Extent of coverage

This indicator measures appropriateness of care by assessing the extent of coverage. Coverage can be achieved by insurance or by market mechanism. It includes the following levels:

(1) percentage of population covered by primary care services;
(2) percentage of population having access to secondary care services;
(3) percentage of population having access to tertiary care services.

Comprehensiveness of coverage

This is a departure from the previous indicator and the two indicators should be studied simultaneously. Comprehensiveness of coverage includes the following levels:

(1) comprehensiveness of coverage in primary care services (the score is 'high' if coverage includes preventive and dental care, 'medium' if only

one type of the above care is provided, otherwise countries are scored 'low');

(2) comprehensiveness of coverage in institutional care (the indicator scores 'high' if institutional coverage includes long term care and mental care; If only one type of extended care is provided, the score is 'medium', otherwise 'low').

The ratio of health professionals per capita

This indicator can be used as a proxy to measure the appropriateness of care qualitatively. It includes the following levels:

(1) primary care physicians per capita;

(2) secondary care physicians per capita;

(3) tertiary care physicians per capita.

In countries where physicians have hospital privileges, it is more meaningful to use the rate of general practitioners or of specialists per capita as an alternative to the three levels listed above.

Since there are no real standards for appropriate ratios of this sort, the normative method is the most useful approach. It consists of computing these ratios for each indicator and for several regions or nations and then testing for outliers. Outliers then represent systems where the supply of health care manpower is inappropriate. Obviously, when there is an oversupply of manpower, the ratios are too high; when there is an undersupply, the ratios are too low.

The balance between health professions

Of all the concepts related to the appropriateness of care, the most difficult concept to operationalize is the balance between health professions. The difficulty arises because the mere calculation of ratios between physicians and nurses or other health professionals cannot account for the legal and administrative differences between countries. Thus, comparisons are restricted to areas or regions of a single country, or to two countries which have adopted similar legal and administrative health manpower policies like the US and Canada. Following are some useful indicators for cross-national or cross-regional comparison of the balance between health professionals:

- the rate of physician assistants per capita;
- the ratio between physician assistants and primary care physicians (or general practitioners);
- the rate of nurse practitioners per capita;
- the ratio between nurse practitioners and primary care physicians (or general practitioners).

Dimension 7 The accountability of a health system

Accountability in a health system can be seen in two ways. First, the accountability of health-care providers is reflected by the appropriateness of use of information in organizational processes. Second, the accountability of consumers is reflected by the ways that consumers can influence directions and policies in their health system.

Provider accountability

The ability of a health system to withstand critical evaluation of its processes of information gathering can be called provider accountability. This accountability can be evaluated by examining the information as it is transferred from level to level up and down the hierarchy of the health system. The process of evaluation addresses the basic role of information systems rather than the content of the messages themselves. In operational terms, the transfer of information may be considered a continuum, limited at one extreme by the absence of information to be transferred. In such a case, decision-makers can be mislead by lack of information, which may cause them to minimize the magnitude of a problem thus hindering the decision-making process. At the other extreme there is a danger of over-collection of information that may be irrelevant or inaccurate. Excess data collection is expensive; it may not even be used at all. Worse, by providing contradictory information it can hamper the decision-making process. For instance data on health services utilization can be gathered either directly from providers or from population surveys. There may be considerable inconsistencies in the data from these two sources. Providers often have an incentive to report higher utilization, and consumers often under-report on the number of doctor visits because of 'recall bias', that is they have forgotten certain details of their utilization.

Since the major functions of organizational development, planning, evaluation, and control, require appropriate information, adequate accounting systems are crucial to the functioning of health care services. The following analysis of accountability is based on general control theory (Anand 1984), and is specifically adjusted for assessing health systems. There are two types of analyses: the first type is called structural accountability because it emphasizes the system's predetermined elements of accountability. The second type of analysis, called action accountability, involves following up the activities of decision-makers.

Structural Accountability

At the basic level, structural accountability is an evaluation of the system's data collection method. In an appropriate information system data will be valid, reliable, sensitive, and specific. Validity is the extent to which the information being collected actually represents reality. In international or cross-regional comparisons, validity can be secured by strictly adhering to accepted criteria. Indeed, WHO statistical publications elaborate criteria for the measurement of either structural data like health manpower, or of outcome data like birth rates or mortality rates (use of ICD-8 or ICD-9 systems) (see WHO publications). While vital statistics are fairly standardized, inconsistencies remain, however, for some input variables such as rates of allied health professions or types of hospital beds.

Reliability is the extent to which a measurement tool will produce the same result when used for multiple measurements of a given item. Failure to report, inaccurate processing, or merely lack of information all threaten the data's accuracy. Examining data from WHO publications can illustrate these concerns. For example, the WHO reports that in 1973 there were 10 625 physicians in Columbia, or 1 physician per 2180 persons. In 1975, it reports 13 000 physicians in Columbia, or 1 physician per 1810 persons, an increase of more than 20 per cent in 2 years (WHO 1979)! Similarly, WHO publications report a spectacular 25 per cent increase in the number of physicians in Uruguay in just 3 years between 1972 and 1975. There are similar discrepancies in reports of outcome measures. For instance, what is the true meaning of the fantastic 21 per cent decrease in infant mortality in El Salvador between 1979 and 1980 (WHO 1983)? Is this simply inaccuracy in reporting, or is it really a reflection of an amazingly rapid improvement in infant care? There is no theoretical way to answer this question, so we must consider empirical means for such an evaluation. Empirical criteria can be developed by identifying 'outlier countries' (for international reporting systems) or 'outlier regions' (for national reporting systems). These empirical criteria suggest that countries can be classified according to the consistency of their reporting on health measures, called the 'stability of data'. Countries with great fluctuations in data reporting over time are thus classified into a 'suspected low accountability' group.

To strengthen the validity of this approach, a companion criterion to stability can also be developed by examining 'data feasibility' which is the extent to which longitudinal data is available from a region or country. For example, we carried out a ten-year survey (1975–1984) in WHO Statistical Annuals (WHO publications) focusing on reports of mortality according to cause. In Switzerland these data were reported ten times, once each year. Figures for the US were reported nine times, once for each year but the last, due to a consistent lag in US reporting. Australia reported data only eight times. On the other hand, there was only one report from Brazil and one from Sri Lanka. Several countries, including the USSR, India, and Kenya, failed to report at all.

At a more sophisticated level, data accountability may include standards and criteria for determining resource allocation (input standards), standards and norms for health activities (process standards), and criteria for recommended health outcomes (outcome standards). Other forms of structural accountability relate to the evaluation of the financial and managerial functions of health organizations like appropriate budget preparation and use or the extent of adherence of health organizations to their stated objectives. This last is often studied by using managerial techniques such as Management by Objectives—MBO (Kaluzny *et al.* 1982, pp. 251–2).

Action accountability

The second type of analysis for the study of provider accountability is action accountability. This type of accountability is based on a feedback control system in which decision-makers are held accountable for their actions. Using this concept for comparative analysis requires defining the limits of acceptable behaviour. We must track the actual behaviour of decision-makers, compare this with their previous behaviour in light of our knowledge of past developments, and then measure deviations from accepted standards for good management practice. This task is not always easy, but it may be rewarding when the analysis is restricted to a limited group of top decision-makers.

Consumer accountability

Consumer accountability, also called 'consumer participation', involves the relationship between provider systems and the recipients of care. It has long been accepted that consumers should be educated to increase their responsibility for their own health, and that they 'should be involved in decisions regarding the provision and evaluation of health care' (Institute of Medicine 1976). However, only a handful of health systems have successfully achieved a significant level of consumer accountability. In Britain, since 1974, Community Health Councils (CHC) have represented the interests of the public in the health system. Reasonable criteria have been developed for ascertaining the interaction between the CHC and health districts within the NHS (DHSS 1974). These arrangements are meant to guarantee that each planning initiative or any change in the health care delivery policy requires consultation with the CHC. The NHS administration, however, has often considered this process 'unnecessary and time-consuming' (Royal Commission 1979). In other countries, particularly those with a market-oriented, free enterprise health system, public opinion generally views the organizing of consumers into a 'scrutineering lobby' as unnecessary because consumers can choose freely among health care providers (Bates 1983).

Indicators of accountability

Structural accountability

Measures of structural accountability include:

Frequency of data reporting This indicator can be based on WHO sources. The *World Health Statistics Annual* (WHO publications) is a particularly useful source for comparisons. A dichotomous variable can be constructed: its value is one when there is regular reporting; otherwise its value is zero. Reporting is considered regular when the country has reported on 50 per cent or more of the required periods. Note that the frequency of regular reporting varies considerably for various types of information. Some measures, like vital statistics, require annual reporting. Other measures, like structural characteristics or the incidence of infectious diseases, require far less frequent reporting.

Consistency (reliability) of data The frequency of regular reporting is a necessary but insufficient indicator of data accountability. Even if reports for consecutive years are available, the figures must be examined carefully for their reliability. This can be done for tracer conditions such as representative age/sex specific mortality rates. For each country studied, consecutive yearly rates are compared and are evaluated for their reliability.

Action accountability

Action accountability is an indirect measure of data accountability. It relates to the investigation of the major administrative processes in a health system. We suggest the evaluation of 'controlled processes' as an indicator. The existence of controlled processes in a health system can be studied by using a proxy like the examination of the budget process. If a detailed annual budget is presented to the public by means of a parliamentary system, and if financial operations are carried out and monitored according to the budget lines, then action accountability is 'high'. This is commonly achieved in western democracies. If there is a budget that was not approved by parliamentary decision, and there is no open monitoring of financial operations, then action accountability is medium, as is typical in socialist countries. When the budget for the health system is not adequately presented, then action accountability of the system will score 'low'. This is typical of most developing countries.

Consumer accountability

If there are formal mechanisms for consumer participation in decision-making within the health system, as is typical in Britain (CHCs), then consumer accountability is 'high'. If there are no such established mechanisms, then the value of this indicator is 'low'.

References

Aday, L. A. and Andersen, R. (1974). A framework for the study of access to medical care. *Health Services Research*, **9**, 208–20.

Aday, L. A., Andersen, R., and Fleming, G. V. (1980). *Health care in the US: equitable for whom*. Sage, Beverly Hills.

Alan Dever, G. E. (1980). *Community health analysis*. Aspen, Germantown, Maryland.

Anand, D. K. (1984). *Introduction to control systems*. Pergamon Press, Oxford.

Andersen, R., Anderson, O., and Kravitz, J. (1975). *Equity in health services: empirical analysis in social policy*. Ballinger, Cambridge, Massachusetts.

Bacon, T. J. and Kotkin, S. Z. (1983). The health professions: policies and issues. In *Policy issues in personal health services* (ed. C. J. Sagar and J. E. Paul), Chapter 11. Aspen, Rockville, Maryland.

Bates, E. (1983). *Health systems and public scrutiny—Australia, Britain and the United States*. Croom Helm, London.

Berliner, J. S. (1988). The comparison of social welfare systems. In *State and Welfare USA/USSR*. (ed. G. W. Lapidus and G. E. Swanson). Institute of International Studies, University of California, Berkeley.

Blum, L. H. (1974). *Planning for health—development and application of social change theory*. Human Sciences Press, New York.

Breemer ter Stege, C. P. (1980). Hospital response to a changing organization environment: the regionalization of hospital care in the Netherlands. *Social Science and Medicine*, **14A**, 445–52.

Crampton, K. R., Weiner D. S., and Regina V. (1978). Matrix structure in a large hospital ambulatory service. *The Journal of Ambulatory Care Management*, **1** (July), 65–74.

Davis, C. M. (1988). The organization and performance of the contemporary Soviet Health Service. In *State and welfare USA/USSR* (ed. G. W. Lapidus and G. E. Swanson). Institute of International Studies, University of California, Berkeley.

DHSS (Department of Health and Social Security) (1974). *Democracy in the National Health Service*. HMSO. London.

Donabedian, A. (1980). *Definition of quality and approaches to its assessment, Explorations in quality assessment and monitoring*. Vol. 1. Health Administration Press, Ann Arbor, Michigan.

Ellencweig, A. Y. (1983). The new Israeli health care reform: an analysis of a national need. *Journal of Health Politics, Policy and Law*, **8**, 366–86.

Ellencweig, A. Y. and Grafstein, O. (1986). Inequities in health care—a proposed model. *Journal of Management in Medicine*, **1**, (3), 206–39.

Ellencweig, A. Y. and Rosen, B. (1989). *Reimbursement of the hospital sector in Israel—pitfalls and prospects*. Unpublished.

Enthoven, A. (1980). *Health plan: the only practical solution to the soaring costs of medical care*. Addison-Wesley, Reading, Massachusetts.

Evans, R. G. (1984). *Strained mercy*. Butterworths, Toronto.

Fein, R. (1972). On achieving access and equity in health care. *Milbank Memorial Fund Quarterly*, **50**, 157–90.

Fried, C. (1976). Equality and rights in medical care. *Hastings Centre Report*, **6**, (1), 29–34.

Glaser, W. A. (1987). *Paying the hospital*. Jossey-Bass, San Francisco.

Gottlieb, S. R. (1974). A brief history of health planning in the US. In *Regulating health facilities construction* (ed. C. C. Havinghurst), pp. 7–26. American Enterprise Institute for Public Policy Research Washington, DC.

Heidenheimer, A. J., Helco, H., and Teich Adams, C. (1983). *Comparative public policy*, (2nd edn). MacMillan, London.

Hyman, H. H. (1976). *Health planning: a systematic approach*. Aspen Systems, Bolder, Colorado.

Iglehart, J. K. (1986). Kaiser, HMOs and the public interest: a conversation with James A. Vohs. *Health Affairs*, **5**, 44–9.

Institute of Medicine (1976). *Assessing quality in health care: an evaluation*. National Academy of Sciences, Washington, DC.

Kaluzny, A. D., Warner, D. M., Warren, D. G., and Zelman, W. N. (1982). *Management of health services*, Prentice Hall, Englewood Cliffs, New Jersey.

Kleczkowski, B. M., Elling, R. H., and Smith, D. L. (1984*a*). *Health system support for primary health care*, Public Health Papers, No. 80. World Health Organization, Geneva.

Kleczkowski, B. M., Roemer, M. I., and van der Werff, A. (1984*b*). *National health systems and their orientation towards health for all*, Public Health Papers, No. 77. World Health Organization, Geneva.

Klein, R. (1983). *The politics of the National Health Service*. Longman, London.

Kurian, G. T. (1984). *The new book of world rankings*, pp. 65–6. Fact on File Publication, New York.

Lane, D. S. and Kelman, H. R. (1975). Assessment of maternal health care quality: conceptual and methodological issues. *Medical-Care*, **8**, (10), 791–807.

Luft, H. S. (1981). *Health maintenance organizations: dimensions of performance*. Wiley—Interscience, New York.

Machiavelli, N. (1988). *The Prince*. (ed. Q. Skinner and R. Price). Cambridge University Press, Cambridge.

Marmor, T. R. and Bridges, A. (1980). American health planning and the lessons of comparative policy analysis. *Journal of Health Politics, Policy and Law*, **5**, (3), 419–30.

Maxwell, R. J. (1981). *Health and wealth: an international study of health care spending*. Lexington Books, Lexington, Massachusetts.

Mechanic, D. (1986). *From advocacy to allocation. The evolving American health system*. The Free Press, New York.

Musgrove, P. (1986). *Measurement of equity in health*, World Health Statistic Bulletin 39, pp. 325–35.

Neuhauser, D. (1972). The hospital as a matrix organization. *Hospital Administration*, **17**, (4), 8–25.

Numerof, R. (1982). *The practice of management for health care professionals*, p. 67. Amacom, New York.

Roemer, M. I. (1977). *Comparative national policies on health care*. Marcel Dekker Inc., New York.

Roemer, M. I. (1986). *An introduction to the US health care system*. (2dn edn), Chapter 7. Springer Publishing Company, New York.

Roemer, M.I. (1989). National health systems as market interventions. *Journal of Public Health Policy*, **10**, (1), 62-77.

Roemer, M.I. and Roemer, R.J. (1981). *Health care systems and comparative manpower policies*, Chapter 2. Marcel Dekker Inc., New York.

Roos, L.R., Nicol, P.J., and Cageorge, S.M. (1987). Using administrative data for longitudinal research: comparisons with primary data collection. *Journal of Chronic Diseases*, **40**, (1), 41-9.

Royal Commission of the National Health Services (1979). *Report*, Cmnd. 7615. HMSO, London.

Ryan, M. (1978). *The organization of Soviet medical care*. Blackwell, Oxford.

Shuval, J. (1979). Primary care and social control. *Medical Care*, **17**, 631-8.

Shuval, J. (1987). Health in Israel: patterns of equality and inequalities in health. Paper prepared for meeting on Inequality in Health. WHO, Regional Office for Europe, Lisbon, 28-30 September.

Sloan, F. and Bentkover, J.D. (1979). *Access to ambulatory care and the US economy*. Lexington Books, Lexington, Massachusetts.

Smith, D.M. (1973). *The geography of social well-being in the US*. McGraw Hill, New York.

Sofaer, S. (1988). Community health planning in the US: a post mortem. *Family Community Health*, **10**, 1-12.

Starkweather, D. and Cook, S.K. (1988). Organization-environment relation. In *Health care management—a text in organizational theory and behavior*, (2nd edn) (ed. S.M. Shortell and A.D. Kaluzny), Chapter 10. John Wiley, New York.

Stein, L.I. (1967). The doctor-nurse game. *Archives of General Psychiatry*, **16**, 699-703.

Taylor, M.G. (1978). *Health insurance and Canadian health policy*. McGill-Queen's University Press, Montreal.

Thompson, J.D. (1967). *Organizations in action*. McGraw-Hill, New York.

Torrens, P.R. (1984). Historical evolution and overview of health services in the US. In *Introduction to health services*, (2nd edn) (ed. S.J. Williams and P.A. Torrens). Wiley, New York.

Townsend, P. and Davidson, N. (1982). *Inequalities in health—the Black Report*. Penguin, Harmondsworth.

Van de Ven, A.H. and Ferry, D.L. (1980). *Measuring and assessing organizations*. Wiley, New York.

Vanhanen, T. (1979). *Power and the means of power: a study of 119 Asian, European, Asian and African States, 1850-1975*. University Microfilm International, Ann Arbor, Michigan.

Webber, J.B. and Peters J.P. (1983). *Strategic thinking. New frontiers for hospital management*. American Hospital Association, Chicago.

Weiner, J.P. (1987). Primary care delivery in the United States and four Northwest European Countries: comparing the 'corporatized' with the 'socialized'. *Milbank Memorial Fund Quarterly*, **65**, (3), 426-61.

WHO (World Health Organization) (1979). Health personnel and hospital establishments, 1978. *World Health Statistics*, Vol. II, 1978a, Geneva.

WHO (World Health Organization). *World Health Statistics Annual*. WHO, Geneva. (Various years.)

World Bank (1980). *Health Sector Policy Paper*. Washington, DC.

Wyszewianski, L. and Donabedian, A. (1981). Equity in the distribution of quality of care. *Medical Care*, **19**, (suppl.), 28-56.

6. The process of health care delivery—direct and indirect determinants

Though the goal of health systems is to improve the health status of the population, outcomes are frequently forgotten due to the complex and turbulent process of care. Only a few sceptics, like Illich (1977), have dared to question the role of hospitals, for example, in shaping health status. As Illich put it, it is possible that instead of improving health, hospitals may rather sustain 'iatrogenesis'. By 'iatrogenesis' Illich means the production of disease and sickness by the hospital system itself. Yet, for most people in modern societies, Illich's view is unacceptable. Though hospitals and other health services are only *means* to improve the *ends* —which are the health of the population—the use of health services is so generally acceptable in modern societies that justifying the *ends* is no longer required.

People in our modern society may take advantage of the health system for ends not obviously associated with improving their health. In this way, they are involved in the process of health care without any concern for the health system goals. Consider a little story about three old ladies who used to have their regular daily meeting at their physician's clinic. One day, one of the ladies failed to show up. 'Where is Ruth?' asked one of her counterparts, 'Oh!' answered the other one, 'she couldn't make it today because she's sick!' Ruth clearly viewed the health system as central to her social life and peripheral to her physical health. Had she come to meet her friends even though she were ill, her proximity to her doctor might have launched her into a complex process of health care.

Let us explore the major components of this process. There are two principal groups of attributes for describing the process: direct attributes and latent or indirect attributes. Direct attributes are characteristics directly related to the process of care, like:

(1) utilization measures;

(2) accessibility to health care systems;

(3) acceptability of the health services by the recipients of care;

(4) patients' compliance to the instructions given by the providers of care;

(5) the appropriateness of the process itself, which also includes ethical and moral characteristics of care.

Latent attributes significantly affect the process of care, though they are not directly related to it. Latent attributes include:

(1) the level of professional autonomy;

(2) labour relationships within the health system;

(3) process-oriented components of the quality of care;

In the following discussion, we shall discuss the many concepts of the health care process at the conceptual level and then describe the appropriate indicators for each of the concepts.

The direct attributes

Utilization

Descriptive utilization

The usage of health care services is the most obvious manifestation of the process of care. Usage of services is often called 'utilization'. The concept of 'utilization' is so broad that it is advisable to distinguish between its various aspects. Various groups of theorists have thoroughly studied patterns of utilization from the patient perspective. Andersen and his colleagues (Andersen and Newman 1972; Andersen *et al.* 1975) have identified three different groups of factors affecting individuals' decisions to use the health care delivery system. These consist of needs factors, predisposing factors like age, sex, and ethnicity, and enabling factors like income, health insurance, and community resources. In a recent account of patient perspectives in utilization, Hulka and Wheat (1985) emphasized perceived health status (e.g. need) as the single major factor motivating a patient to utilize health services. They also found that other factors such as demographic characteristics, physician availability, organizational characteristics, and financing mechanisms also play some role in patients' behaviour. This study also provides a comprehensive review of other published articles on this topic. In contrast to Hulka and Wheat, Mechanics's view on the multivariate measurement of physician utilization is more pessimistic (1989). Mechanic thinks that an evaluation of cultural and social psychological processes must also be considered for the improvement of predictions of utilization.

In the previous paragraph we have been discussing usage of health systems at the individual level. Our goal in this chapter is rather to evaluate usage at the system level. We shall focus on aggregate attributes that explain the usage of health care services within an entire population. We shall divide our discussion into an examination of descriptive patterns of utilization and an examination of the more analytical facets of health services usage within populations. We can refine such a descriptive analysis of utilization by dividing crude utilization figures into specific categories. By such a stratification of the data we can control for the effects of several variables. These variables may include the type of services, age, sex, type of provider, and type of disease (diagnoses and symptoms).

In terms of the type of service, descriptive utilization measures are particularly easy to obtain for the hospital sector. Figures on admission and hospital days are occasionally available through the WHO annual statistical publications, (see for example WHO 1983). More elaborate information is provided by WHO regional office in Europe (1981) and by the Pan American Health Organization (PAHO), the Regional WHO office for the Americas (for example, PAHO 1986 p. 146). Other comprehensive sources are the excellent OECD report *Measuring Health Care* (1985) and its data extension of 1989 (OECD Secretariat 1989). Illustrative figures are given in Table 6.1.

Table 6.1 In-patient care admission rates: by country; selected years between 1960 and 1987, percent of population.

Country	1960	1965	1970	1975	1980	1987
Australia	–	–	19.8	–	20.1	21.6
Austria	14.1	14.5	15.5	17.0	19.5	22.6
Belgium	–	8.0	9.3	11.8	13.8	–
Canada	15.0	15.9	16.5	16.5	14.9	14.5
Denmark	–	12.7	14.4	17.7	18.3	20.5
Finland	13.1	15.0	18.2	18.9	21.0	22.6
France	–	–	7.4	16.5	20.0	21.2
Germany	13.3	13.8	15.4	16.9	18.8	21.1
Greece	–	8.9	10.5	10.8	11.8	12.1
Iceland	–	12.7	16.2	19.5	20.9	–
Ireland	–	–	12.4	15.6	17.2	16.9
Italy	7.8	10.5	13.8	15.4	16.0	15.0
Japan	3.7	4.6	5.4	5.5	6.0	7.5
Luxembourg	11.6	12.8	13.4	13.7	16.6	–
Netherlands	–	9.0	10.0	11.0	11.7	11.0
New Zealand	7.9	8.7	9.3	12.5	13.3	13.0
Norway	–	12.1	13.2	14.7	15.5	16.3
Portugal	4.2	4.9	5.9	7.2	9.2	9.3
Spain	–	–	–	8.1	9.3	–
Sweden	13.4	14.5	16.6	18.1	18.3	20.0
Switzerland	12.4	13.5	13.1	11.4	12.6	13.2
Turkey	3.4	3.8	4.4	4.3	3.9	5.5
United Kingdom	9.1	10.1	10.9	11.6	13.6	15.8
United States	13.9	14.8	15.5	16.7	17.1	14.7

Adapted from *Health Care Financing Review*, Annual Supplement, 1989. OECD (1989).

There are also two valuable regional compendia, one for Europe (*Eurohealth* 1985) and one for Asia and the Pacific (*Health Care Profiles* 1986).

Cross-regional utilization measures are also available for many countries. For the US, the National Center for Health Statistics (NCHS) provides data on average length of stay (Health, United States, for example, USDHHS, 1985) while patient days and admissions are recorded in the AHA *Hospital Statistics Annual* (AHA publications). In the US, The Health Care Financing Administration is another source for data on hospital utilization by regions. It provides yearly estimates on the dollar values of hospital utilization across the various states and is a very useful tracer for trends in hospital utilization (see for example, the USDHHS *Health US* 1986). In Canada, routine data on regional variations in hospital use is published in the *Canadian Hospital Directory* (CHD publications). An account of inter-regional variations in hospital use for the European countries is provided by *Eurohealth* (1985). There are separate reports for each country and the uniform format used in this resource book allows for easy cross-country comparisons of admission rates, average length of stay, hospital days and occupancy rates. International data on utilization of services other than hospitals are less available. One exceptional example for international comparison is undoubtedly the classic 7 country–12 site comparison carried out in the late 1960s by Kohn and White (Kohn and White 1976). This carefully planned study shows up to 80 per cent variations in the volume of physician-contacts across regions studied. Another survey reported in PAHO's *Health Conditions in the Americas* (1986, Vol. 1, p. 146) reports the number of consultations per inhabitant per year for countries in the American continent. In a recent comparison for OECD countries, the Canadian province of Quebec had the lowest physician utilization. As seen in Fig. 6.1, Japan, the country with the highest physician utilization, had a three-times higher utilization than Quebec (Sandier 1989). More general indicators like the mean number of reported symptoms by age are found in other international comparisons (Anderson and Smedby 1979). There are also regional variations in the usage of ambulatory services. Using the monetary values for services rendered to patients in ambulatory settings as a tracer for actual utilization, it has been shown that there are wide variations in the usage of physician services in Canada and France (Andreani *et al.* 1987).

In recent years, researchers in many countries have become increasingly interested in examining utilization by type of disease or procedure, particularly with the growing efforts to link reimbursement with disease conditions. In the pioneering work in the 1970s and 1980s, for example, considerable variations in the rates of surgical and diagnostic procedures among England, Canada, the US, and Norway were reported. For most procedures, the utilization rates in the US ranked high above the rates for other countries (Bunker 1970; Vayda 1973; Wennberg *et al.* 1980;

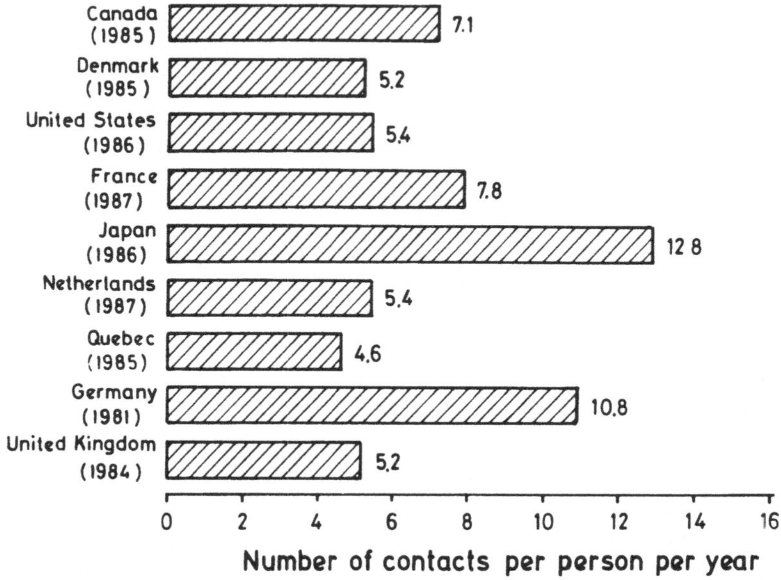

Fig. 6.1 Utilization of physician services: selected countries; selected years between 1981 and 1986. (From Sandier (1989), with permission.)

McPherson *et al.* 1981; McPherson *et al.* 1982). These differences were generally, but not always, explained by varying levels of the availability of physicians or of hospital beds. Even within the US there were spectacular variations in carrying out hospital procedures (Chassin *et al.* 1986). These variations could not be attributed either to resource-availability or to differences in the quality of care (Chassin *et al.* 1987). In a summary of recent research, McPherson (1989) shows that these variations in carrying out hospital procedures are a function of those procedures varying the most. In such cases, these great variations were due to a great uncertainty about the medical indication leading to those procedures. Thus we see in Table 6.2 (McPherson 1989) that the rate of tonsillectomies in the US is ten times higher than in Britain. However, for inguinal hernia repair, the highest rate, in the US, is less than four times greater than the lowest rate, in Japan.

These and other studies were prompted by the remarkable progress in reporting on utilization. For example, in the early 1980s, disease-oriented classification schemes in the form of Diagnosis Related Groups (DRGs) were introduced in the US for facilitating in-patient reimbursement for medical clients (Fetter 1983). The use of these DRGs promised good prospects for the future analysis of disease-based utilization. Parallel strategies in other countries, like the CMG system in Canada, have been similary successful (McGeorge *et al.* 1985).

Among countries with differing systems of physician remuneration, there

Table 6.2 Reported admission rates for selected procedures: selected countries for which data were reported, 1980

Country	Tonsillectomy	Coronary bypass	Cholecystectomy	Inguinal hernia repair	Prostatectomy	Hysterectomy
Australia	115	32	145	202	183	405
Canada	89	26	219	224	229	479
Denmark	229	–	21	–	234	255
Ireland	256	4	91	100	124	123
Japan	61	1	2	67	–	90
Netherlands	421	5	131	175	116	381
New Zealand	102	2	99	211	191	431
Norway	45	13	30	78	238	–
Sweden	65	–	140	206	48	145
Switzerland	51	–	49	116	–	–
United Kingdom	26	6	78	154	144	250
United States	205	61	203	238	308	557

Source: OECD, 1989.

were large variations in the number of physician office visits per capita (Reinhardt and Sandier 1983). There were also remarkable differences in the use of ancillary services. For example, Epstein *et al.* (1984) compared ambulatory test-ordering for hypertensive patients in the US and England. They found that for each of 13 tests, utilization was either equal or higher in the American system than in England.

Demographic factors in utilization have also been compared on international and interregional bases. In their pioneering work, Kohn and White (1976) showed discernible variations across age and sex. They found that females in their child-bearing years (ages 15–44) tended to use health care services more than males. They observed this trend in each of the regions that they studied. In his summaries of evidence from developing countries Nathanson (1977) found similar trends. In fact, Doty (1987) found that even more commonly than in developed countries, in developing countries health service utilization is much higher by females than by males.

Utilization analysis

In previous sections we have examined the descriptive aspects of utilization; now we shall discuss its analytical aspects. Many policy concerns, and much academic research deal, with utilization analysis. Because it means different things to different people and can encompass a variety of activities, an elaborate definition of utilization analysis is needed.

Comparative utilization analysis is an extremely broad area. It includes the examination of the determinants, composition, volume, and trends in health care services provided in a set of given geographic areas during a given period of time. The analysis may be undertaken for a number of purposes including evaluating the appropriateness of care, accounting for trends in expenditures and practice patterns, monitoring the adoption and utilization of specific health care technologies, and testing specific hypotheses about the behaviour of health care providers and consumers. In Part III of this book we shall show that these objectives can be reached by applying the modular approach. Here we are concerned with identifying the major approaches for measuring utilization trends.

One analytical approach in the analysis of utilization is the longitudinal study of time-trends in utilization. Trend analysis, also called time-trend analysis, is the method of choice when data on long-term utilization are available for many countries or regions. A simple time-series analysis consists of longitudinal sequences displayed in graphic or tabloid form. Another approach involves the use of cross-sectional designs for assessing utilization profiles in cross-national studies. This approach has been extensively used by Bridgman in his international study on hospitals (1979). In his study he compared demand for hospitalization services with consumption of hospital days. He used discharge rates as a proxy variable for demand

and bed day rates as a proxy variable for consumption. He compared demand and consumption across sex, age, geographical location, type of settlement, and type of service. He then superimposed the resulting utilization profiles on each other to determine interregional trends in utilization. Figure 6.2 displays a typical utilization profile for one region as suggested by Bridgman. This profile includes distributions of discharge rates and distributions of bed day rates across age and sex.

Pfaff and Nagel (1986) show longitudinal trends in the average length of stay and in hospital admission rates for 18 European countries. They conclude that while average stays decreased in all the countries studied, admission rates increased because populations are ageing. Using data compiled by the OECD (1985) for 19 developed countries, Poullier (1988) showed that at the one-digit level of the International Classification of Diseases, for several disease categories, length of stay is three or four times longer in countries with the highest average hospital stay than in countries with the shortest hospital stay. However, he did not observe any substantial differences in the classic health status indicators, like mortality and morbidity profiles, among these countries.

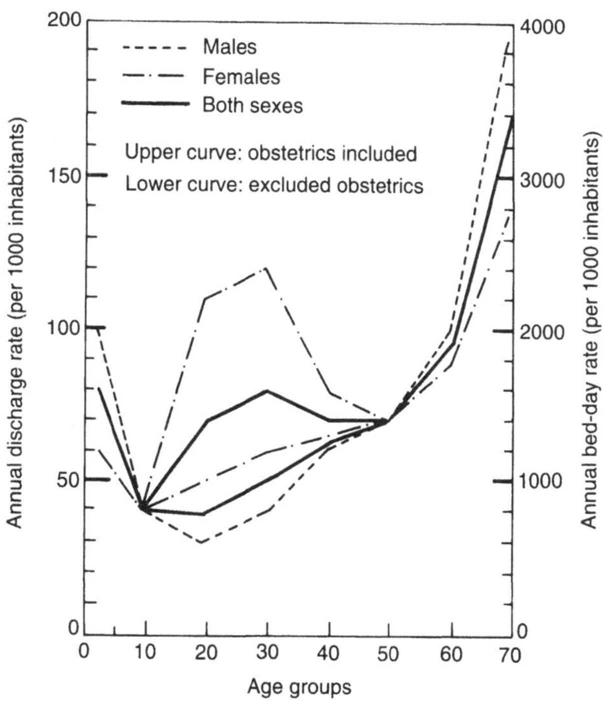

Fig. 6.2 Hospital utilization profile: single region. (From Bridgman (1979), with permission.)

Let us now turn to comparisons of primary care utilization. Weiner (1987) compared average annual ambulatory care visits to physicians in the US, in the UK, and three Scandinavian countries. He argued that the definition of 'a visit to a physician' varies across countries. Thus, though some rough comparisons can be made, the validity of cross-country comparisons is not assured. The rates of physician-contacts per individual per year are substantially higher in the US, the UK, and in Denmark (5.0, 5.3, and 8.0, respectively) than in Finland and Sweden (3.6 and 3.7, respectively). In Weiner's 1987 study, the higher rates were found in countries where most visits take place in the physicians's office. The lower rates were found in countries where most physician-contacts were at health centres or other organized settings. However, organized settings are definitely not a solid factor in the containment of primary care utilization. In Israel, where an overwhelming majority of visits occur in polyclinics, the average rate of physician contacts per individual per year approaches 12 (CBS 1983).

In another analytical approach to explain utilization, a variety of explanatory variables are used in a multivariate regression technique. This approach permits the analysis of relative or of partial effects on utilization caused by each of several contributing factors. For instance, researchers have studied a wide range of explanatory variables to explain geographic variations in hospital use. These variables include socio-economic status, age-related characteristics, organizational factors of health care delivery, need factors, variables related to provider behaviour, and epidemiological variables (Rothberg 1981, Chapter 1). Regression techniques have been used, for example, to account for differences in surgical rates throughout the US. Mitchell and Cromwell (1982) showed that need factors and accessibility to health care, affect utilization the most.

The advantage of multivariate analyses is that it is possible to control for the effects of each single contributory variable while maintaining the effects of other explanatory variables constant. The major disadvantage is that longitudinal trends are not dealt with explicitly in the analysis. To remedy this problem, one can either use a series of cross-sectional regression analyses for different points in time or include *time* as *one* of the independent variables in the multiple regression model.

None of the approaches cited here, however, can provide a thorough explanation of trends in utilization, as the following quote from Campbell and Stanley (1963) illustrates:

> Small area approaches enable the investigator to capture the nuances embedded in physician behavior and to make more precise estimates of supply and demand. However, it is difficult to generalize from findings generated via the small area approach, in that knowledge of local physician norms and local fluctuations in supply and demand do not necessarily help explain utilization dynamics at the larger regional or societal level.
>
> Researchers employing the cross-sectional approach and using large geographic

units of observation can make some generalizable statements about health-care delivery in large geographic regions; yet the broad-based approach obscures subtle dynamics that occur within large geographic areas.

Longitudinal or time-series designs rely on historical data and enable researchers to test the stability of their findings; yet historical data rarely capture important variables that are difficult to measure (such as physician norms) nor do they normally allow the researcher to attain the level of specificity achievable in cross-sectional designs. Moreover, longitudinal analyses usually rely on 'hard' secondary-source indicators such as census data, and such data often present the investigator with special validity and reliability problems of a maturational and historic nature.

Indicators of utilization

Indicators of utilization: primary care

Indicators for utilization can be categorized by type of service. The three major categories are primary care, acute hospital care, and long-term care. Indicators often used in primary care services are listed below.

Rate of physician contacts per person per year When there is a documented source of information, annual rates are used most frequently. For sources other than documentary, particularly for patient information collected in surveys, a much shorter recall time is chosen (e.g. two weeks). It has been determined from national health surveys in the US and elsewhere that longer recall periods may result in biased reports due to selective reporting of the data. As a general indicator, physician-contacts can be subdivided into rate of specialist contacts, the rate of surgical contacts, the rate of dental contacts, the rate of preventive contacts, contact rates with allied health professionals, and so on. Comparative data on the average rates of physicians' contacts over time is available in the OECD (1985) and in its data extension (OECD Secretariat 1989).

Percentage of population per year not seeing a physician As an important measure of health services utilization, this indicator not only reflects utilization (process) but also provides a direct estimate of equity of access. Unfortunately, updated data on regional or international variations in the level of this indicator are scarce. Documentary sources are generally available only where data are routinely collected for reimbursement purposes as in the Canadian provinces. Otherwise, it is necessary to gather information through surveys like the National Health Survey in the US.

Total number of referrals to a laboratory or X-ray procedures per person per year There are also other categories of primary care, such as laboratory tests, X-rays, and other testing procedures, for which data on utilization are available. Information on per capita per year utilization can be collected.

Average number of medicines per person per year This kind of information is available in OECD (1985). This indicator can also be translated into monetary terms, that is, the total dollar value of drugs consumed in a specific country or area over a defined period.

All these indicators can be further subdivided by demographic variables, by type of provider, or by disease categories when data are available. In general, national health surveys provide information on utilization of the general population and also by age and sex. Utilization by the type of provider is less routinely reported by regular sources. Data on utilization by disease-category is seldom available for primary care.

Indicators of utilization: hospital care

Indicators used in hospital care are more easily available and generally more reliable than indicators used in primary care. This is because in-patient services have more organized information systems. There are also more and stricter regulatory mechanisms in the hospital sector requiring mandatory reporting. Finally, hospital reimbursement schemes requiring detailed reporting in exchange for hospital funding guarantee that data will be available. Indicators frequently used in the acute hospital care are listed below.

Admission or discharge rates These rates (per 1000 population) are easily available from international sources, for instance, *Eurohealth* (1985) or OECD (1985).

Hospital days Hospital days indicate the total number of days of hospitalization for all patients during one year; either admission or discharge days are counted. This indicator can be expressed in absolute terms but is more useful when expressed as rates of hospital days per 1000 population.

Average length of stay in acute care hospitals (ALOS) ALOS has become the most popular indicator used in hospital statistics. It is the number of hospital days divided by the number of discharged patients per year. Comparative ALOS are available in Eurohealth (1985) and OECD (1985, 1989). These comparative rates are given by disease categories and over time for several developed countries. It is remarkable that ALOS is very short in The US and Canada, much longer in West Germany and the Netherlands and in other central European countries, and very long in Japan. OECD also provides some cross-country comparisons according to detailed diagnoses; these comparisons share the trends mentioned previously.

Occupancy rate A companion indicator to ALOS, occupancy rate, is the percentage of all beds occupied during one year. Since occupancy is largely affected by local conditions, this indicator is less significant than ALOS in cross-regional or cross-national comparisons.

Bed turnover Bed turnover is another companion to ALOS; it is expressed by the following equation:

$$\textit{Bed turnover} = \frac{\text{occupancy rate} \times 365}{\text{ALOS} \times 100}$$

This equation indicates the average number of cases treated per hospital bed per year. Data are available in OECD (1985, 1989). As expected, higher turnover rates are associated with lower ALOS. For instance, turnover rates in the US are much higher than in France, Germany or the Netherlands.

For several indicators, hospital use by age and sex categories is often available; hospital use by disease *categories* is reported whereas reimbursement schemes are based on the *type* of disease—as in Canadian provinces or for clients reported by the DRG system in the US.

Indicators of utilization: long-term care

For the most part, comparative indicators used for long-term care are generally similar to those used for acute hospital care, though the range of values recorded differs significantly. Typical values of ALOS are within the range of hundreds of days which makes ALOS too long for useful comparisons. Bed turnover rates are similar to ALOS and are also rarely used. The more meaningful indicators for the measurement and comparison in studies of long-term care reflect utilization in a population perspective, like admission rates by type of long-term care delivery system.

Accessibility

In our discussion on equity in Chapter 5, we concluded that equity of access to health services is a precondition to equity of care. However, we have not yet specified what we mean by 'access' or what are the operational definitions required for determining this access. Here we distinguish between access and accessibility. Accessibility is defined as 'the number or proportion of a given population that can be expected to use a specific facility, service, etc., given a certain barrier to access' (Micovic 1984). By this operational definition accessibility can be measured while access can only be discussed at the conceptual level. Though there have been attempts to remove barriers to access, they are still common all over the world, especially in the developing countries. As seen in Fig. 6.3, conditions of child-care during the first year of life, a period characterized by a very high need for health services, are globally unsatisfactory. The figure shows that there are general barriers to access, particularly in the developing countries.

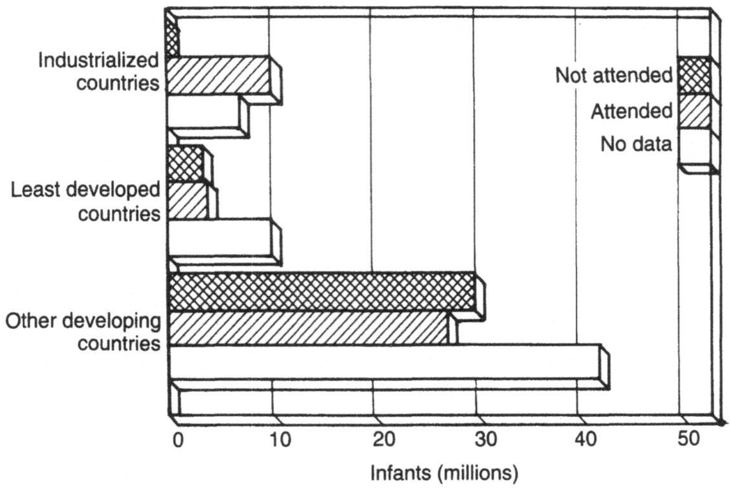

Fig. 6.3 Infants attended during their first year, according to development level of countries, 1986–1988. (Based on information reported to WHO by Member States.)

In the following sections we shall analyse the various barriers to access to health care in detail. These barriers to access can be determined as physical barriers (distance, travel time, waiting time), as economic barriers (fee charges, co-payments, travel cost), or as social and cultural barriers (denial of care). These social and cultural barriers reflect the extent to which a recipient of care is likely to accept and use a given health service.

Physical accessibility

The concept of physical accessibility is oriented to the recipient of care. This concept reflects the extent that health services can be reached and used by a particular patient or by the community as a whole. A discussion of physical accessibility includes several components. We shall review each component separately beginning with the study of effects of distance from the source of care as a measure of physical accessibility.

The effect of distance from the source of care has been extensively examined by medical geographers. The main thrust of these researchers and planners was the characterization of the variations across space in the accessibility of health services to groups or populations. This problem can be examined on two levels. At the resource level it is just a comparison of the regional (or national) distributions of the supply of health services versus the demand for them. The supply of a particular health service, like hospital services, is reflected by a specific indicator, for example the number of hospital beds within each region. The demand for a service is reflected by a population indicator, like the absolute size of the population. The ratio of the demand to the supply is a measure of availability which can be used here as a proxy for accessibility. The concept of availability is indeed a close companion of the concept of accessibility. While physical accessibility is oriented to the recipient of care, availability is oriented to the provider of care and reflects the volume of active services in an area available to the population. When existing health services are available to an entire population, availability equals accessibility. Roos and co-workers (1976) used the demand/supply ratio for physicians to evaluate accessibility to physician services in Canada. In his international study on hospital utilization, Bridgman (1979) considered several catchment areas with hospitals in each one. Then he examined the distribution of patients from the several catchment areas among these hospitals. Bridgman called the resulting measure the 'attraction rate.' The attraction rate can be represented as the percentage of patients admitted to hospitals in their own catchment areas in comparison to the percentage population that were admitted to hospitals outside their area of residence. We shall discuss the use of the 'attraction rate' in a later section on indicators. Weiner used a similar approach for estimating access to primary care in the US and in four European countries (Weiner, 1987). He concluded that access is satisfactory in Europe and in the US-HMO systems due to the carefully planned availability of services and the careful attention to maintaining ease of entry to the system. However, in the US when reimbursement is based on Fee For Service (FFS), access to care is much less satisfactory.

Measuring physical accessibility at the analytical level requires a more thorough analysis of regional accessibility. This requires understanding the interaction between resources and their potential users (Joseph and Philips 1984). In its simplest form this approach can be used to evaluate the empirical evidence of the effects of distance on the decay in utilization. As Joseph and Philips argue, these effects can be aggregated to show how increasing distances from sources of care cause the diminished utilization of services.

The common dependent variable characterizing the two other components of physical accessibility, travel-and waiting-time, is time elapsed between the expression for the demand for health services and the moment of their receipt. Measuring travel- or waiting-time in small regions is not problematic, but measured in large areas, these variables are essentially averages of the measures in the smaller areas aggregated to make the larger areas. Such averages reduce the sensitivity of the measurements. This is seen in the work of Kohn and White (1976). They found that the differences in waiting- or travel-time for ambulatory facilities are often manifested in smaller areas. For example, a rural dweller may require a high travel-time while an urban dweller is likely to require a lower travel-time. We can see that taking the average of travel-times for rural dwellers with that of urban dwellers would reduce the sensitivity of their separate measurements. When considering large areas, the most promising strategy is to deal only with those services that can be used as 'tracers' for general physical accessibility. For these services, there will still be large variations in their measures among these large regions and countries. Waiting periods for specific types of surgery are among the best 'tracers' for comparisons of the time component in physical accessibility. For example, for several types of surgery, waiting-times were longer in England and Wales than in Canada and the US (McPherson *et al.* 1981).

Economic accessibility

Economic accessibility reflects the ability of an individual in the community to cover the cost of his health care. Basically, it addresses the eligibility of individuals for modern medical care. In developed health systems where health services are readily available to the population, the issue is confined to the assessment of two components, coverage and comprehensiveness. Practically, by coverage we mean insurance coverage since such insurance plans are the most common kind of coverage in Western health markets. By measurement of levels of insurance, a well-documented indicator, we can operationalize the concept of coverage. Indeed this has been done in most European countries where universal insurance—and consequently universal insurance coverage—prevails (WHO, *Eurostat* 1989). However, caution is warranted here. The use of insurance as a proxy for coverage can be somewhat misleading: it is often wrong to assume that the non-insured population is also not covered for medical care services. For under-privileged populations it is usually true that being non-insured means non-coverage. However, for wealthy and relatively young non-insured individuals this is no longer true in modern health systems. It was shown that this group manages to meet limited needs for health services by using market mechanisms (Aday *et al.* 1980). Non-insurance is often found in the US where health insurance is not mandatory. Since the size of the non-insured population is relatively small compared to the insured population (even in the US only about 15 per cent of the population is non-insured), we shall assume for the rest of our discussion that levels of insurance are fairly representative of coverage. This assumption is even stronger in developing countries where insurance coverage is an excellent predictor of health service utilization. Gish (1990) reported that even in developing countries, levels of utilization are surprisingly high among individuals having relatively easy access to health services, that is, the insured population.

With the increasing levels of coverage in modern health systems, researchers have increased their attention to the comprehensiveness of coverage. It is more and more evident that cost-containment strategies affect the comprehensiveness of coverage in health care systems. With respect to cost-containment, the most threatening strategy is cost-sharing.

By cost-sharing we mean that part of the costs of medical or health treatment is transferred by the health system to the recipient of care. For some recipients this transfer creates a financial barrier to utilization. Several studies have dealt with how cost-sharing may diminish the use of health services. These studies generally show a negative relationship between levels of utilization and individual costs of ambulatory care services in the US (Scheffler 1984; Lohr *et al.* 1986; Hennelly and Boxerman 1979) and in Canada (Beck and Horne 1980). For instance, the randomized clinical trial conducted by RAND (Lohr *et al.* 1986) disclosed substantial differences in the rates of utilization by recipients of care having alternative coverage plans. In these studies, cost-sharing generally reduced the probability of the use of medical care across a wide spectrum of clinical conditions. The effects of other co-variates in affecting levels of utilization were not ruled out, but it was emphasized that economic accessibility plays a prime role in explaining the variations in use. Assessing economic accessibility in comparative cross-national studies of the process of care is fortunately possible because information on co-payments and other cost-sharing arrangements is available for national health systems. For example, compound information is given in the research report '*Social security programs throughout the world*' (USDHHS 1986).

Acceptability (social and cultural accessibility)

There are several caveats in determining acceptability and its companion concept, compliance. Though they both represent social and cultural accessibility these two concepts are slightly different. Acceptability is encountered at an earlier and often preliminary stage of the contact between providers and recipients of care. When clients have declined a medical treatment or a health care programme it may reflect lack of acceptability. Compliance refers to the adherence of a patient to the instructions of health care providers *during* the process of care. We consider compliance only when there has been an initial contact with the health system.

The difficulty in operationalizing these two concepts is in their strong behavioural components. The problem is that they are normally measured at the individual, but not at the population, level. In the absence of population-based models for determining acceptability and compliance, we shall review the various elements of the individual-based socio-behavioural model and consider the relevance of these elements to the population as a whole. In Becker and Maiman's socio-behavioural model, also called the health belief model (1975), there are two major components for explaining compliant (or accepting) behaviour. As shown in Fig. 6.4, there is a predisposing factor of concern about health matters in general, followed by a readiness to behave compliantly. The predisposing factor is accompanied by an enabling factor which includes prior experience with the health system, source of advice to medical care, etc.

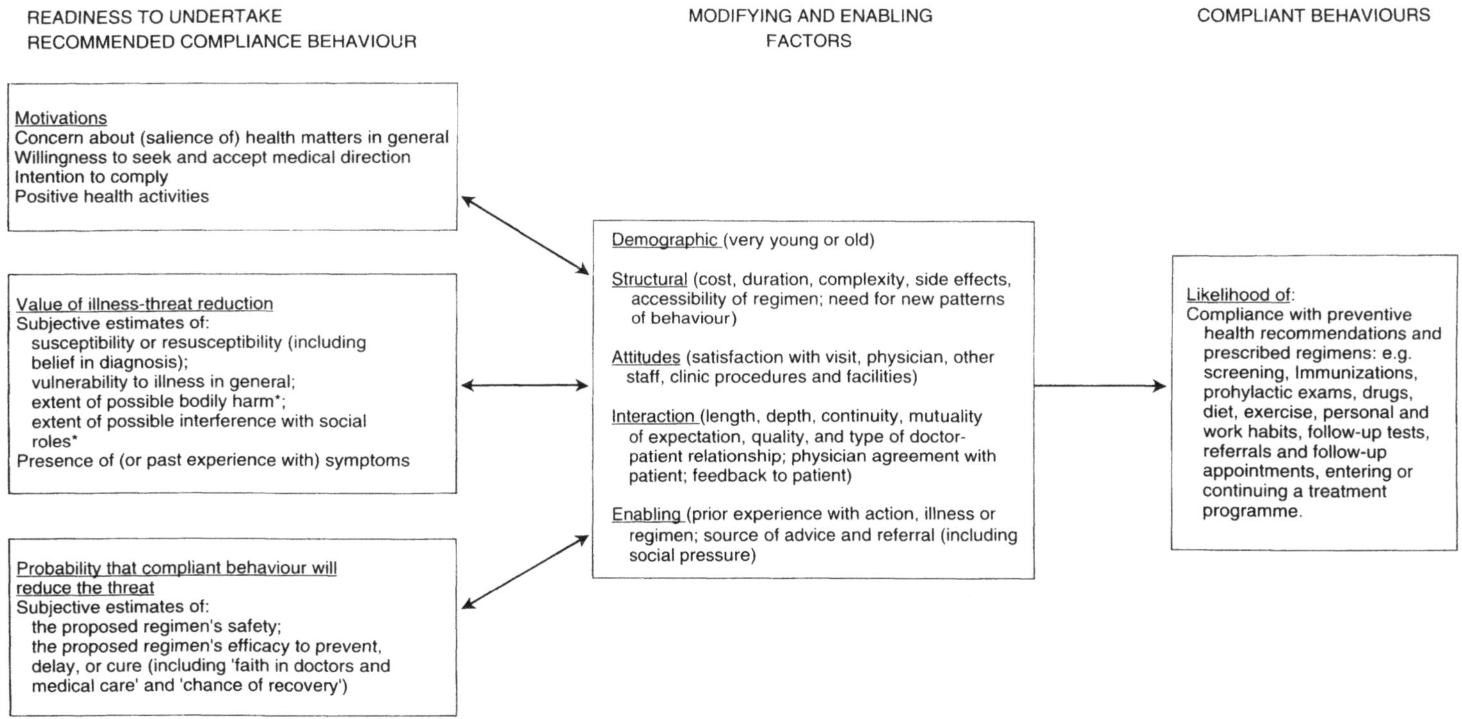

Fig. 6.4 Model of patient behaviour. (From Becker and Maiman (1975), with permission.)

At the population level, there are several predisposing elements that may be measured. These are motivation to seek medical care, differences in sick-role behaviour, and perception of higher odds for successful treatment reflecting faith in the medical system. Among individual groups these variables may be shared in common, but they differ considerably among populations of different regions and countries. Suchman (1964, 1966) considered various ethnic and cultural groups in New York. He found that the ethnic group of an individual affected his health orientation and value systems. Individuals in 'cosmopolitan' groups tended to seek medical services in an early stage of an illness. These groups included massive numbers of highly compliant individuals. Individuals in more 'parochial' groups avoided extensive contacts with the medical system. In a similar approach, Zola (1963, 1964) compared patients of Italian and Irish Anglo-Saxon ancestry. Zola defined trigger mechanisms affecting patients' acceptability. There were different 'triggers' for different ethnic groups for the decision to seek medical care. For most Italians, social interactions affected their acceptance of care while the acceptance of care by Anglo-Saxons was related to 'the nature and quality of their symptoms.' Similar conclusions were reached in other studies that focused on the socio-psychologic approach in studying acceptability (McKinlay 1972; Becker and Maiman 1983).

For population-based studies, the effect of enabling and modifying factors is larger than that of predisposing factors. Enabling and modifying factors are suitable for population-based analysis because they are mostly ecological variables. The single most extensively reviewed modifying variable is age (Kohn and White 1976). The effect of age on acceptability is supported by the observation that higher levels of non-compliance are seen at the two extremes of the lifespan. This is consistent with symptoms of social and psychological disorientation that are particularly evident in ageing populations. With respect to other modifying effects, Salkever (1976) found that females and more educated people are the most compliant with the health care delivery system, especially regarding the use of preventive services.

In the context of the physician–patient contact, the enabling factors most influencing patients' compliance are attitudes towards health personnel, the personal interest of the physician in the patient, physician-availability in the community, and lack of stigma in seeking a particular type of service. All these factors affect the patient's decision to use health services (Mechanic, 1982). In particular, Salkever (1976) analysed periodic screening examination, a tracer condition which is mostly affected by acceptability, by studying the findings of the WHO International Collaborative Study of Medical Care Utilization (Kohn and White 1976). The utilization pattern seen in this study supports the assumption that enabling factors play a central role in explaining variations in use. This study also provides simple readily-available indicators for measuring attitudes (see the section on indicators in this chapter). Finally, continuity of care is another important enabling factor explaining acceptability. Having a regular source of care is clearly a positive factor for improving compliance (Salkever 1976, Becker *et al.* 1972).

Regarding the issues of acceptability and compliance, a word of caution is advised. We have not yet addressed the concept of patient satisfaction with care. Though strongly associated with acceptability and with compliance, we can justify distinguishing satisfaction from acceptibility and compliance if we consider the basic components of the Modular Approach. These components are inputs, processes, and outcomes. Because satisfaction has long been recognized as a typical outcome factor, we shall deal with it later. It should be emphasized that any discussion of acceptability and compliance would not be complete without including the issue of satisfaction.

Indicators of accessibility

Indicators of physical accessibility

Ratios of resources to population Several ratios can be calculated and compared among regions or countries. Typical ratios consist of beds per 1000 population, primary care physicians per 1000 population, and nursing personnel per 1000 population. While all these ratios reflect availability, their usefulness as proxies for accessibility is based on the ease of data collection. The validity of these ratios is relatively high due to a general consensus among health administrators and researchers on operational definitions for these ratios. Besides this, the well accepted definitions of resource-related indicators guarantee the relatively high reliability of data collection.

Attraction rates Attraction rates were originally developed to assess how patients are assigned to hospitals in respective catchment areas. The primary function of this indicator is thus for planning purposes in an individual region or country. However, attraction rates can also be used as proxies for comparing accessibility in various areas. The method consists of assessing the percentage of the population living in a given geographic region that is cared for within the boundaries of that region. This percentage can be compared across regions or countries provided that health systems in these countries are similarly configured as in the Scandinavian countries.

Continuity of care This is another proxy for assessing accessibility. Operationally, continuity of care as a proxy measure for accessibility is restricted to easily measured phenomena. For example, there is continuity of primary care if a 'regular' source of primary care (e.g. a family physician) can be formally identified for all consumers. On a national scale one can distinguish between countries for which this condition prevails, as in the UK and the Scandinavian countries and countries for which continuity-accessibility seldom prevails for the general population, as in Canada and the US.

Time-based indicators This series of indicators is based on the use of time-scales as criteria for comparisons between countries or regions. Since there are no universal criteria for waiting time, for example, such comparisons can be made only on a normative basis. For example, in England performance measurement requires data on waiting lists per 1000 population. These indicators are available for several districts in England and can serve as comparative inter-regional measures of access for several medical and surgical procedures (Harly 1988).

Indicators of economic accessibility

Coverage of health care One way of measuring the extent of coverage is the percentage of the population covered by health insurance when co-payments or deductibles are minimized but regardless of the form of payment. For OECD countries, the OECD (1985) provides a comprehensive set of comparative indicators reflecting various aspects of health coverage as follows:

(1) coverage for hospital care risks;
(2) coverage for ambulatory medical services;
(3) coverage for pharmaceutical products.

Qualitative information delineating population groups for which health insurance is available in most countries is provided by a publication of USDHHS (1986).

Range of services Comprehensiveness of care can be studied by examining the range of services available to people *already having* health coverage. The range of services generally includes all or part of the following:

(1) ambulatory coverage
    (a) general physician care
    (b) specialist physician care
    (c) dental care
    (d) maternity care
    (e) laboratory and other diagnostic services
(2) hospital coverage
    (a) acute care hospitalization
    (b) maternity care
    (c) long term care
    (d) mental care

(3) coverage for special services, for example:
  (a) drugs for chronic patients
  (b) other drugs
  (c) medical appliances
  (d) special services for the elderly like home nursing, homemaker, and handyman for repairs.
  (e) transportation.

The USDHHS (1986) compendium is a very useful source of information for this indicator.

Cost-sharing Cost-sharing can take the form of a co-payment, where a recipient of care pays a certain percentage of the actual cost of treatment or diagnosis, or of a deductible where the recipient of care pays a constant lump sum for any particular treatment performed. Because out of pocket payments can potentially reduce or even hinder the use of health services, the level of cost-sharing may be regarded as a proxy for comprehensiveness of care. Indeed, recent evidence from health maintenance organizations (HMOs) in the US shows that introducing a co-payment for each visit to the doctor significantly decreases rates of screening examinations in a given population (Cherkin *et al.* 1990). The USDHHS (1986) provides a wide range of co-payments and deductibles prevailing in several countries.

Indicators of acceptability (social accessibility)

As we suggested previously, we shall mostly discuss modifying and enabling factors appropriate for use as proxy indicators for measuring acceptability. Among the useful modifying factors are the following:

Age distribution The age distribution of the population in the countries or regions studied. The percentage of the population aged 65 and over, can be used as a supplementary indicator. Where there are high proportions of elderly people it is likely that acceptability will be lower.

Proportion of females This is the proportion of females within each age group, particularly for those aged 65 and over. Where the percentages of females in the population are high one finds better acceptability and compliance with health care.

Educational status Proportion of population having at least twelve years of schooling. As mentioned before, well educated individuals presumably show a more accepting and compliant behaviour with respect to the health care delivery system.

Among the enabling factors, a few tracer conditions can be used to assess acceptability and compliance.

The use of non-urgent services Some services are important but not perceived as urgent. Such services require high acceptability on the part of the recipient of care. Screening procedures are a typical example of such services. The comparative assessment by Kohn and White (1976) of the frequency of use of screening procedures in seven countries is a useful example how this indicator served for cross-national comparisons.

Continuity of care This indicator can be used for assessing acceptability and compliance as we suggested above for the assessment of physical accessibility.

Ethical Issues in Utilization

The enormous progress in medical care has created difficult moral choices; abortion, human experimentation, organ transplantation, euthanasia— the right of a patient to terminate his own life, informed consent, and so on, all involve delicate choices. These choices are often between two or more alternatives, each supported by serious moral arguments. These choices must be made either by an individual or by an entire society. Society's reaction to these moral questions is crystallized through discussion, into a consensus. Only then, the general acceptance of such a consensus may lead to a formal public policy. Such policy is made through the legislative and judicial actions of the Government. In the context of health system analysis, we are interested in a rather narrow perspective, the approaches of various governments for the formulation of these public policies. Since it is difficult to determine universally accepted operational definitions for ethical issues, we shall consider some specific moral issues in utilization as tracers. Clearly, for any given issue selected as a tracer condition, we must first distinguish between countries that have formulated an accepted policy on the issue and those countries without any formal policy. The two formal stands of governments on the ethical issues of health systems are:

(1) the role of government in the allocation of resources or, 'Who shall live?';
(2) the regulation of procedures and therapies or, 'Who shall decide?'.

There is an extensive literature on this topic for those interested in broader ethical issues affecting societies (see for example van de Veer and Regan 1987; Harris 1985; Winslade and Ross 1986).

Indicators on Ethics

Operationally, to compare the behaviour of health systems on ethical and moral issues we must examine tracer conditions highlighting them. Let us consider organ transplantation as a tracer condition for which comparative indicators may be developed as shown below. Note that for each of the two issues, allocation and regulation, there are two indicator levels.

Organ transplantation (resource allocation)

1. With respect to resource allocation, the indicator level is '1' when there is government intervention in deciding on population eligibility.
2. The indicator level is '0' when the government does not intervene in the decision on population eligibility. In this case, physicians have full professional autonomy for such decision making.

For example, because organs are in short supply, the law on organ allocation in Argentina provides mechanisms for fixing priorities. The law requires that health authorities set up a co-ordinating centre for managing organ procurement and allocation. In most countries, however, there is no legislative intervention in allocative decisions, and the choice is left to physicians. (Abdussalam 1985).

Organ transplantation (regulatory mechanisms)

1. The government may create legislation on several ethical and moral issues. Among such issues can be enumerated organ procurement, the definition of the moment of death, and regulations regarding donors and recipient. When such legislation exists, the health system is judged to be formally involved in organ transplantation and the indicator is '1'. This is the case for nearly all developed and several developing countries, like India, Algeria, Malaysia, and the Philipines (Abdussalam 1985).
2. In countries lacking such regulations, the indicator level is '0'. In such cases, there is constant fear that ethical issues are not treated appropriately (Abdussalam 1985).

The indirect attributes

Professional autonomy

Medical professionals, particularly physicians, value individual autonomy and peer consideration. Sociologically, it is precisely this legitimately organized autonomy that distinguishes between occupations that are also professions and those that are not. The medical profession is distinguished from others in the great dominance of its practitioners over their sphere of work (Freidson 1961). To quote Freidson (1970):

> Unlike other occupations professions are deliberately granted autonomy including the exclusive right to determine who can legitimately do its work and how the work should be done.

Fuchs (1974) noted that physician behaviour is motivated by patient approval and by the 'instinct of workmanship', that is the desire to practice the best medicine possible. Because of this, physicians may reject administrative authority in clinical areas (Freidson 1975). To preserve their professional autonomy, physicians established professional guilds, called medical associations. Like other guilds, a medical guild is a closed order whose members pursue quality, prestige and profit to their mutual benefit (Parsons 1964). These guilds provide physicians with a protective environment that encourages them to protect one another from 'harmful influences.' Protective measures may range from the rejection of criticism against the medical community to the establishment of active opposition to restrictive legislation affecting the medical profession. Surprisingly, the increasing involvement of governments in the provision of medical care has not been very threatening to the professional autonomy of physicians because governments are usually reluctant to restrict physician autonomy directly. Restrictive measures may be indirect and can take several forms as we describe in the following sections.

Rationing utilization

The most straightforward control on professional autonomy is rationing utilization. It controls the volume and the nature of medical tasks by controlling diagnostic tests, procedures, and drug prescriptions (Schulz and Harrison 1986). Rationing can be done at both the level of the individual practitioner and at the institutional level. However, efforts to ration individual practitioners, particularly physicians, have often been unsuccessful (Morgan *et al.* 1985). A notable example is the failure of the NHS in England in 1984 to fix a budgetary limit to the amount spent in prescribing drugs. General Practitioners (GPs) were furious with this NHS policy (Day and Klein 1989). However, in some other countries of centralized planning, rationing prescriptions was successful. At least until the recent political changes, drug prescription review has been common in some East European countries. In Czechoslovakia, the German Democratic Republic, and Yugoslavia, there have been special pharmaceutical committees to examine at least some prescriptions; various averages were calculated and the appropriateness of individual prescriptions was assessed. Although punitive sanctions were rare, these health systems were successful in controlling drug prescriptions (Vuori 1982).

Particularly in the United States, rationing institutions by the imposition of collective constraints on the use of medical procedures were generally more successful. These institutional constraints can be administrative or financial or both. Administrative constraints can take the form of the substitution of one type of service for another. In the US, HMOs were particularly effective in substituting expensive hospital utilization by cheaper ambulatory use (Luft 1981). Financial constraints are encountered when utilization is restricted to specific population groups. For example, recent efforts in the UK to curb utilization costs were concentrated on restricting the provision of care by the NHS to citizens of Britain only. However, on a macro scale, rationing utilization in general was not successful. As Schulz and Harrison (1986) note in their cross-national comparative study, rationing utilization was confined to a few large scale intervention efforts, and these efforts yielded only moderate effects. Examples include the use of reimbursement disincentives in the US, the constraints imposed on the general level of public expenditure on health in Britain, and the distinction between hospital based and community based physicians in Germany, Britain and Israel. This distinction would preclude, for example, that a primary care physician would examine hospital patients. In this way, the physician's professional autonomy is limited to his normal place of practice.

Physicians autonomy and the State

We suggest, however, that the intensive involvement of the State in the health sector does not necessarily imply an erosion in physician autonomy. This is the case in Britain (Larkin 1988; Schulz and Harrison 1986) and in Italy (Krause 1988) where physician dominance has been strengthened with the proletarianization of medicine. In both of these countries, and also in Australia (Willis 1988), the doctors' personal autonomy was not affected by increased state interference. It is surprising to note that physicians were rather used as an instrument to increase the State's control over the health sector. In return, physicians received even more power and autonomy (Long *et al.* 1985). These examples show that bureaucracy as such need not threaten professional autonomy in democratic societies. However, what may threaten professional autonomy are government control mechanisms for curtailing the cost of medical care. Consider the treatment protocols typical in Scandinavian countries. These protocols are a set of general guidelines for health personnel for the promotion of efficiency and quality of care. However, by their nature, these protocols constrain physicians' judgement and independence (Vuori 1982).

Opposing trends are seen in socialist systems where bureaucracy can affect clinical autonomy though its role in restricting physicians' decisions is often exaggerated (Field 1988). Control in socialist systems is hierarchic. It is achieved by granting high level medical institutions the responsibility for the medical performance of those lower level institutions within their jurisdiction. For example, in the USSR, the chief of surgery in a regional hospital is in charge of all surgeons working in district hospitals and in polyclinics within his region. He carries out his responsibility by making routine 'control visits' to all health care institutions in his region (Vuori 1982).

The increasing professionalization of the paramedical and nursing professions is another serious challenge to medical autonomy (Morgan *et al.*

1985). There are several examples of health occupations whose workers can practice without having their patients referred by doctors. This is typical for many nurse practitioners, paramedics and physio-therapists. The autonomy gained is at the expense of the autonomy previously exercised by physicians, and thus create a new situation. Presently, professional autonomy is often granted by the State to the personnel of several health occupations. By doing this, the State creates professions of these occupations thus facilitating the decline of the strength of the medical hegemony (Armstrong 1976).

Quality assurance—a process-oriented perspective

Process evaluation

Quality assurance programmes can be regarded as another approach undertaken by the Government or by other ownership to control the process of health care delivery. Very often, such programmes also interface with physicians' autonomy, thus limiting the clinical freedom of practitioners. Formally, quality assurance is defined as the:

> measurement of the actual level of the quality of services rendered, plus the effects to modify when necessary the provision of these services in the light of the results of the measurement.
>
> (Vuori 1982).

However, common procedures for quality assurance are not generally suitable for cross-comparisons. As Vuori (1982) put it:

> Routine quality assurance programmes virtually never provide conclusive evidence for comparing various systems of providing care. They may suggest that differences exist but, since they do not aim at controlling intervening variables, there is no way of telling whether one system should be preferred to another in planning for the future—a question often posed by decision-makers.
>
> The question "Is A better than B" has to be supplemented by a host of more specific questions such as "In which respect?", "From whose point of view?", "Within which time frame?" and "With what costs?" The decision-maker also wants to know whether the differences between two systems are due to factors that are amenable to manipulation by legislative, administrative, educational or some other means. To be able to tell that, the researcher has to design a controlled trial with appropriate experimental and control groups. The difficulties involved in conducting rigorously controlled experiments in the field of social policy are well known. They do not, however, justify jumping to premature and untenable conclusions on the basis of the results of routine quality assurance programmes designed for other purposes.

Since controlled trials are generally beyond the scope of cross-comparisons, an alternate strategy for comparing system A and B is needed. For example, a monitoring system for measuring the performance of health professionals within the system may be introduced. In the next section we survey the available procedures for quality assurance in terms of the process of care.

For a quality assurance procedure, the most important element is the selection of a yardstick as a measure of good care. Such a 'yardstick' (or criterion) can be either disease-specific or general, and either explicit or implicit. Kessner (1978) provided the following description of these criteria:

> Process or outcome criteria that are based on a physician's judgment but not codified before review are known as judgmental or implicit criteria, and those that are specified before review are known as predetermined or explicit.
>
> When judgmental criteria are used, physicians review patient records or interview and examine patients and judge the quality of the process and outcome. This method is subject to observer variation and to the economic and logistic problems of employing highly skilled professionals but it is widely used for inpatient and ambulatory-care assessment.
>
> Predetermined or explicit criteria can be more easily and inexpensively applied. To establish these standards, the clinical judgment of an outside panel of experts or of the physicians to be evaluated or both, may be used. The criteria may reflect common local practice, data from case studies or information derived from well controlled clinical trials.

The selection of procedures for quality assurance

The two most popular quality assurance procedures for comparative analysis are utilization reviews and medical audits. Utilization reviews consist of a formal critical examination of appropriate use in the health care system. Medical audits consist of the screening of medical records for inappropriate or irrelevant medical procedures. Thus, medical audits are most suitable at the micro-level than are utilization reviews.

Utilization review is mostly carried out by a peer committee for reviewing physician performance and mandating corrective action. In the US, these peer committees were first established as Professional Standard Review Organizations (PSROs). PSROs were designed to control health care costs and to improve the quality of medical care. Instead, however, PSROs intervened directly with physician practice by 'monitoring physician performance and taking corrective action' (Snyder 1975). After the introduction of DRG's in 1984, the US Federal Government introduced Profession Review Organizations (PROs) to replace PSROs. PROs are responsible for evaluating the quality of care and the appropriateness of hospital admissions and discharges of patients whose hospitalization is financed by federal and state governments. Now, non-government insurers or payers in the US also offer utilization review services. Even private clients may request utilization reviews by PROs or by independent companies (Field and Gray 1989). This again is an intrusion on physician autonomy with respect to care. Moreover, recent developments in utilization review point to the increased use of explicit criteria in assessment procedures. For example, the American Medical Association (AMA) is co-operating with the Rand Corporation to develop comprehensive guidelines for deciding the appropriateness of diagnostic procedures or treatment regimens (Findlay 1989). The results of this collaboration will be a computerized tool for evaluating physicians' judgment and assessing the appropriateness of their decisions. In summarizing the effects of the PSROs and PROs, Lieske (1985) wrote:

> Many physicians see the PSRO/PRO mandate as an effort by the government to intervene in the currently self-regulated practice of medicine. The professional autonomy afforded physicians through specialized knowledge and skill and ultimate control of the health care decision-making process is jeopardized as medical practice moves from the private arena into the public sector with its accompanying close scrutiny by the consumer. This change will necessarily result in public input regarding decisions related to the allocation of resources and the respective roles of health professionals and patients.

Labour relationships

In the course of modern history, professional unions in the health field have been strengthened through collective bargaining. Their power is dramatically expressed when crises in the health care field are evoked by these unions. Though a crisis can take many forms, strikes are among its most potent manifestations. During the last several decades, the health scene of democratic countries has provided a multitude of situations which have led to doctors' strikes. Some of the more remarkable examples are described below.

In 1962 in Saskatchewan, Canada, doctors withheld their services following the implementation of a province-wide health reform (Tollefson 1963). In April 1964 in Belgium, some 90 per cent of the doctors held an unprecedented strike because of a political compromise between Belgian political parties concerning the organization of health care. Belgian doctors considered the proposed legislation threatening to their conditions of work and income. This long and bitter strike lasted for 17 days until negotiations between the Government and the doctors finally led to a compromise (Lancet 1964). Several doctors' strikes in the US have also been reported in the literature (McNamara and Green 1979; Jones 1979). In December 1975, in Britain, a dispute over pay scales for junior hospital doctors and the rights for private practice for senior consultants brought the Labour Government and the doctors to a confrontation (Lancet 1975). And for 118 days from March to June 1983, Israel experienced one of the most prolonged doctors' strikes ever recorded (Ellencweig 1987). Strikes are also common for other health personnel, particularly nurses.

These examples suggest that modern health systems are characterized by varying, but substantial levels of unrest often leading to strikes. Whether these trends are localized and sporadic or whether they constitute a generalized phenomenon is yet unanswered. The indirect effects of labour unrest on the process of care are seldom reported systematically enough to be used in international cross-comparisons. The level of labour unrest in a health system must be estimated by the use of proxies. We shall elaborate on the use of these proxies in the following section on indicators.

Indicators for the indirect process

Constraints on utilization: rationing

The rationing of utilization is commonly undertaken by health systems at a time when cost containment is a major regulatory instrument for the Government or for other funding organizations. However, it is inherently difficult to rank rationing measures hierarchically because these measures are often so ill-defined that both their application and effects are hard to evaluate. A plausible alternative is to use a nominal scale to categorize countries into groups according to the method used for the rationing of utilization.

Rationing methods Various monetary and non-monetary constraints may be imposed in order to ration utilization:

1. *Budgetary constraints* By setting a ceiling on expenditures these contraints restrict the volume of utilization for providers as a group. This is seen for the budget limitations for districts in England, the contracts between physicians and provincial governments in Canada, and the sanctions imposed by central government in Finland when hospitals overspend their budgets.
2. *Constraints on reimbursement* These constraints also limit individual utilization as found in prospective payment systems (DRGs) in the US where providers are reimbursed a fixed amount for each episode of care.
3. *Non-monetary constraints* Here are included administrative constraints affecting utilization, like the limits on the right of hospital-based physicians in England or in Israel to practice privately. Alternatively, sometimes regulatory mechanisms state explicitly who is authorized to perform procedures and which therapies are to be used. This is another form of constraint restricting the rights of health professionals to practice.
4. 'Rationing' through *market competition* Market competition has long been considered an alternative to legislative regulation (Enthoven and Kronick 1989). Recent developments in several European countries have revealed that stimulating competition may involve self-regulatory containment mechanisms (HMSO 1989).

Indicators for process-oriented quality assurance

Utilization review Whether a utilization review is performed on a large scale or not, it can serve a health system as an indicator for distinguishing between those systems heavily involved in quality assurance and those in which quality assurance activities are performed sporadically or locally. The US system which has established several mechanisms for utilization review as discussed in the previous system is an example of the first group. The NHS in England can be considered as a system in which utilization review played little role. The proposal of the British Government to elicit a competitive market in the hospital sector also addresses quality assurance and urges for establishing mechanisms for utilization review (HMSO 1989).

Indicators for labour unrest

The information on labour unrest in the health sector is generally too scacre and incomplete to be used comparatively. Instead, labour unrest must be measured using proxy variables. These proxies are based on information routinely collected and published by the International Labour Office (ILO) (ILO publications). By definition, all the available data reflect levels of general labour disputes rather than disputes specifically in the health field. When labour disputes are reported by industry, the health sector is included as part of the larger group of community, social, and personal services. Though this reduces its usefulness for comparisons, it can still aid in elucidating the understanding of the effects of an unstable labour market on health care. Country indicators on specific industries reported by the ILO (ILO publications) include:

Industrial disputes These are reported as the total number of disputes per year over several years. Since in most countries there is no distinction made between strikes and lock-outs it is permissible to count them in a single category.

Volume of disputes Number of workers involved in industrial disputes per year over several years.

Working days lost The total number of days lost in industrial conflicts per year over several years. These are based on approximations calculated by the ILO. Because the reliability of these data is hard to establish, they should be used very carefully.

References

Abdussalam, M. (1985). Organ substitution therapy in the developing world: from corneal grafting to renal dialysis. In *Health policy, ethics and human values—an international dialogue*. Council for International Organizations of Medical Sciences, Geneva.

Aday, L.A. and Andersen, R. (1975). *Development of indices of access to medical care*. Health Administration Press, Ann Arbor, Michigan.

Aday, L.A., Andersen, R. and Fleming, G.V. (1980). *Health care in the US. Equitable for whom?*. Sage, Beverly Hills, London.

AHA *Hospital Statistics Annual*. Chicago, Illinois. (Various years.)

Andersen, R. and Newman, J.F. (1972). Societal and individual determinants of medical care utilization in the United States. *Milbank Memorial Fund Quarterly*, **51**, 95-124.

Andersen, R., Kravitz, J. and Anderson, O. (1975). *Equity in health services: empirical analyses in social policy*. Ballinger, Cambridge.

Anderson, R. and Smedby, B. (1979). Changes in response to symptoms of illness in the United States and Sweden. In: *Health handbook*, (ed. K. Chacko), Chapter 51. North Holland, Amsterdam.

Andreani, S., Mizrachi, A. and Tornellier, F. (1987). Geographical disparities in health economics: the case of France. *World Health Statistics Quarterly*, **40**, (4), 304-12.

Armstrong, D. (1976). The decline of medical hegemony: a review of Government reports during the NHS. *Social Science and Medicine*, **10**, 157-63.

Barer, M. and Evans, R.G. (1986). Riding north on a south-bound horse? Expenditures, prices utilization and incomes in the Canadian health system. In *Medicare at maturity: achievements, lessons & challenges*, (ed. R.G. Evans and G.L. Stoddart). The Banff Centre, the University of Calgary Press, Calgary.

Beck, R.G. and Horne, J.M. (1980). Utilization of publicly insured health services in Sasketchewan, before, during and after co-payment. *Medical Care*, **18**, 787-806.

Becker, M.H. and Maiman, L.A. (1975). Socio-behavioural determinants of compliance with health and medical care recommendations. *Medical Care*, **13**, (1), 10-24.

Becker, M.H., Drachman, R.H. and Kirscht, J.P. (1972). Predicting mother's compliance with pediatric medical regimens. *Journal of Pediatrics*, **81**, 843-50.

Bridgman, R.F. (1979). *Hospital utilization, an international study*. Oxford University Press, Oxford.

Bunker, J.P. (1970). Surgical manpower: A comparison of operations and surgeons in the United States and in England and Wales. *New England Journal of Medicine*, **282**, 135-44.

Campbell, D.T. and Stanley, J.C. (1963). *Experimental and quasi-experimental designs for research*, p. 56. Rand McNally, Chicago.

CBS (Central Bureau of Statistics) (1983). *Use of health services survey, 1981*, CBS Special Series No. 717. Jerusalem, Israel.

Chassin, M.R., Brook, R.H., Park, R.E., Keesey, J., Fink, A., Kosecoff, J. *et al.* (1986). Variations in the use of medical and surgical services by the Medicare population. *New England Journal of Medicine*, **314**, (5), 285-90.

Chassin, M.R., Kosecoff, J., Park, R.E., Winslow, C.M., Kahn, K.L., Merrick, N.J. *et al.* (1987). Does inappropriate use explain geographic variation in the use of health care services? A study of three procedures. *Journal of the American Medical Association*, **258**, (18), 2533-37.

CHD (Canadian Hospital Directory). Canadian Hospital Association, Ottawa. (Various years.)

Cherkin, D.C., Grothaus, L. and Wagner, E.H. (1990). The effect of office visit co-payment on preventive care services in an HMO. *Inquiry*, **27**, (1), 24-38.

Day, P. and Klein, R. (1989). The politics of modernization: Britain's National Health Services in the 1980s. *The Milbank Quarterly*, **67**, (1), 1-34.

Doty, P. (1987). Health status and health services use among older women: an international perspective. *World Health Statistics Quarterly*, **40** (3), 279-90.

Ellencweig, A.Y. (1987). Modern dilemmas in health care: the Israeli's doctors' strike. *Industrial Relations Journal*, **18**, 117-29.

Enthoven, A. and Kronick, R, (1989), A consumer choice health plan for the 1990s. *New England Journal of Medicine*, **320**, (1), 29-37.

Epstein, A.M., Hartley, R.M., Charlton, J.R. Harris, C.M., Jarman, B., and McNeil, B.J. (1984). A comparison of ambulatory test ordering for hypertension patients in the United States and England. *Journal of the American Medical Association*, **252**, 1723-26.

Eurohealth Handbook (1985). Robert S. First Inc. New York.

Fetter, R.B. (1983). *The new ICD-9-CM diagnosis-related group classification scheme*, HCFA Publication No. 03167. US Government Printing Office, Washington, D.C.

Field, M.G. (1988). The Position of the Soviet physician: the bureaucratic professional. *The Milbank Quarterly*, **66** (suppl. 2), 182-201.

Field, M.J. and Gray, B.H. (1989). Commentary—should we regulate utilization management? *Health Affairs*, **8**, (4), 103-12.

Findlay, S. (1989). *Looking over the doctor's shoulder*. US News and World Report, January, p. 30.

Freidson, E. (1961). *Patient's views of medical practice*. Russell Sage Foundation, New York.

Freidson, E. (1970). *The profession of Medicine*. Dodd Mean and Co., New York.

Freidson, E. (1975). *Doctoring together: a study of professional social control*. Elsevier, New York.

Fuchs, V.R. (1974). *Who shall live*. Basic Books, New York.

Gish, O. (1990). Some links between successful implementation of primary health care interventions and the overall utilization of health services. *Social Science and Medicine*, **30**, (4), 401-05.

Harly, M.J. (1988). Performance indicators in the management process. *Health Services Management Research*, **1**, (1), 29-42.

Harris, J. (1985). *The value of life*. Routledge & Kegan Paul, London.

Health Care Profiles (1986). Asia-Pacific. Bachman, Favereau, Glover Assoc.

Hennelly, V.D. and Boxerman, S.B. (1979). Continuity of medical care: its impact on physician utilization. *Medical Care*, **17**, 1012-18.

HMSO (Her Majesty's Stationery Office) (1989). *Working for Patients*. HMSO, London.

Hulka, B.S. and Wheat, J.R. (1985). Patterns of utilization, the patient perspective. *Medical Care*, **23**, (5), 438-60.

Illich, I. (1977). *Limits to medicine*. Penguin Books, Hamondsworth, Middlesex.

ILO. *Year-Book of Labour statistics*. International Labour Office, Geneva. (Various years.)

Jones, J.J. (1979). Impacts of medical malpractice slowdown in LA County: January 1976. *American Journal of Public Health*, **66**, 437-43.

Joseph, A.E. and Phillips, D.R. (1984). *Accessibility and utilization. Geographical perspective on health care delivery*. Harper & Row Publishers, New York.

Kessner, D.M. (1978). Quality assessment and assurance: early signs of cognitive disonance. *New England Journal of Medicine*, **298**, (7), 381-86.

Kohn, R. and White, K.L. (1976). *Health care, an international study*. Oxford University Press, Oxford.

Krause, E.A. (1988). Doctors, partitocrazia, and the Italian State. *The Milbank Quarterly*, **66** (suppl. 2), 148–66.

Lancet (1964). Notes and news. *Lancet*, No. 11, pp. 838, 883, 927.

Lancet, (1975). Editorial, much in jeopardy. *Lancet* Vol. **ii**, p. 1194.

Larkin, G.V. (1988). Dominance in Britain: image and historical reality. *The Milbank Quarterly*, **66** (suppl. 2), 117–32.

Lieske, A.M. (1985). Standards: the basis of a quality assurance program. In *Quality assurance* (ed. C.G. Meisenheimer). Aspen, Rockville, Maryland.

Lohr, N.L., Brook, R.H., Kamberg, C.J. Goldberg, G.A. Leibowitz, A., Keesey, J. *et al.* (1986). *Use of medical care in the Rand Health Insurance Experiment*, R-3469-HHS. Rand, Santa Monica, California.

Long, A.F., Harrison, S. and Mercer, G. (1985). Comparative perspectives on performance. In *Health services performance, effectiveness and efficiency* (ed. A.F. Long and S. Harrison). Croom Helm, London.

Luft, H.S. (1981). *Health maintenance organizations.* Wiley, Interscience, New York.

McGeorge, K.R., de Mora, J.A. and Legros, G.L. (1985). A case mix management system. *Health Management Forum*, **6**, (2), 53–64.

McKinlay, J.B. (1972). Some approaches and problems in the study of the use of services—an overview. *Journal of Health and Social Behavior*, **13**, 115–52.

McNamara, J.J. and Green, M. (1979). An evaluation of emergency room services during the New York City house officers' strike. *American Journal of Public Health*, **66**, 135–8.

McPherson, K. (1989). International differences in medical care practice. *Health Care Financing Review*, 1989 Annual Supplement, pp. 9–20.

McPherson, K., Strong, P.M., Epstein, A. and Jones, L. (1981). Regional variations in the use of common surgical procedures: within and between England and Wales, Canada and the United States of America. *Social Science and Medicine*, **15A**, 273–88.

McPherson, K., Wennberg, J.E., Hovinol, O.B., and Clifford, B. (1982). Small area variations in the use of common surgical procedures: an international comparison of New England, England and Norway. *New England Journal of Medicine*, **307**, (21), 1310–14.

Manning, W.G., Newhouse, J.P., Duan, N., Keeler, E.B., Leibowitz, A. and Marquis, H. (1987). Health insurance and the demand for medical care: evidence from a randomized experiment. *American Economic Review*, **77**, (3), 251–77.

Mechanic, D. (1982). The epidemiology of illness behavior and its relationship to physical and psychological distress. In *Symptoms, illness behavior and help-seeking* (ed. D. Mechanic). Prodist, New York.

Mechanic, D. (1989). *Painful choices—research and essays on health care*, Chap. 9. Transaction Publishers, New Brunswick.

Micovic, P. (1984). *Health planning and management glossary*, SEARO Regional Health Papers, No. 2. WHO/SEARO, New Delhi.

Mitchell, J.B. and Cromwell, J. (1982). Variations in surgery rates and the supply of surgeons. In *Regional variations in hospital care.* (ed. D.L. Rothberg), Chapter 5. Lexington Books, Lexington, Massachusetts.

Morgan, M., Calnan, M. and Manning, N. (1985). *Sociological approaches to health and medicine*, Chapter 4. Croom Helm, London.

Nathanson, C.A. (1977). Sex, illness and medical care: a review of data, theory and method. *Social Science and Medicine*, **11**, 13–25.

OECD (Organization for Economic Co-operation and Development) (1985). *Measuring health care, 1960–1983*, Social Policy Study, No. 2. Paris.

OECD (Organization for Economic Co-operation and Development) Secretariat (1989). Health care expenditure and other data. *Health Care Financing Review*, 1989 Annual Supplement, pp. 111–94.

PAHO (Pan American Health Organization) (1986). *Health conditions in the Americas, 1981*–1984, Scientific Publication No. 500. Washington, D.C.

Parsons, T. (1964). *Introduction to Max Weber, the theory of social and economic organization*, pp. 58–60, The Free Press, New York.

Pfaff, M. and Nagel, F. (1986). Consequences for hospitals resulting from demographic, social and morbidity changes: A European perspective. *International Journal of Health Planning and Management*, **2**, 311–33.

Poullier, J.P. (1988). The cathedrals of Twenty-First Century. Some economic reflections of the reduction of excess capacity in hospitals. In *The future of health and health care systems in industrialized societies*, (ed. Bui Dang Ha Don), Chapter 17. Praeger, New York.

Reinhardt, U.E. and Sandier, S. (1983). *Alternative methods of physician remuneration and their effects on physician activity: an international comparison.* CREDOC, Paris.

Roos, P.N. and Shapiro, E. (1981). The Manitoba Longitudinal Study on Aging. Preliminary findings on health care utilization by the elderly. *Medical Care*, **19**, (6), 644–57.

Roos, N.P., Gaumont, M. and Horne, J.M. (1976). The impact of the physician surplus on the distribution of physicians across Canada. *Canadian Health Policy*, **2**, 161–91.

Rothberg, D.L. (1981). *Regional variations in hospital use*, Chapter 1. Lexington Books, Lexington, Massachusetts.

Salkever, D.S. (1976). Accessibility and the demand for preventive care. *Social Science and Medicine*, **10**, 469–75.

Sandier, S. (1989). Health services utilization and physician income trends. *Health Care Financing Review*, 1989 Annual Supplement, pp. 33–48.

Scheffler, R.M. (1984). The United Mine Workers' Health Plan: an analysis of the cost sharing program. *Medical Care*, **22**, 247–54.

Schulz, R. and Harrison, S. (1986). Physician autonomy in the Federal Republic of Germany, Great Britain and the United States. *International Journal of Health Planning and Management*, **2**, 335–55.

Shimmura, K. (1988). Effects of different remuneration methods on general medical practice: a comparison of capitation and fee-for-service payment. *International Journal of Health Planning and Management*, **3**, 245–58.

Snyder, R.C. (1975). Professional self regulation in the public interest: the intellectual politics of PSRO. In *Proceedings, Conference on Professional Self Regulation*. Health Resources Administration, Department of Health, Education and Welfare, Washington, D.C.

Suchman, E.A. (1964). Socio-medical variations among ethnic groups. *American Journal of Sociology*, **70**, 319–31.

Suchman, E.A. (1966). Health orientation and medical care. *American Journal of Public Health*, **56**, 97–105.

Tollefson, E.A. (1963). *Bitter medicine—the Saskatchewan medicine feud.* The Modern Press, Saskatoon.

USDHHS (United States Department of Health and Human Services) (1985).

Health, United States, DHHS publication. No. PHS 87-1232, 1986. US Government Printing Office, Washington, D.C.

USDHHS (United States Department of Health and Human Services) (1986). *Social security programs throughout the world*. US Social Security Administration, Washington, D.C.

van de Veer, D. and Regan, T. (1987). *Health care ethics—an introduction*. Temple University Press, Philadelphia.

Vayda, E.A. (1973). A comparison of surgical rates in Canada and in England and Wales. *New England Journal of Medicine*, **289**, 1224-29.

Vuori, H. (1982). *Quality assurance of health services*, Public Health in Europe, No. 16. World Health Organization, Copenhagen.

Weiner, J.P. (1987). Primary care delivery in the US and four north west European countries: comparing the 'Corporatized' with the 'Socialized'. *Milbank Fund Quarterly*, **65**, (3), 426-61.

Wennberg, J.E., Bunker, J.P., and Barnes, B. (1980). The need for assessing the outucome of common medical practices. *Annual Review of Public Health*, **1**, 277-95.

WHO (World Health Organization) (1981). *County reviews and statistics. Health Services in Europe*. Vol. 2, (3rd edn). Regional Office for Europe, Copenhagen.

WHO (World Health Organization) (1983). *World Health Statistics 1983*. Geneva.

WHO (World Health Organization) (1989). *Eurostat* (HFA—Indicators) HFA/PC software package. Regional Office for Europe, Copenhagen.

Willis, E. (1988). Doctoring in Australia: a view at the bicentenary. *The Milbank Quarterly*, **66**, (suppl. 2), 167-81.

Winslade, W.J. and Ross, J.W. (1986). *Choosing life and death. A guide for patients, families and professionals*. The Free Press, New York.

Zola, E.A. (1963). Problems of communication, diagnosis and patient care: the interplay of patient, physician and clinic organization. *Journal of Medical Education*, **38**, 829-38.

Zola, E.A. (1964). Illness behaviour of the working: implications and recommendations. In: *Blue collar world* (ed. A.B. Shostak and W. Gomberg). Prentice Hall, Englewood Cliffs, New Jersey.

7. Assessing the outcomes of health systems

Outcomes

The unequivocal ultimate goal of any health system is the improvement of the health of populations of a given region or country. For overall goals, there is general agreement with the World Health Organization 'Health for all' policy. However, at the population level, definitions of health outcomes, methods for outcome measurement, and the cause and effect relationships between factors and their effects on outcomes are characterized by confusion and disagreement. As we already mentioned in Chapter 2, there is disagreement about both the definition of health and the boundaries of the health system. In systems where there is a comprehensive welfare strategy, health is only one dimension in a multifaceted array of social networks. Thus, positive health outcomes depend not only on the health system but on society's success in the general social and psychological arenas. This relationship reflects the WHO definition of health, in which social and psychological well-being are equal to physical health. Nevertheless, in many countries there are narrower boundaries for the national social systems, for health, welfare, and education, and thus they are strictly separated. Because in some countries the social systems are interrelated, and in some strictly separated, it is not feasible to standardize these boundaries. The picture is made even more complex by the modern definitions of health in which factors shaping up health outcomes but external to the health care system, are emphasized. These factors are societal norms, environmental factors and biological phenomena. (See for example De Miguel 1975; Alan Dever 1980; Blum 1981).

The problems in defining health outcomes and the boundaries of health can be resolved by using two different approaches. In one, health outcomes are examined in a broad macro perspective. Outcomes are considered separately without any reference to causality. In fact, the underlying assumption for this approach is that each category of health outcomes is affected by multiple causes. Outcomes are defined in terms of specific measurable indicators: Field's five Ds: death, disease, disability, discomfort, and dissatisfaction (1973). These five Ds are measures of health outcomes as empirical quantities; but they cannot explain cause and effect relationships. The second approach is much narrower and is confined to specific micro conditions which suggest causal relationships. This second approach can be applied only to limited situations where significant interdependence between structures, processes, and outcomes can be shown.

If a relationship between cause and effect is suspected, one may ask if the effect is within the health care system or whether it results from external factors like life styles or the environment. In fact, many health outcomes are stimulated by external factors, like the cause and effect relationship between tobacco intake and cancer. In general, there is an extensive epidemiological literature examining causal associations between outcomes and external factors. (For further details see textbooks on epidemiology e.g. Lilienfeld and Lilienfeld 1980).

If we compare these two approaches, the macro perspective can provide a better overview of the actual 'state of the art' of health outcomes, but it provides little or no information about specific causal and confounding effects. On the other hand, while the micro causal approach provides an in-depth perspective of systems' behaviour, the view of the actual health outcomes may be incomplete. Because each approach is insufficient in itself, we shall compare them in a stepwise procedure. First we screen several trends at the macro level to identify differences and unexplained gaps. Then, we focus on specific findings warranting further attention. As we shall see, this stage may involve a more analytical approach at the micro than at the macro level of causal associations; it may be regarded as the modern approach to health outcomes.

The macro approach

Mortality

By and large, mortality has long been the most extensively studied of the various elements constituting the macro approach. As Uemura and Pisa (1985) put it:

> One of the main reasons for the frequent use of mortality data, as compared with morbidity data, is the availability of reliable data for comparisons among countries. Death is a distinct, objectively recognized and extremely serious event which makes it much easier to record than the occurrence of illness *per se*.

In industrialized countries, and in some of the more advanced developing countries, there is complete or nearly complete registration of death. At national and international levels, mortality statistics are readily available particularly in the WHO Statistics Annual (WHO publications). This series of publications is extremely useful for characterizing a large number of countries reporting mortality uniformly and annually. The frequency of the reports contributes to the reliability of the data, because data for consecutive years can thus be aggregated and used to stabilize possible periodic fluctuations. Strict adherence to well-defined definitions of various mortality-related variables enhances the validity of the WHO reporting system. Commonly used variables include crude mortality rates, age-specific mortality rates, and cause-specific mortality rates. As we describe in Chapter 9, most countries have adopted the newest International Classification of Diseases Scheme (ICD-9CM), though some countries are still using an earlier version (ICD-8). Developing countries tend to report less frequently than developed countries, or may not report at all, as we discussed in Chapter 5. For example, Mauritius is the only country reporting in the African region in 1983–5 (WHO 1986). A thorough description of various classification schemes can be found in WHO publications (WHO 1977) and in various reports on international information systems (e.g. Weber 1982). In Europe, the WHO Regional Office has compiled mortality data from several countries on its Eurostat Health for All Personal Computer Package (WHO Eurostat 1989). This Package provides mortality data longitudinally in tabloid, map, and graphic forms. For example Fig. 7.1 provides data on infant mortality rates per 1000 live births in several European countries for 1970 (first year), and for 1984 to 1987 (last year).

At national or regional levels vital statistics are generally disseminated by national ministries of health or by other government agencies. For example, the National Centre for Health Statistics of the US Department of Health and Human Services (US-DHHS) publishes geographically-based mortality statistics which includes comparisons by age, sex and ethnicity (NCHS 1987). In Canada, similar interregional comparisons are available through the annual publications of vital statistics issued by Statistics Canada (see for example *Mortality—summary list of causes—1988*, by Statistics Canada 1988). In Britain, similar information is obtained through the *Annual*

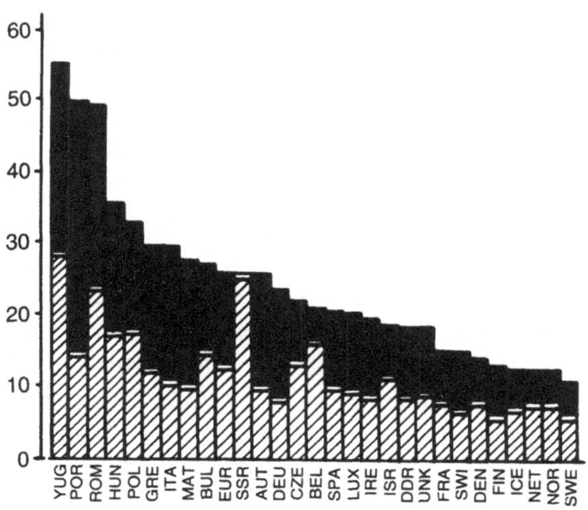

First available year: full bars, 1970.
Last available year: dotted bars, 1984–1987 according to the country

Fig. 7.1 Infant mortality rate per 1000 live births for member countries of the WHO European Region. (Data from WHO Eurostat (1989).)

Abstracts of Statistics (Central Statistics Office publications). Another source of information on regional differences in mortality is the *Eurohealth Handbook* (1985) which includes mortality data for several European countries on a regional basis. Twentieth century mortality trends for European and other selected countries are found in Alderson's International Mortality Statistics (1981). This book is particularly helpful for those wishing to conduct longitudinal comparisons by sex, calendar period, cause of death, and country.

Along with cross-sectional reports on mortality, some investigators have also studied longitudinal trends in overall mortality and in cause-specific mortality rates. For example, Uemura and Pisa (1982, 1985) published a series of data on trends in mortality due to all causes and particularly due to cardiovascular diseases for 27 industrialized countries. They report two interesting findings:

1. In cross-sectional comparisons, there are surprisingly large differences, sometimes amounting to two fold differences among countries.
2. An escalating rate of cardiovascular death in industrial socialist countries in Europe and a corresponding decrease in rates over time for Western European countries have caused an increasing gap in mortality trends over time.

Marmot (1985) reached similar conclusions in his analysis of age-adjusted data on mortality from coronary heart disease (CHD) for the age group 35–74 years. Of all Western countries, age-adjusted mortality rates increased between 1968 and 1982 only in Sweden. On the other hand, an increase in CHD was found in all the Eastern European Countries.

Several international comparisons on mortality have focused on specific age groups. Naturally, the groups that attracted most attention are those at the two age extremes, the neonates and the elderly. A constant gradual increase in life expectancy was seen in longitudinal comparisons of mortality rates among the elderly, that is in the probability of survival among the old and the very old (Lopez and Hanada 1982; Heikkinen 1984, 1987). A comparison of trends in the probability of survival between the ages of 75 and 84 in five Scandinavian countries is shown in Fig. 7.2 (Heikkinen 1987). Though there are absolute differences among countries, with prolonged life span there is a demonstrable tendency to find compressed differences in life expectancy. This phenomenon was ascribed by Fries and Crapo (1981) to the 'rectangularization of mortality' at higher ages. Similar work has been done on infant mortality, particularly on perinatal mortality. Perinatal mortality includes the deaths that occurred during the first week of life and during the late fetal stages. With the sharp fall in mortality rates in developed societies, perinatal mortality has become a major indicator for the evaluation of pregnancy outcome. Several international comparisons on the connection between perinatal mortality and low birth-weight have been

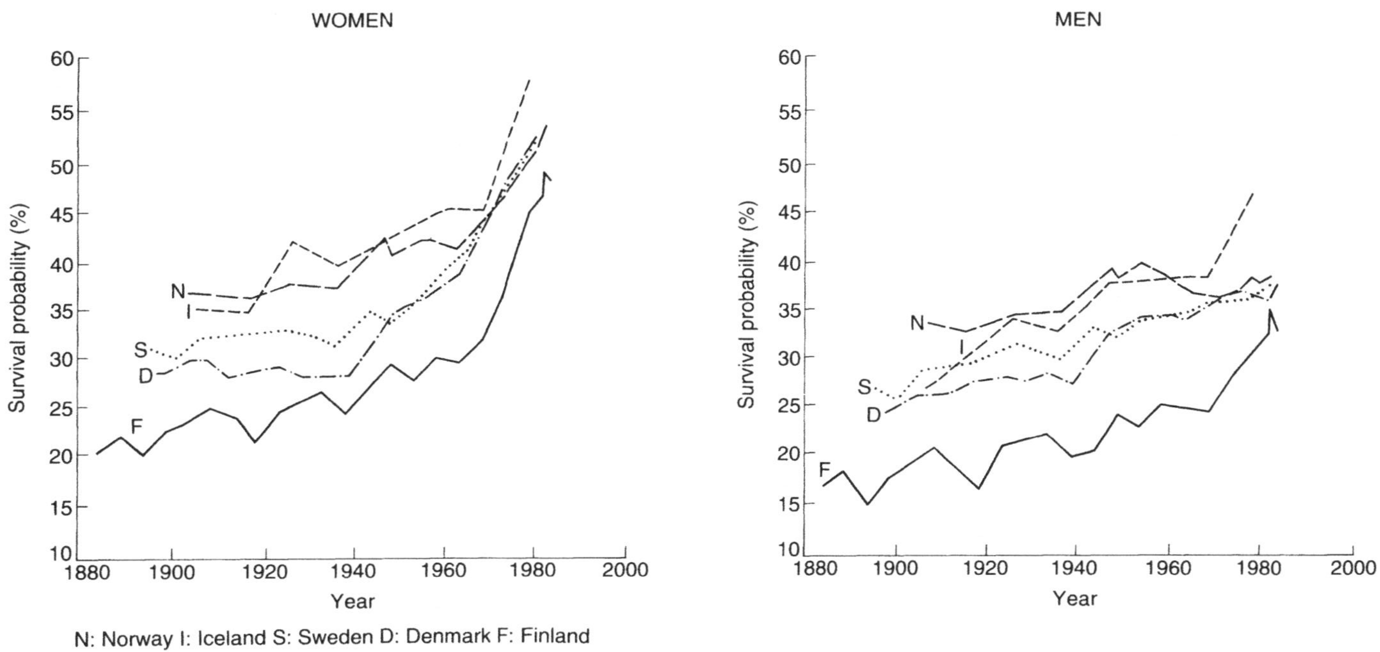

Fig. 7.2 Trends in the probability of survival between ages 75 and 84 in the Nordic countries. (From Martelin and Volkonen, unpublished material.)

carried out. Consider, for example, the comparative international study involving eight countries by Foster (1981). Though practical difficulties in the definition of the measured attribute and lack of consistency and reliability across systems (Edouard 1985) may interfere with these studies, the sensitivity of this indicator suggests that it will be extensively used in the future.

In recent years, international comparisons of age- and cause-specific mortality have departed from straightforward comparisons and tended to concentrate on comparisons of excess death rates across several countries. As Plaut and Roberts (1989) state 'mortality cannot be prevented but it can be postponed', so it is important to estimate 'excess' or 'premature' death in several countries and then to draw conclusions on how and where the health system can intervene in postponing death. Researchers in ten European countries collaborated to compile the *European Community Atlas of Avoidable Death* (Holland 1988). This Atlas provides Standardized Mortality Ratios for several age- and cause-specific groups.

Mortality data, through easily accessible, is somewhat problematic because of the validity of the definition of mortality. As Elling (1980, p. 148) put it:

> Custom, tradition, or knowledge-production arrangements determined by socio political conditions of the past may be frozen into current usage which can vary remarkably between countries. France, for example, counts a birth as "live" only after the first 24 hours, while most other countries report a live birth when the baby has breathed on its own for some short period. This has some effect on infant mortality rates, since, as one study in West Germany showed, close to one-third occurred during days two to six, and the rest thereafter in the first year of life. To get accurate comparisons, one would have to include stillbirths and late fetal deaths with infant mortality. But this would not lend perfect comparability—even assuming accuracy or at least comparable approaches in registration systems and agents responsible for informing, coding, and tabulating information—since definitions of when life begins and information on when gestation started is variable and difficult to obtain.

Another problem frequently encountered in longitudinal comparisons is that measurement tools are regularly, though infrequently, updated. At the end of the 1970s, many countries adopted ICD-9 in place of ICD-8. This change affected the comparability of statistics gathered before and after this change. In some countries, notably the US, the comparability of the two ICD versions was examined by coding a sample of death certificates in each one. While overall comparability was good, for some specific groups there were some significant deviations. For instance, the assignment of ischaemic heart disease as a cause of death measured by ICD-9, corresponded only to 88 per cent of the cases as measured by ICD-8 (USDHEW 1980).

In view of the difficulties encountered in comparing health outcomes, Chase (1972) carefully evaluated criteria for including countries in comparative studies on mortality. He suggested using inclusion criteria like self-governance, population above one million, not excluding groups of cases from mortality records as is sometimes the case for mortality in rural areas in some developing countries, and so on. Using these criteria, the list of the 220 countries reporting to the UN was reduced to only 41 eligible for comparisons of infant mortality rates. Though successful in establishing inclusion criteria for the most basic indicators, one may fail to do so for more sensitive indicators like cause-specific mortality rates. This may happen when a given condition like AIDS or suicide may carry a social stigma. Furthermore, severity of illness may be differently interpreted in various nations (Sidel 1981).

Because descriptive statistics on mortality are readily available, investigators have attempted to explain the differences in mortality rates among countries or regions. In several studies they concentrated on the effects of health systems on changes in mortality patterns. We shall address this topic more thoroughly in Chapter 10.

Clearly, mortality and longevity are also affected by factors external to the health system. Though the effects of such external factors on health outcomes are beyond the scope of this book, we cannot avoid making at least a concise overview of typical studies on the effects of external factors on mortality in an international context.

Let us consider life-style as an example of such an external factor. As described in Keys' obesity study (1970), life-style may have a decisive role both literally and conceptually in determining an individual's shape and size. As Keys notes:

> . . . more American men were obese – 63 percent – than were men in any of the other national samples examined. Subjects from the other countries – the Netherlands, Italy, Yugoslavia, Finland, Greece, and Japan – exhibited a decreasing frequency of obesity (in order listed), with only 2 percent of Japanese men being obese. It is no coincidence that Japanese men have the world's lowest mortality rates and that US males rank nineteenth. The other countries fall between the United States and Japan with respect to mortality rates.

Marmot and colleagues (1975) related cardiovascular disease to dietary customs. They studied groups of Japanese who migrated to Hawaii and to California. The cardiovascular disease rates for migrants who had adopted the dietary habits of their new neighbours approached the rates for native Hawaiians and Californians and were much higher than those rates in Japan. Jones and colleagues (1985) linked the prevalence of teenage pregnancies to infant mortality and morbidity. Compared with some European countries, rates of teenage pregnancies in the US were much higher, which accounts for the substantially increased mortality and morbidity in the US. The variations may be explained by differences in sex education and in the frequency of the use of birth control. Another life-style factor, life-endangering accidents, was also extensively studied. Age-specific rates for mortality due to motor vehicle accidents were analysed by Havard (1979), and rates due to all types of accidents for children, adolescents, and young adults, by Taket (1986). It was shown that in industrial countries, the highest risk group for motor vehicle accidents were young male adults and adolescents. Rates were higher in developed countries outside Europe than for the countries of the European continent (Havard 1979). Mortality due to accidents other than road accidents had lower rates but similar trends. A longitudinal data analysis showed that for most developed countries there is a decreasing or an eventually decreasing trend in mortality rates. In contrast, trends for developing countries like Mexico and Thailand showed an increase in mortality rates due to accidents, especially motor vehicle accidents (Taket 1986).

Some comparisons of environmental influences on health across various geographical regions are also available. In Canada, the results of one study suggest that high cadmium concentrations in ground water cause an increase in both the incidence and the mortality rates due to carcinoma of the prostate (Bako *et al.* 1982). In the US, Comstock (1979) found an association between regional variations in the quality of drinking water and cardiovascular mortality. His results strongly suggest that there are lower mortality rates in regions with hard water. Similarly, mortality rates can be

Table 7.1 Suicide rates per 100 000 for selected countries (1978 and 1980)

Country	Men	Women	Ratio (Men/Women)
Hungary[a]	64.5	26.5	2.5
Finland[b]	41.9	9.7	4.3
Denmark[a]	41.1	22.3	1.8
Austria[a]	37.8	14.9	2.5
Switzerland[a]	36.7	15.2	2.4
France[b]	24.7	10.0	2.5
Japan[a]	22.2	13.1	1.7
Canada[b]	22.3	7.3	3.1
United States[a]	18.6	5.5	3.4
Norway[a]	18.3	6.6	2.8
Australia[a]	16.4	5.6	2.9
England and Wales[a]	11.0	6.7	1.6
Italy[b]	9.3	3.8	2.4
Israel[ac]	8.1	3.8	2.1
Ireland[b]	6.4	3.5	1.8
Spain[b]	6.1	2.2	2.8

[a]1980 [b]1978 [c]Jewish population only
Source: Adapted from WHO (1981; 1982). *World Health Statistics Annual.*

substantially affected by the social environment as well as by the physical environment. Consider deaths due to suicide, as shown in Table 7.1. The large international variations may be only partly explained. For example, one explanation for high suicide rates is the disintegration of culture as in Hungary under the socialist regime. Another explanation valid for the Scandinavian countries is based on the harmful side effects of extensive substance abuse.

Indicators of Mortality

In the voluminous literature on mortality there is a broad spectrum of indicators for its measurement. Direct indicators, produced by a single measurement can be distinguished from composite indices made up of several indicators. A concise analysis of the different types of mortality indicators is given in Table 7.2. For a thorough analysis of mortality indicators and their utility, the reader is referred to the excellent review by Murnaghan (1981).

Table 7.2 Basic mortality indicators

Indicator	Numerator	Denominator	Comments
1. Crude death rate	Total number of deaths reported during a given time interval	Estimated mid-interval population	
2. Cause-specific death rate	Number of deaths assigned to a specific cause during a given time-interval	Estimated mid-interval population	
3. Proportional mortality ratio	Number of deaths assigned to a specific cause during a given time-interval	Total number of deaths from all causes during the same period	
4. Case fatality rate (ratio)	Number of deaths assigned to a specific disease during a given time-interval	Number of new cases of that disease reported during the same time-interval	

Table 7.2 *continued*

Indicator	Numerator	Denominator	Comments
5. Fetal death rate	Number of fetal deaths of 28 weeks or more gestation, reported during a given time-interval	Number of fetal deaths of 28 weeks or more gestation, reported during the same time-interval plus the number of live births occurring during the same time-interval	Sometimes 20 weeks gestation is used as the cut-off point
6. Fetal death ratio	Number of fetal deaths of 28 weeks or more gestation, reported during a given time-interval	Number of live births reported during the same time-interval	
7. Perinatal mortality rate	Number of fetal deaths of 28 weeks or more gestation, reported during a given time-interval, plus the reported number of infant deaths under seven days of life during the same time-interval	Number of fetal deaths of 28 weeks or more gestation, reported during the same time-interval plus the number of live births occurring during the same time-interval	Sometimes 20 weeks gestation and infant death under 28 days of life are used as cut-off points
8. Infant mortality rate	Number of deaths under one year of age reported during a given time-interval	Number of live births reported during the same time-interval	
9. Neonatal mortality rate	Number of deaths under 28 days of age reported during a given time-interval	Number of live births reported during the same time-interval	

Table 7.2 *continued*

Indicator	Numerator	Denominator	Comments
10. Post-neonatal mortality rate	Number of deaths from 28 days of age up to, but not including, one year of age, reported during a given time-interval	Number of live births reported during the same time-interval	
11. Maternal mortality rate	Number of deaths assigned to causes related to pregnancy during a given time-interval	Number of live births reported during the same time-interval	Singled out in developed societies

Adapted from Alan Dever (1980)

Basic indicators

Basic indicators may be absolute numbers, rates, or ratios. There are three classes of basic indicators:

(1) crude indicators;

(2) specific indicators;

(3) adjusted (standardized) indicators.

Crude indicators include the absolute number of deaths during a year in a population, or mortality rates in a population. For specific indicators, specificity can be related to age, sex, disease, ethnicity, area, or any combination of these like age-specific mortality rates or cause- (disease-related) specific mortality rates. Adjusted indicators are hypothetical rates based on the fiction that two or more populations to be compared have a similar composition with respect to a given confounder variable. Common confounder variables are age and sex and the use of adjusted indicators may account for the differences caused by such confounders. For those interested in the adjustment procedure see, for example, Fleiss (1973).

Table 7.2 provides a wider variety of mortality indicators than may be potentially used in cross-comparative studies. However, selecting an appropriate indicator mix for measuring health outcomes for cross-comparisons may be problematic because the definition of mortality indicators, for example, are not standardized across countries. Indeed the

European region of the WHO has taken the lead for developing criteria for standardizing these indicators. This effort may be seen in the broader context of the formulation of a regional strategy for attaining the goal of 'health for all'. The European approach included the identification of 38 targets, of which 12 are identified with generally desirable changes in health status. Practically, the 38 targets can be divided into essential and optional indicators. Essential indicators are relevant for all countries and thus are important at the regional level. Optional indicators are more detailed and specific than essential indicators; data on optional indicators would be useful but are not always available (Brzezinski 1986).

In Table 7.3 are listed the essential and optional indicators recommended for cross-national comparisons by the WHO European Regional Office.

Table 7.3 Mortality indicators in relation to regional targets for 'Health For All'. WHO European Region

Target	Essential regional indicators	Optional regional indicators
Life expectancy	Life expectancy at birth by sex Life expectancy at ages 1, 15, 35, and 65, by sex	Number of years of life lost due to deaths occurring before age 65
Infant mortality	Infant mortality rate	Neonatal mortality rate (first 4 weeks of life) Post-neonatal rate (second to eleventh month of life) Perinatal mortality rate
Maternal mortality	Maternal mortality rate	
Cardiovascular diseases	Mortality rates, by sex and age from diseases of the circulatory system (ICD 390–459); with special reference to: ischaemic heart disease (ICD 410–414) or cerebrovascular diseases (ICD 430–438)	Incidence of ischaemic heart disease Incidence of cerebrovascular diseases
Cancer	Mortality rates, by sex and age, from malignant neoplasms (ICD 140–234) (more detailed	Incidence of cancer of the cervix

Table 7.3 *continued*

Target	Essential regional indicators	Optional regional indicators
	information by site recommended)	
	trachea, bronchus and lung cancer (ICD 162)	
	cancer of cervix uteri (ICD 180)	
Accidents	Mortality rates, by sex and age from external causes of injury	Incidence of motor vehicle traffic accidents, accidents and poisoning occurring in the home, accidents related to work
	poisoning (ICD E800-E999)	
	motor vehicle traffic accidents (ICD E810–E819)	
Suicide	Mortality rates, by sex and age, from suicide (ICD E950–E959)	Incidence of attempted suicide

Adapted from Brzezinski (1986)

Composite indices

Crude data on mortality rates are relatively easy to collect. As a result, many investigators have been encouraged to develop comprehensive measures permitting health status to be viewed from several angles. Here we shall discuss only those composite indices that are internationally accepted.

Standardized Mortality Ratio (SMR) Of the composite indices, *SMR* is perhaps the most widely used. It is the ratio of the observed number of deaths to the expected number of deaths. SMR_a, the Standardized Mortality Ratio in region a is calculated as follows:

$$SMR_a = \frac{D_a}{1000\sum_{i=1}^{n} M_i P_i}$$

where: D_a = observed number of deaths in region a;
M_i = standard specific death rate per 1000 population in age group i (for region a);
P_i = size of the population in age group i (for region a).

In a comparative perspective, SMRs for several regions or countries may be calculated and compared.

Years of Life Lost Index (YLL) Particularly among health economists, *YLL* is a popular index. It permits the estimation of the total years of life lost per population in a given area, based on the known number of deaths at various ages. This indicator can also be used to study the effects of specific causes of death. For example, it can be used in a comparative study of *YLL* due to acute myocardial infarction in various areas. The general equation is:

$$YLL = \frac{1}{1000}\left\{\frac{\sum_{i=1}^{n} D_i(70 - Y_i)}{\sum_{i=1}^{n} M_i P_i (70 - Y_i)}\right\}$$

where: D_i = observed deaths in age group i;
M_i = standard age-specific death rates per 1000 population in age group i (for specific causes);
P_i = area population in age group i;
Y_i = the midpoint of each age interval i (age 70 is taken as the upper limit for the calculation).

The indicator YLL was recently applied in cross-national comparisons between Spain and Portugal. Analysis revealed that in the Iberian Peninsula the most contributing causes to premature death were malignant tumors and violent deaths as due to accidents (Rodriguez and Cayolla da Motta 1989).

Excess Mortality Ratio (EMR) The indicator *EMR* is based on the idea that a low level of mortality can be chosen as a norm, or standard reference, for mortality. The lowest age-sex-specific death rate in a given country or region is called a 'Minimal Death Rate'. Once the minimal death rate is determined for a given country/region, an increase in mortality rate beyond this minimum in other regions or in other countries is considered 'Excess Mortality', that is δD:

$$\delta D = D - D_s$$

where: D = the actual total number of deaths in a country per year;
D_s = the expected number of deaths in a country based on the norm of the Minimal Mortality Rate.

Now,

$$\delta D = \sum_{i=1}^{n}\sum_{j=1}^{m} P_{ij} M_{ij} - \sum_{i=1}^{n}\sum_{j=1}^{m} P_{ij} - M_{ijs}$$

where: P_{ij} = the population for age group i and sex j;
M_{ij} = observed age-sex-specific death rate;
M_{ijs} = standard age-sex-specific death rate.

Finally:

$$EMR = \frac{\delta D}{D_s} = \frac{D - D_s}{D_s}$$

$$= \frac{\sum_{i=1}^{n} \sum_{j=1}^{m} P_{ij} M_{ij} - \sum_{i=1}^{n} \sum_{j=1}^{m} P_i M_{ijs}}{\sum_{i=1}^{n} \sum_{j=1}^{m} P_i M_{ijs}}$$

Uemura (1989) used the indicator *EMR* in cross-national comparisons. First, he identified the lowest age-sex-specific rates in the world—these rates were found for children in northern European countries and for middle-aged people in Japan, Israel, and Greece. These calculations were done for the year under study and for historical data. Second, he identified the computed data comprising the lowest death rates ever recorded since 1950. He used both current and historical data to compute cross-sectional and longitudinal changes in *EMR* for selected countries, as shown in Fig. 7.3.

Morbidity

Morbidity is an ill-defined concept. Lack of standard definitions makes it difficult to use in international comparisons. Except for a few diagnoses like neoplasms in countries with hospital-based cancer registries, the WHO does not routinely publish morbidity statistics. Instead, special analyses based on morbidity statistics are collected by individual countries and published frequently in the *World Health Statistics Quarterly* (previously called the *World Health Statistics Report*). These morbidity statistics are also used in several technical and scientific publications and in documents issued by the Headquarters and the Regional Offices of the WHO. Besides this, additional data is collected routinely on an *ad hoc* basis by several other WHO programmes. For instance, information on cases of infectious disease and on immunization programmes is collected and analysed by the Expanded Programme on Immunization.

Inadequate data collection systems, possibly invalid diagnoses, and unreliable case-reporting make the use of morbidity-related measures in cross-comparisons problematic. The inherent ambiguity in the operational definition of disease may cause invalid diagnoses and unreliable case-reporting. The validity of diagnoses is particularly affected by the subjective nature of disease resumption. As seen in Chapter 3, illness can be subjectively perceived by an individual though this perception may not be

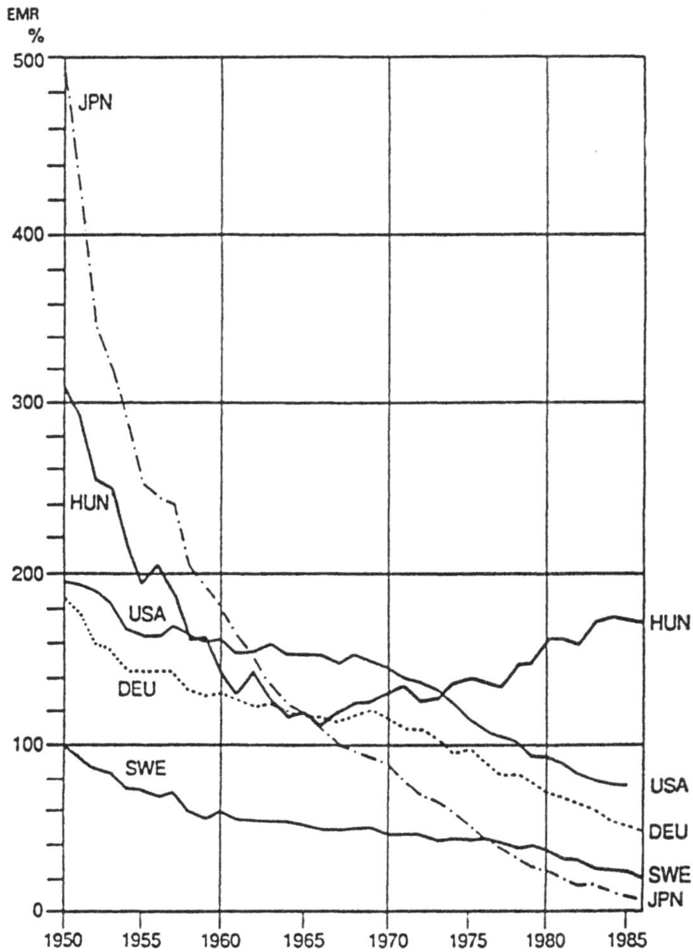

Fig. 7.3 Trends in Excess Mortality Ratio (EMR) with reference to the historical minimum death rates (as of 1986), both sexes under 65 years, selected countries. (From Uemura (1989), with permission.)

supported by an objective medical examination. Alternatively, diseases in the asymptomatic or mild symptomatic staging, can easily go unnoticed by the patient though later the disease may become more severe.

Illnesses have a duration, can recur, and have various degrees of severity. The epidemiologic indices of incidence and prevalence are specifically designed to resolve the ambiguity of the notion of duration. A point prevalence measurement is an indication of illnesses present at a point in time; similarly, a period prevalence measurement, for a given period. On the other hand, measurement of incidence is an indication of illnesses diagnosed during a defined period. Unfortunately, similar progress cannot be shown for evaluating the severity of disease as for chronic conditions.

Inappropriate data collection methods further complicate the methodological and practical difficulties in defining and measuring morbidity. Generally speaking, there is no morbidity databank like the comprehensive reporting on mortality. For example, only 5 European countries routinely report the incidence of ischaemic heart disease while 18 do not report it at all (Nossikov *et al.* 1990). This limits international comparisons to relatively unambiguous chronic and acute conditions that are high in the public awareness. With this in mind, let us now explore the potential sources for information on morbidity. The first group of data is for several infectious communicable diseases for which most countries require notification to health authorities. Mandatory notification by statute implies that all cases must be reported. Indeed, 23 European countries report regularly on the incidence rates of infectious diseases while only 2 do not report at all (Nossikov *et al.* 1990). In fact, however, reporting is grossly incomplete: often mild cases are not reported due to diagnostic inexactitude or negligence. Social and cultural stigma associated with sexually transmitted diseases or with gastro-intestinal epidemics are also cause for underreporting. In spite of this, the WHO provides international comparisons on morbidity for selected communicable diseases (for example WHO 1983, 1984) and more recently on AIDS (WHO 1987). In Europe, information is available through the WHO, Regional Office. For example. Fig. 7.4 provides longitudinal data on incidence of hepatitis in several European countries in the beginning of the 80s (1979–1982, year according to the countries) and in the middle of this decade (1984–1987, year according to the

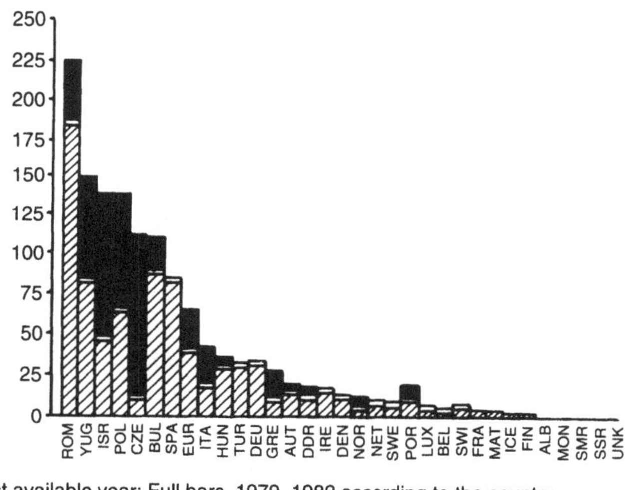

Fig. 7.4 Incidence of hepatitis: total per 100 000, for member countries of the WHO European Region. (Data from WHO Eurostat (1989).)

countries). The figure shows large variations among countries, but generally, incidence rates decrease over time (WHO Eurostat 1989). Population registries are yet another source for international comparisons of morbidity. These are particularly useful for incidence and prevalence studies of chronic conditions. Most useful for international comparisons are the registries on several types of cancer which are the most reliable and the most frequently recorded. And even these registries are incomplete, as some mild cases of cancer, like localized skin cancers, may not be included. Maintaining the validity of the cancer registries has been largely achieved by international standardization, as strongly advised by WHO experts (WHO 1976).

The sentinel model is another successful approach used in international comparisons of morbidity. In the sentinel model, either some physicians or some health care facilities are designated as sentinel sites. Sentinel sites may be entire cities or one or more major or specialized institutions within a city. In international comparisons, a sentinel network is of a number of sentinel sites or of physicians operating in a given group of countries. A prime example of such a network is the MONICA project (MONItoring of trends and determinants in CArdiovascular disease) which was started in 1983 as an international network. MONICA was designed to measure trends in cardiovascular mortality and morbidity, and to relate them to etiological factors. It involves 40 centres in 26 countries and covers a population of 11 million (WHO MONICA 1987). Another example of a sentinel system includes physicians rather than institutions: it consists of regional networks of volunteer physicians who report the numbers of cases of certain specified diseases and conditions seen in their practices every week. These networks are not operational internationally. However, in Europe, there are a number of networks operating efficiently within countries, including the UK, the Netherlands, Belgium, France and Switzerland. Usually, each network includes a few hundred reporting physicians. The geographical distribution of sentinel sites is based on population size, age, sex, and type of medical practice. The information collected within each country's network can then be compared across countries (Woodall 1988). Occasionally, morbidity is assessed through a special global effort, generally supported by the WHO, to evaluate a given disease or condition. An interesting example is the study on the world incidence of low birth-weight. This focus on low birth-weight was due to its importance as a prime measure for the health and nutritional status of the mother, and also for the probability of the survival of the newborns (Division of Family Health 1980).

Routine utilization data can also be used as a 'tracer condition' for assessing comparative morbidity. This is advantageous because in most developed countries, hospital discharge charts are readily available and are commonly processed either on-line or in a relatively expeditious off-line process. Particularly within the European community there is a constant effort to standardize information in the form of minimal basic data sets (MBDS) (Roger

1982). However, utilization data should be used cautiously. First, it is fairly limited to hospital data because ambulatory systems lag far behind in documenting diagnostic and treatment data. Second, though in most countries the validity of data is established by the use of the ICD system (ICD-8 or ICD-9), reporting is often unreliable. Objectively, this is due to the non-standardized reporting processes; subjectively, this is also due to the vested interests of the reporters. For example, suppose that reporting of diagnoses and the severity of disease could affect the level of hospital reimbursement: in such cases, one must always suspect that hospital personnel may occasionally upgrade the interpretation of the severity of a disease. Then one should question whether hospital charts include cases for which the diagnosis is interpreted in more severe terms than warranted.

The use of crude morbidity data is also limited because these data reflect neither differences in age/sex distribution nor differences in the characteristics of health systems like the availability of services and the access to health care. Comparisons of morbidity data can be facilitated by age- and sex- adjusted rates since they act as a control for demographic differences. However, differences due to systems' characteristics are harder to correct. Moreover, several kinds of comparisons are based on aggregate rather than individual data, making comparisons difficult to interpret. For instance, the OECD (1985) provides differences in average lengths of hospital stay by disease categories for several developed countries. This information has also been updated for later years (OECD 1989). While this information is interesting, its suspect validity limits its suitability for analysis (Poullier 1987).

By comparing levels of perceived morbidity in the population we can potentially overcome some of the shortcomings mentioned above. This approach is based on the belief that planning should be grounded on sound epidemiological principles and on needs-assessment strategies. Bice and White (1969) argue that perceived morbidity responds to community needs better and is thus superior to the use of calculated incidence rates. They show that there are frequent variations in use of the health services in areas with similar incidence rates but with significant differences in levels of perceived morbidity. Kohn and White (1976) used perceived morbidity for international comparisons in their WHO-supported international collaborative study on medical care utilization. Perceived morbidity is seen as a needs assessment variable to explain utilization. Since perceived morbidity levels depend on population surveys, this method differs from the other methods based on documentary or professional sources. Because of this, perceived morbidity should not be used for the primary assessment of comparative morbidity, but rather as a supplementary instrument.

Indicators of morbidity

Morbidity data is the measurement of the occurrence of specific diseases, conditions, or symptoms. Incidence and prevalence rates are most often reported, some of which are shown in Table 7.4.

The data in Table 7.4 on the incidence or prevalence of specific diseases or conditions must be based on the existence of frequent notifications, surveyance systems, or plausible 'tracers' for the diseases and conditions described.

Table 7.4 Basic morbidity indicators

Indicator	Numerator	Denominator
Incidence rate	Number of new cases of a specified disease reported during a given time period	Estimated mid-interval population
Attack rate	Number of new cases of a specified disease existing at a given point in time	Total population at the same point in time
Point prevalence rate (ratio)	Number of current cases, new and old, of a specified disease existing at a given point in time	Estimated population at the same point in time
Period (case load) rate (ratio)	Number of current cases, new and old, of a specified disease occurring during a given time interval	Estimated mid-interval population

Adapted from Alan Dever (1980)

The 'morbidity list'

This indicator, suggested by Murnaghan (1981), may be used both for cross-country comparisons and as a means to direct public attention and intervention to the most critical health problems in a country or a region. For this indicator, the 10 or 15 most commonly reported health problems in a given population are listed in order of their frequency. The 'morbidity list' thus compiled provides decision-makers and health-planners with a systematic outline of the patterns and trends or morbidity in their regions and can be used as a basis for comparison with other countries or regions.

Disability

Though they have no predictable linear relationship, for many health professionals the concept of disability often coincides intuitively with the concept of morbidity. However, on a more formal basis, the two concepts differ. While morbidity is relatively easy to define, it is difficult to define disability because its definition depends on one's subjective perception. In an effort to overcome these difficulties, Wood (1983) focuses on the *origin* of disability. In Wood's perception, disability can be measured by its three major causes:

(1) developmental disability caused by congenital incapacities or by malnutrition;
(2) acute disability caused by injury or communicable disease;
(3) chronic disability caused by noncommunicable disease, by alcohol and drugs, or by mental illness.

Alternatively, disability can be defined according to the severity of the health condition, as expressed in the following WHO classification as reported by Hogarth (1978).

- Impairment: Loss of structure and/or function (organ or system level).
- Disability: Restriction or lack of ability to perform a function; consequence of an impairment; affects function of the person, but does not necessarily lead to handicap.
- Handicap: Disadvantage, resulting from impairment or disability; limits or prevents fulfillment of role in society.

The need for standard definitions for disability encouraged Wood to publish an International Classification of Impairments, Disabilities and Handicaps (ICIDH), called the 'Wood Classification'. This index, issued by the WHO in 1980, records in detail the patient's impairments and consequent disability and handicap on institutional admission or discharge. In ICIDH, numerical codes are assigned to predetermined categories of all forms of incapacitating conditions; ICIDH is thus complementary to the ICD system for the classification of mortality and morbidity. ICIDH covers particular health conditions, but is not concerned with the general health status of the individual. Because the general health status of disabled individuals is also of great concern to health authorities, there was a parallel effort to develop a variety of measurement scales for assessing their physical, social, and behavioural health states. A thorough review of those measurement scales is beyond the scope of this book. For an extensive review the reader is referred to the excellent textbook by Kane and Kane (1987) and to a recent world report (Kane *et al.* 1990).

Earlier attempts to assess disability levels in cross-national comparisons suffered from the lack of unanimity in definitions of disability, and from variability in data collection methods. For both these reasons, the validity and reliability of early studies were unsatisfactory (Haber 1973). The first effort to standardize the definition of disability was made in the *WHO International Collaborative Study on Medical Care Utilization*. In this study, self-reported occurrences of acute and chronic disabling conditions were standardized for 12 sites in 7 countries (Kalimo and Rabin 1976). More recently, in a socio-medical survey carried out by the WHO in its European region, the health of the elderly was compared in eleven countries across the European continent (Heikkinen *et al.* 1983). The aim of this survey was to produce standardized comparable data on the health and functional abilities of elderly people from representative population samples. The use of health and social services by the elderly was also reported. In each country, data were collected from cross- sectional interviews by standard protocols. As expected, among elderly subjects both impairment and disability were fairly common and increased with age. However, striking variations were found among countries. For instance, in semi-rural Leuven, Belgium, only 16 to 21 per cent illness was reported, increasing with age, while the corresponding figures for all age groups in Kiev, USSR, were 72 to 88 per cent. A possible explanation for these differences is that ill-health is always reported subjectively and thus reflects cultural and societal attributes. Even after these effects were considered, there were still remarkable variations among countries. It is not known whether these variations resulted from methodological drawbacks, patients' subjective perceptions, or somatic and/or psychosocial differences.

In another study, cross-national comparisons were made of disabled persons in Denmark, Israel, Poland, the UK, and the US (Shanas 1971). There were large variations among countries in this study also. For instance, in Israel 53 per cent of a matched sample reported incapacitating illness as compared with only 26 per cent in the US. The rates for physician-contacts were similarly different. Cross-national variations in disability rates are also very large: a recent survey of 49 countries shows that the percentage of the total population that is disabled varies between 0.2 and 20.9 per cent (Chamie 1989)! This range is not only caused by actual differences in disability but also by differences in methods of data collection and analysis. In answer to the need for standardizing data collection methods and analytical instruments, national definitions of concepts on disability were presented in a case study of five countries (UN 1986). Statistical instruments for data collection like censuses, civil registration systems, and national household surveys, were also presented for each country. This five-country study was followed up by the development of the International Disability Statistics Data Base (DISTAT), now available on personal computer diskettes (UN 1988). DISTAT now includes statistics on disability for 55 countries which will shortly be published as a compendium.

Some comparisons on disability rates by regions within countries are also available. A recent national survey in Canada shows that age-adjusted disability rates vary across the Canadian provinces: there is a low of 10.8 per cent in Prince Edward Island and a high of 14.4 per cent in Sasketchewan (Statistics Canada 1986). Though these data are based on individual responses and may therefore be biased, they may be suggestive of the origin of such inter-regional differences.

The problem of chronic medical conditions has mostly been considered in relation to the evaluation of disability. However, some comparative data on chronic conditions are also available in relation to acute dysfunctioning (OECD 1985) of which absenteeism from work is perhaps the most popular indicator. Because compensation practices are highly variable across various countries, this indicator suffers from wide variations. We have already discussed these problems in Chapter 6.

Indicators of disability

Disability may be measured in a variety of ways each relating to the underlying cause for its measurement. Loss of employment may be sufficient for insurance purposes while disease-staging processes, reduction of physical activity, increase in mental disorders, and social disintegration may be necessary for health research. Comparing data on disability is difficult because there is such a broad range of problems. For cross-national comparisons we follow Murnaghan (1981) who determined that only a few universally accepted indicators be used, as shown in Table 7.5.

The last two disability indicators in Table 7.5 can be further subdivided

Table 7.5 Disability indicators

Indicator	Numerator	Denominator	Comments
Acute Disability: Persons	Persons with sick days during past 14 days	Estimated mid-interval population	Highly dependent on definition of a sick day
Acute Disability: Days	Volume of sick days during past 14 days	Estimated mid-interval population	Highly dependent on definition of a sick day
Persons with chronic disability or impairment	Persons with chronic disabling condition—prevalence rate	Estimated mid-term population over 65	
Persons in Long-Term Care (LTC) institutions	Persons residing in LTC institutions	Estimated mid-term population over 65	

Adapted from Murnaghan (1981)

according to the ICIDH nomenclature. This would provide condition-specific rates for the most common impairments and disabilities.

The 'modern' approach—positive health

The modern approach is based on the Health Field Concept as suggested by Lalonde (1974) or by Alan Dever (1980). It may be regarded as a concept of holistic health, which we discussed in Chapter 2. The basic targets of the Health Field Concept are positive health targets also known as targets of well-being. The philosophy of positive health outcomes is that outcomes must be related to their causal effects and that the examination of outcomes is only a step in an on-going procedure of improving health status. However, it is both methodologically and practically problematic to define the indicators of 'positive health' operationally. Because health systems are still characterized by the traditional concept of health as measured by death, disease, and disability, reporting and documentation on health outcomes are largely based on these indicators. As a result, mortality and morbidity are regularly reported while the positive indicators are rarely and often inconsistently reported.

Methodologically, little has been done to standardize positive health into accepted sets of operational indicators. Notable exceptions are the 12 WHO global indicators for monitoring progress toward 'health for all' (Uemura 1987) which are divided into four groups. The group of interest to us here focuses on health status. Health status includes nutritional status, primary health care status (safe water supply, immunization status), life expectancy, infant mortality rates, and adult literacy rates. Operational definitions for the indicators describing these concepts are given in the following sections on indicators of positive health. Indicator values for several countries can be found in the more recent editions of the *World Health Statistics Annual* (for example WHO 1986 and later). Another source for information on positive health indicators which provides indicators of lifestyle is OECD (1985, 1989). In particular, this source provides data on tobacco and alcohol consumption.

Indicators for positive health

Indicators on positive health may be divided in three categories:

(1) general well being;
(2) life styles;
(3) environmental factors.

For a more thorough discussion of these indicators the reader is referred to Catford (1983) or Abelin (1986).

General well-being indicators

For the purposes of our study, we are interested in indicators for general well-being at the population level.

Life expectancy Life expectancy is commonly estimated separately for males and females at birth, but it can be estimated at any age. The traditional source of data on life expectancy is the *World Health Statistics Annual* (WHO publications). An alternative source of data for the European countries is a micro-computer data system (WHO Eurostat 1989).

Levels of health awareness It is difficult to measure this indicator for well-being—education for health. As a proxy measure, we can use adult literacy rates measured for males and females separately or combined. Such data is available in *World Bank World Development Reports* (World Bank publications).

Lifestyle indicators

There are several lifestyle indicators available providing information on consumption and behaviour patterns. Here is a partial list.

Death rates from accidents Death rates from accidents can be computed in several modalities specific for age, sex, and cause. Data for cross-national comparisons are available from the *World Health Annual Statistics* (WHO publications).

Alcohol consumption Alcohol consumption in many of the WHO European member states was reported by Walsh (1982) in a WHO-EURO report. Later, Walsh and Grant (1985) published a global scale showing great variations among countries. Highest alcohol consumption was seen in developed countries; unfortunately, there are alarming signs that alcohol consumption is increasing in developing countries too.

Daily calorie intake This indicator may be a measure of either the total daily calorie intake or specifically of the daily protein intake. The indicator is useful in cross-national comparisons. It is particularly valuable in developing countries as a tracer for malnutrition. Data are available in *World Bank World Development Reports* (World Bank publications).

Cigarette smoking The proportions of regular cigarette smokers, other smokers, ex-smokers, and non-smokers by age and sex is given for 48 regions in 25 countries in the report of the WHO MONICA project (Multinational Monitoring of Trends and Determinants in Cardiovascular Disease). Particularly for women, MONICA reports more than ten-fold variations in prevalence of smoking among regions (WHO *Statistics Annual* 1989, p. 137).

Indicators of environmental factors

Here are some useful examples; several other indicators may be also delineated.

Water supply The regularity of water supply is a common proxy for assessing the quality of water supplies. It is measured as the percentage of households with water supplied regularly to their homes. In most developed countries the value of this indicator is close to 100 per cent: thus, it is more useful for discerning differences in safe water supply in developing countries. Data on the percentage of population with safe water supplies are available in the 1986 WHO *Statistics Annual.*

Coverage with adequate sanitary facilities This is another common indicator for measuring environmental effects. Data are available in the 1986 WHO *Statistics Annual.*

While these two indicators are the most frequently used in the reporting of physical environmental conditions, the operational definitions of 'safe water' and 'adequate sanitation' are ambiguous. Furthermore, the reports from several countries are lacking. These shortcomings limit our ability to use environmental influences to produce more than a rough estimate of the actual environmental conditions.

Suicide rate Suicide rate is a proxy for evaluating the effects of psychological and social factors in the environment. Cross-comparisons are possible because data are reported annually by age- and sex-specific groups in the *World Health Statistics Annual* (WHO publications).

References

Abelin, T. (1986). Positive indicators in health promotion and protection. *World Health Statistics Quarterly*, **39**, 353–64.

Alan Dever, G.E. (1980). *Community health analysis.* Aspen, Germantown, Maryland.

Alderson, M. (1981). *International mortality statistics.* Facts on File Inc., New York.

Bako, G., Smith, E.S.O., Hanson, J., and Dewar, R. (1982). The geographical distribution of high cadmium concentration in the environment and prostate cancer in Alberta. *Canadian Journal of Public Health*, **73**, 92–4.

Bice, T.W. and White, K.L. (1969). Factors related to the use of health services—an international comparative study. *Medical Care*, **7**, 124–33.

Blum, H. (1981). *Planning for health*, (2nd edn). Human Sciences Press, New York.

Brzezinski, Z.J. (1986). Mortality indicators and health-for-all strategies in the WHO European region. *World Health Statistics Quarterly*, **39**, 365–78.

Catford, J.C. (1983). Positive health indicators—towards a new information base for health promotion. *Community Medicine*, **5**, 125–32.

Central Statistics Office. *Annual Abstract of Statistics*, London. (Various years.)

Chamie, M. (1989). Survey design strategies for the study of disability. *World Health Statistics Quarterly*, **42**, (3), 122–40.

Chase, H.C. (1972). The position of the United States in international comparisons of health status. *American Journal of Public Health*, **62**, 581–5.

Comstock, G.W. (1979). Water hardness and cardiovascular disease. *American Journal of Epidemiology*, **110**, 375–400.

de Miguel, J. (1975). A framework for the study of national health systems. *Inquiry*, **12**, (2) (suppl.), 10–24.

Division of Family Health (1980). The incidence of low birth-weight—a critical review of available information. *World Health Statistics Reports*, **33**, 113–224.

Elling, R.H. (1980). *Cross national study of health systems—political economics and health care*. Transaction Books, New Brunswick.

Edouard, L. (1985). The epidemiology of perinatal mortality. *World Health Statistics Quarterly*, **38**, 289–301.

Eurohealth Handbook (1985). Robert S. First Inc., New York.

Field, M. (1973). The concept of 'health system' at the macro-sociological level. *Social Science and Medicine*, **7**, 763–85.

Fleiss, J.L. (1973). *Statistical methods for rates and proportions*. Wiley, New York.

Foster, F.H. (1981). Trends in perinatal mortality. *World Health Statistics Quarterly*, **34**, (5), 138–46.

Fries, J. and Crapo, L.M. (1981). *Vitality and ageing: implications of the rectangular curve*. W.H. Freeman, San Francisco.

Fulop, T. and Reinke, W.A. (1981). Statistical analysis of interdependence of country health resource variables, with special regard to manpower-related ones. *Bulletin of the World Health Organization*, **59**, (1), 129–41.

Haber, L.D. (1973). Some parameters for social policy in disability: A cross-national comparison. *Milbank Memorial Fund Quarterly*, **51**, 319–40.

Havard, J.D.J. (1979). Mortality from motor vehicle accidents in the 15–24 year age group. *World Health Statistics Quarterly*, **32**, (3), 225–41.

Heikkinen, E. (1984). Implications of demographic changes for the elderly population. In *Demographic trends in the European region* (ed. A.D. Lopez, and R.L. Cliquet), European Series No. 17. WHO, Regional Office for Europe, Copenhagen.

Heikkinen, E. (1987). Health implications of population ageing in Europe. *World Health Statistics Quarterly*, **40**, 22–40.

Heikkinen, E., Waters, W.E., and Brzezinski, Z.J. (1983). *The elderly in eleven countries, a socio-medical survey*, Public Health in Europe, No. 21. World Health Organization, Copenhagen.

Hogarth, J. (1978). *Glossary of health terminology*, Public Health in Europe. No. 4. WHO Regional Office for Europe, Copenhagen.

Holland, W.W. (1988). *European Community Atlas of Avoidable Death*. Oxford University Press, Oxford.

Jones, E.F., Forrest, J.D., Goldman, N., Henshaw, S.K., Lincoln, R., Rosoff, J.I. *et al.* (1985). Teenage pregnancy in developed countries: determinants and policy implications. *Family Planning Perspectives*, **17**, 53–63.

Kalimo, E. and Rabin, D.L. (1976). Relationships among indicators of morbidity: cross-national comparisons. *Journal of Chronic Diseases*, **29**, 1–14.

Kane, R.L. and Kane, R.A. (1987). *Long-term care: principles, programs and policies*. Springer Publishing Company, New York.

Kane, R.L., Grimely Evans, J., and MacFayden, D. (ed.) (1990). *Improving the health of older people—a world view*. WHO and Oxford University Press, Oxford.

Keys, A. (1970). Coronary heart disease in seven countries. *Circulation*, **41** (suppl.), 1-198.

Kohn, R. and White, K.Z. (1976). *Health care, An international study*. Oxford University Press, Oxford.

Lalonde, M. (1974). *A new perspective on the health of Canadians*. Government of Canada, Ottawa.

Lilienfeld, A.M. and Lilienfeld, D.E. (1980). *Foundations of epidemiology*, (2nd edn). Oxford University Press, New York.

Lopez, A.D. and Hanada, K. (1982). Mortality trends and patterns among the elderly in development countries. *World Health Statistics Quarterly*, **35**, (3/4), 203-24.

Marmot, M.G. (1985). Interpretation of trends in coronary heart disease mortality. *Acta Medica Scandinavica*, (suppl.), **701**, 58-65.

Marmot, M.G., Syme, S.L., Kagan, A., Kato, H., Cohen, J.B., and Belsky, J. (1975). Epidemiologic studies of coronary heart disease and stroke in Japanese men living in Japan, Hawaii and California. *American Journal of Epidemiology*, **102**, 514-25.

Melia, R.J. and Swan, A.V. (1986). International trends in mortality rates for bronchitis, emphysema and asthma during the period 1971-1980. *World Health Statistics Quarterly*, **39**, 206-17.

Murnaghan, J. (1981). Health indicators and information systems for the year 2000. *Annual Review of Public Health*, **2**, 299-361.

NCHS (National Center for Health Statistics) (1987). Mortality. *Vital Statistics of the US*, Vol. I-II. Washington, D.C.

Nossikov, A., Prokhorskas, R., and Shabanah, M. (1990). Using regional indicators: the experience of Europe. *World Health Statistics Quarterly*, **43**, (1), 25-31.

OECD (Organization of Economic Co-operation and Development) (1985). *Measuring health care, 1960-1983*, Social Policy Study, No. 2. Paris.

OECD (Organization of Economic Co-operation and Development) (1989). Compendium health care expenditure and other data. *Health Care Financing Review*, Annual Supplement, pp. 111-94.

Pisa, Z. and Uemura, K. (1982). Trends in mortality from ischaemic heart disease and other cardiovascular diseases in 27 countries 1968-1977. *World Health Statistics Quarterly*, **35**, 11-48.

Plaut, R. and Roberts, E. (1989). Preventable mortality: indicator or target? Applications in developing countries. *World Health Statistics Quarterly*, **42**, (1), 4-15.

Poullier, J.P. (1987). OECD experiences with the initiation and co-ordination of health indicator systems, with special emphasis on inter-institutional co-ordination and comparability. In *Indicators and trends in health and health care* (ed. D. Schwefel). Springer Verlag, Berlin.

Preston, S.H. (1976). *Mortality patterns in national populations, with special reference to the cause of death*. Academic Press, New York.

Rodriguez, L.A.C. and Cayolla da Motta, L. (1989). Years of potential life lost: application of an indicator for assessing premature mortality in Portugal and in Spain. *World Health Statistics Quarterly*, **42**, (1), 50-6.

Roger, F.H. (1982). The minimum basic data set for hospital statistics in the EEC. In *Hospital statistics in Europe* (ed. P.M. Lambert, and F.H. Roger). North Holland Publishing Company, Brussels.

Shanas, E. (1971). Measuring the lone health needs of the aged in five countries. *Journal of Gerontology*, **26**, 37-40.

Sidel, V.W. (1981). International comparisons of health services: How? Who? Why? In *Critical issues in health policy* (ed. R.Z. Straez, M. Lieberman, and A. Sardell). Lexington Books, D.C. Heath & Company, Lexington, Massachusetts.

Statistics Canada and Secretary of State of Canada (1986). *Report of the Canadian Health and Disability Survey* 1983-1984. Ministry of Supply and Services, Ottawa.

Statistics Canada (1988). Mortality—summary list of causes—1986. *Vital Statistics*, Vol. III, Cat. No. 84-206, Ottawa.

Taket, A. (1986). Accidents mortality in children, adolescents and young adults. *World Health Statistics Quarterly*, **39**, (1), 232-56.

Uemura, K. (1987). Application of indicators for monitoring progress towards health for all by the year 2000. In: *Measurement in health promotion and protection* (ed. T. Abelin, Z.J. Brzezinski, and V.D.L. Carstairs), WHO Regional Publications, European Series No. 22. WHO, Copenhagen.

Uemura, K. (1989). Excess mortality ratio with reference to the lowest age/sex specific death rates among countries. *World Health Statistics Quarterly*, **42**, (1), 26-48.

Uemura, K. and Pisa, Z. (1985). Recent trends in cardiovascular disease mortality in 27 industrialized countries. *World Health Statistics Quarterly*, **38**, 142-62.

UN (United Nations) (1986). *Development of statistics of disabled persons*—case studies. Department of International Economic and Social Affairs, Statistical Office, New York.

UN (United Nations) (1988). *United Nations Disability Statistics Data Base* 1975-1986, Technical Manual. Department of International Economic and Social Affairs, Statistical Office, New York.

USDHEW (United States Department of Health Education and Welfare) (1980). *Mortality Vital Statistics Report*, USDHEW Publication No. (PHS) 80-1120, Vol. 28, No. 11 (suppl.). Washington, D.C.

USDHHS (United States Department of Health and Human Services) (1987). Publication No. (PHS) 87-1114. Public Health Service, US Government Printing Office, Washington.

Walsh, D. (1982). *Alcohol-related medicosocial problems and their prevention*. World Health Organization, Regional Office for Europe, Copenhagen.

Walsh, B. and Grant, M. (1985). *Public health implications of alcohol production and trade*, Offset Publication No. 88. World Health Organization, Geneva.

Weber, A.A. (1982). International exchange of hospital data. In *Hospital statistics in Europe* (ed. P.M. Lambert and F.H. Roger). North Holland Publishing Company, Brussels and Luxembourg.

WHO (World Health Organization) (1976). *WHO Handbook for Standardized Cancer Registries*, WHO Offset Publication No. 25. Geneva.

WHO (World Health Organization) (1977). *Manual of the international statistical classification of diseases, injuries, and causes of death*, Vol. I, Geneva.

WHO. *World Health Statistics Annual*. Geneva. (Various years.)

WHO (World Health Organization) (1986). *World Health Statistics Annual*, pp. 92-109. Geneva.

WHO (World Health Organization) (1989). *World Health Statistics Annual*—1989, p. 137. World Health Organization, Geneva.

WHO Eurostat World Health Organization (1989). *Eurostat (HFA/Indicators) HFA/PC Software Package*. Regional Office for Europe, Copenhagen.

WHO MONICA (World Health Organization MONICA Project) (1987). The principal investigators: geographic variation in mortality from cardiovascular diseases. *World Health Statistics Quarterly*, **40**, (2), 171–84.

Wood, P.H.N. (1983). Prospects for control. In *Disability prevention: the global challenge*. (ed. J. Wilson), p. 92. Oxford University Press, Oxford.

Woodall, J.P. (1988). Epidemiological approaches to health planning, management and evaluation. *World Health Statistics Quarterly*, **41**, (1), 2–10.

World Bank. *World Development Report*. Oxford University Press, New York. (Various years.)

8. New horizons for systems outcomes: effectiveness, efficiency, equity, and quality

In Chapter 7 we delineated the concept and measurement of outcomes related to the health status of the population. We primarily discussed implications for better health, selecting only those variables measurable in the context of a population. In fact, all the health status measures described in Chapter 7 could be examined in the absence of a health care system. However, since health care systems are designed to provide their own effects on health status, it is appropriate to study the health systems outcomes, that is, how health care systems were successful in mobilizing their resources and in optimizing their processes for better health. Here we suggest four concepts for the measurement of the outcomes of a health care system: effectiveness, efficiency, equity, and quality. We shall explore possible definitions for these four concepts and consider their relevance to our discussion. After we elaborate on each concept, we suggest appropriate indicators for it.

Effectiveness

First let us explore effectiveness as Holland put it, 'In its simplest form, the effectiveness of an intervention measure can be expressed as a reduction in morbidity and mortality' (Holland 1983). That is to say, when a health outcome is improved by a health intervention measure, that measure is effective. In practice, effectiveness is linked to the production of desired effects which are usually called objectives or targets (Long 1985, p. 11). At this point the reader should be aware that the concept of effectiveness has been subject to an even broader interpretation. For instance, Donabedian (1980) divided effectiveness into two components: technical and psychological. Each of those can be perceived in a context of the system's structure, process, and outcome. Babson (1972) views effectiveness as a process measure which consists of three components: accessibility, quality, and integration. In this book, however, we perceive the term effectiveness as referring only to the end result of the process of care. In this case we should limit our investigation to the effects caused by one or more of the processes performed in a health system.

Effectiveness is measured by two components. First, a health status indicator, or index, is identified as we showed thoroughly in Chapter 7. Second, measuring effectiveness requires that the health system whose effectiveness is to be measured undertakes a medical intervention or an action for health improvement. However, the measurement of the concept of effectiveness is problematic. Consider processes that should be evaluated against clearly stated objectives. Unfortunately, health systems may undertake processes with objectives that are either ambiguous or stated in terms hindering effective measurement. In addition, sometimes one single activity is designed to reach a number of objectives. Alternatively, sometimes a single objective may be reached by a number of different activities. Because it is hard to separate the impact of each activity, all this makes the effectiveness of health system activities difficult to measure. This kind of evaluative problem can be seen for long-term care programmes for the elderly. These programmes have multiple objectives, notably improvement, or at least maintenance, of physical and mental status and of social involvement for the elderly. Similarly, these programmes are characterized by an array of concurrent activities in the fields of acute medical care, social support, assistance in daily living (like homemaker services, handyman services, or meal on wheels), psychological care, housing and transportation. No doubt, the evaluation of programme-effectiveness for such programmes is complex. Some remedy for these difficulties can be found in considering specific measures of effectiveness instead of the broad concept of effectiveness itself. One of these specific measures is the study of *attributable effectiveness*, which is the difference in the health outcomes for a group exposed to a given health care activity compared with a control group given different care, or no care at all. The goal here is in identifying the benefits of the programme. Related to attributable effectiveness is *population-attributable effectiveness* which is the number of persons within a population who would gain from being exposed to a given health activity. In this case we would like to measure either the long-term gains or the impact of an intervention or activity. A third specific measure called, *relative effectiveness*, is the ratio of the outcome for individuals within an intervention programme to those who are not included in it.

Another concern of measurement is that positive outcomes apparently produced by a medical intervention may have been really caused by some other factor altogether. A spectacular example of this problem is in the field of infectious diseases. The prevalence of tuberculosis, once a major societal health problem, significantly declined during the nineteenth and early twentieth century even though no health care intervention had yet been initiated (McKeowen 1976).

It is important to note that the concept of effectiveness as discussed in this chapter is by no means objective. Since different groups share varying interests and concerns in studying effectiveness one must constantly ask: effectiveness for whom? This problem is seen in the interesting profile

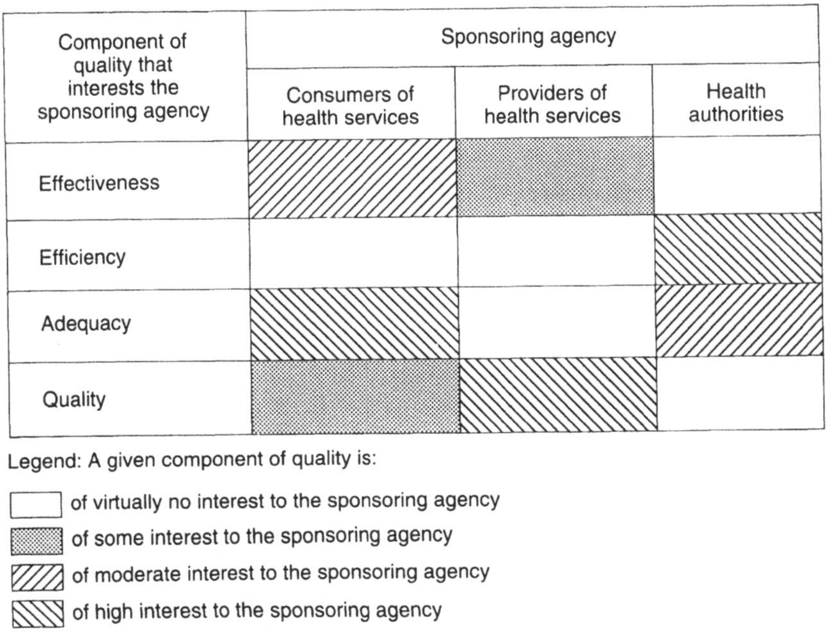

Fig. 8.1 The interest profile of agencies sponsoring quality assurance. (From Vuori (1982), with permission.)

suggested by Vuori (1982) as shown in Fig. 8.1. Vuori argues that although providers are moderately interested in effectiveness and consumers are somewhat interested in it, health authorities are barely interested in effectiveness *per se* at all. As we show later, the indirect interest of health authorities in effectiveness is reflected in their interest in improving efficiency.

Though an evaluation of effectiveness is complex, particularly at the macro level, there are some applications available in the literature. Rutstein and co-workers (1976) outlined a method for counting the cases of unnecessary disease and disability and unnecessary or untimely deaths. They did this by listing all the medical conditions amenable to treatment in a format compatible with ICD-8. The ensuing counts of unnecessary deaths within each ICD-8 category are then transformed into rates comparable across systems. Though the authors have not reported any practical uses of their method, they do indicate that their list is designed to be used in comparative analysis across countries. Charlton and colleagues (1983) used a similar method for studying the variations in death rates for diseases amenable to medical intervention in England and Wales. In the 98 health areas studied, there was considerable variation in avoidable death rates. Adjusting for social factors did not eliminate the significant differences among these areas. The authors suggest that the areas differed in the level of *effectiveness* and that the variations should be examined further in relation to health service inputs.

Indicators of effectiveness

In the following, instead of merely delineating the instruments for measuring effectiveness, we shall discuss the more fundamental issue of what is to be measured. This approach, unusual for us, resulted from the problem of defining effectiveness operationally, particularly at the system level. The following scheme, adapted from Long (1985), clearly demonstrates the process of defining what is to be measured for determining the effectiveness of health care systems.

In conclusion, the implementation of the ideas outlined in Table 8.1 would require the quantification of both the inputs and the outcomes. We can use several of the indicators developed in previous chapters to reach this goal.

When data on the various components in Table 8.1 is made available, one can estimate the effectiveness of a health care system or a region within a health care system for solving a problem or for carrying out a plan, and then compare it with the effectiveness of another health care system or another region in dealing with a similar problem.

A comparative approach for measuring effectiveness is useful only for programmes with specified objectives which are similar to a great degree. For example, the funding and reimbursement schemes in the Scandanavian countries (Brogren and Brommels 1990). One should not, however, underestimate the difficulties encountered in using this approach. Too often, objectives are unclearly stated or difficult to express. Furthermore, since other outcome indicators are scarce, achievements are often measured only by mortality indicators. However, as we will discuss in Chapter 9, mortality indicators are not sensitive to minor changes in health status. For the assessment of current inputs and needs, only few indicators are commonly available. These indicators, like the rates of beds and personnel, are often inadequate for describing the actual contribution of the various inputs to a health system. In addition to these problems, the measurement of effectiveness for cross-comparisons can be hindered by unreliable data collection.

Finally, even when the quantitative evaluation of inputs and outcomes is possible, a causal relationship between inputs and outcomes cannot always be established. When it is difficult to relate changes in outcome to changes in inputs, questions about what actually has been done remain mostly unanswered.

Table 8.1 Key questions for reviewing the effectiveness of a health service/plan

A. Long-term objectives and measures of outcome

1. What are the objectives of the health activity or intervention being reviewed? Identify health and health-related objectives.
2. How can their achievement be assessed? Draw up (quantitative) indicators and measures of health outcome—quantitative measures may consist of traditional health outcome indicators or indices (e.g. mortality, morbidity, disability) or of indicators of well-being.

B. Current service and need

1. What is the level, type, and extent of the current service or activity?
2. Who gets the service or activity?
3. Who needs it?
4. What gaps exist? What limits (financial, manpower, technological) are there on it?

For a multi-service evaluation this procedure can be repeated for each type of service or activity.

C. Comparison of the ideal and the actual

1. What is the impact of the current service on its stated objectives (A.1), or in terms of the indicated measures of outcome (A.2)?
2. What evidence is there for changes in health status as being due to the health activity or intervention? This can be repeated for each service separately.

D. Areas for modification and implementation

1. How can the impacts of the activity/intervention be increased? Identify any wider social or political issues raised (such as professional views, or governmental policy).
2. Who will attempt to implement the recommended activity/intervention changes? How will this be done?

E. Cost

1. What is the cost of the current service, in absolute terms, and in relation to changes in outcome.
2. What will the cost be if the recommended changes are to be implemented.

For multi-service assessment, cost evaluation can be applied for each service separately and then added up to calculate total costs.

Efficiency

Approaches to the concept of efficiency are much more standardized than approaches to the concept of effectiveness. Overall, efficiency is defined as the determination of the ratio of the effects of an activity (or an intervention) over operational costs. While this definition captures the essence of the concept, more refined definitions are needed for elaborate analyses. In the following discussion these refined definitions are presented in the form of four dimensions of efficiency: allocative, distributive, dynamic and managerial.

Allocative efficiency

Allocative efficiency is a measure of the appropriateness of the level of investment in the health care sector. Allocative efficiency can be applied at both the broad societal level and within the health system. At the broad societal level, one can ask whether the resources allocated to the health care sector in a society would be more beneficial if allocated to other sectors. These sectors can be other social sectors like the education system, or economic sectors not representing social concerns like the system of transportation. While choosing the appropriate allocation among sectors may be a matter for philosophers and moralists, selection between alternatives may be more practically accomplished within the health system. Indeed, allocative efficiency can be used to evaluate and compare the appropriateness of priorities set in health systems.

Perhaps the most important evaluative approach for assessing allocative efficiency is cost–benefit analysis (CBA). Cost–benefit analysis is a process of valuing the consequences of alternative programmes. The consequences are presented as benefits and are valued in monetary terms. The ratio of the benefits to the costs is a measure of the value of the programme. This technique allows the worth of a programme to be assessed (do the benefits exceed costs?), as well as for a comparison of competing alternatives. Since CBA uses standardized monetary units, it can be used to facilitate the best investment of public funds whenever they are limited. In other words, it is eminently suitable for measuring allocative efficiency (Drummond 1980).

From a cross-national or cross-regional perspective, however, the use of CBA should be restricted since there is little sense in comparing alternative plans within different systems. In our opinion, in the comparison of systems, the frequency of the use of CBA or similar techniques, rather than the actual priorities determined by these techniques, may become the main interest of such a comparative evaluation. However, the use of CBA cross-nationally or cross-regionally is more promising when comparative allocative efficiency is evaluated within a single health field, like mother and child-care or long-term care. In such cases, costs and benefits within a single field may be comparatively assessed in different regional settings. For example, as Sorkin (1976) describes for several regions in China, cost-benefit analysis was undertaken to estimate the efficiency of barefoot doctors (villagers who performed paramedical tasks). Indeed, he found substantial regional variations in the efficiency of the programmes across the different study sites in China. In another example, as reported by Creese (1983), Ponnighaus compared the costs and benefits of measles immunization in Southern Zambia. He showed that while benefit-to-cost ratios for the immunization were favourable in an urban setting, these ratios were unfavourable in rural areas.

Distributive efficiency

Distributive efficiency can be examined from both the organizational perspective, also called the Supply Oriented Perspective, and the consumer perspective, also called Demand Oriented Dimension (Long 1985). Since the consumer perspective is related to the concept of equity, we shall consider it separately in the section on equity.

With respect to the organization of health systems, distributive efficiency refers to the optimization of the distributional arrangements of goods and services in a health care system. It is an instrument for measuring how successful the structural components, particularly input resources and methods, were for improving the health status of a population.

It may be confusing to compare this definition of distributive efficiency with the definition of effectiveness. Fortunately the two concepts differ in their emphasis. Effectiveness is measured by the comparison of actual performance to objectives. It addresses neither the configuration nor the utilization of resources. Distributive efficiency is high when maximal results are achieved with minimal efforts in organizing and investing in inputs.

Distributive efficiency can be very difficult to measure. Paradoxically, one major difficulty stems from the great efforts made by governments to improve distributive efficiency in their health systems. These efforts may be so considerable that it is extremely difficult to determine a 'base line', that is, a starting point for these efforts. Consequently, comparisons are burdensome and are sometimes quite impossible. In most European systems, an attempt has been made to improve organizational efficiency by making structural changes. The reorganization of the British NHS in 1976 and 1982 and the proposed changes for 1991, are clear examples of government-controlled initiatives that affect organizational structures in an attempt to improve efficiency. In North America, attempts to improve distributive efficiency were more likely to be directed at the configuration of the system than at its structures. In the US a complex mix of reimbursement regulations, certification and tax incentives are intended to enhance efficiency (Long 1985). In Canada, the systems for federal financial support to provincial health plans, plus the reimbursement and certification by provinces at the individual provider level, are meant to achieve these same goals (Evans 1984).

The lack of consistency among systems makes quantitative cross-national comparisons of distributive efficiency almost impossible. A sound alternative, as we show later in the section on indicators, is to compare developments within each system longitudinally. This allows for the assessment over time of the impact of policy changes on the distribution of resources in health systems. The frequency, breadth, and depth of these observed changes can then be compared across systems.

Dynamic efficiency

Dynamic efficiency, also called technological efficiency, concerns the optimization of technologies in a health care system. Financially, ethically, and scientifically this topic is of paramount importance for health systems.

Financially, in most health systems the use of resources for medical care has been increased. This increases the National Expenditure on Health (NEH) to more than the increase in the Gross National Product (GNP). It is believed that a major cause of this rapid increase in the NEH, is the introduction into the health field of new technologies as innovations or as substitutes for existing technologies (Banta and Kemp 1982; Altman and Blendon 1979).

Ethically, the use of technology must be constantly monitored. As an illustration, consider a column written in the 8 August 1983 issue of *Newsweek*. The author, Barbara Hutman is a nurse. She described a cancer patient who spent six months dying in a hospital. During a single month, more than fifty attempts were made to resuscitate the patient. Respecting his family's and his plea to die, Nurse Hutman finally took the responsibility to delay the fifty-third resuscitation attempt. She did so despite early signals indicating the need for resuscitation. The patient died, and Nurse Hutman was accused, by some persons, of murder (Shinn 1986). In this case, the dilemma faced a single health worker. However, such an example can easily be examined at a systems' level by considering the health systems' policy on euthanasia (the right to die).

Finally, scientifically, a technology should be judged for its safety and efficacy. While the meaning of safety is self-evident, efficacy is the measure of the benefits to the individual from procedures or programmes perfectly applied.

From now on, we shall discuss dynamic efficiency from a macro perspective. Due to limits in interpreting individual phenomena at a macro level, we can only reasonably analyse the efficiency of the *diffusion* of medical technologies. In their book, Banta and Kemp (1982) compared the management of health care technology by analysing case studies for each of nine industrialized countries. In the last chapter of their book, Banta and Russell

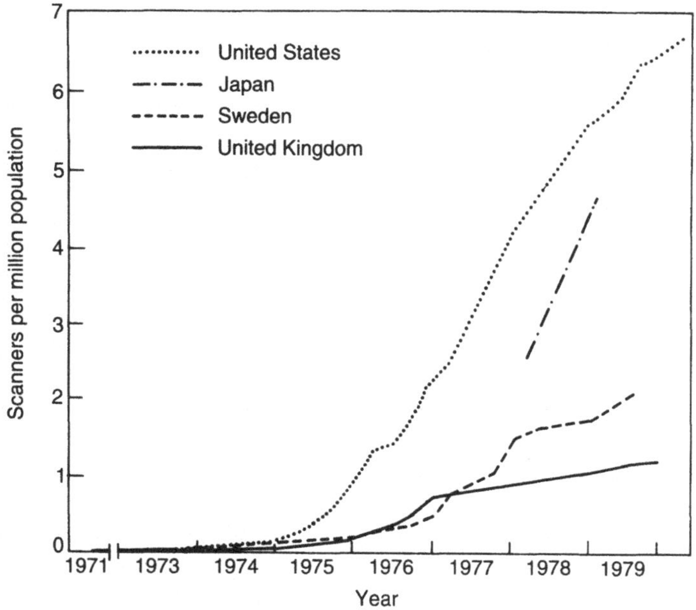

Fig. 8.2 Rates of diffusion for computerized tomography technology: 4 selected countries. (From Banta and Kemp (1982), with permission.)

combine and summarize the evidence from these nine countries. For instance, they calculated the rate per million of population for randomized controlled trials set to study the efficacy and efficiency of gastrointestinal procedures (Banta and Russell, in Banta and Kemp 1982, p. 200). They clearly found that rates vary across countries.

Financially, the level of controls on investments in medical technology can also be indirectly evaluated for comparative purposes. To do this, the rates of the diffusion of technologies over time may reflect the relative success of such controls on investment procedures. As shown in Fig. 8.2, controlling the rate of diffusion for computerized tomography was the most successful in the UK and least successful in the US and probably in Japan.

In two issues of the *International Journal of Technology Assessment in Health Care*, in work similar to that of Banta and Russell (in Banta and Kemp 1982), Anderson (1988) and several co-authors recently compared the diffusion of medical technologies. In the introduction, Anderson suggests four different modes for the spread of technology: adoption, diffusion, financing, and planning. These concepts were elaborated in country reports that were made available and can in turn be contrasted for evaluation. The United States (Russell and Sisk 1988), the United Kingdom (Stocking 1988), Canada (Deber *et al.* 1988) and Israel (Ellencweig 1988) were among the countries for which country reports are available.

Managerial efficiency

At the macro level, managerial efficiency addresses systems' performance, and can be quantified as the ratio of inputs to outputs. Inputs are traditionally expressed in either physical or in monetary terms, while outputs can be approached from various perspectives. The most popular expression of output is in terms of effectiveness. In fact, several studies outlined in Chapter 7 implicitly provide a basis for evaluation of managerial efficiency. Various health status attributes like mortality indices, morbidity measures, or disability scales, can be considered as the output indicators. These output indicators are then contrasted with the input indicators, including a variety of socio-economic indicators like literacy and educational levels (Fulop and Reinke 1981; Ceresto and Waitzkin 1988), financial indices like GNP and health expenditure per capita (Cochrane *et al.* 1978; Fulop and Reinke 1981; Ceresto and Waitzkin 1988), or resource-oriented indicators like physicians per capita (Cochrane *et al.* 1978; Fulop and Reinke 1981).

While these articles are valuable as case studies, a more thorough approach requires a formal analysis of the interaction between inputs and outputs. To that end, a special technique, Cost Effectiveness Analysis (CEA) has been developed (Drummond 1980). CEA involves calculating the costs of a health intervention and then evaluating its consequences in non-monetary terms. CEA can also be described as an evaluation of the relative costs of alternative programmes for achieving a given goal. The effectiveness of the health intervention is measured by the successful attainment of its goal rather than by the monetary value of its consequences. When benefits are hard to measure directly or when the expression of outputs in monetary terms is undesirable, CEA is used and no attempt is made to place a monetary value on outputs. In this case, other outcome units are used, for example 'years of life saved'. A typical example of a non-monetary value of outputs is seen in the study of the effectiveness of alternate programmes for extending life spans. Though immeasurable in monetary terms, longevity is an excellent measure of effectiveness.

Since in CEA the focus is on alternative courses for reaching a given objective, it can not be used to prioritize among different programmes. Quite paradoxically, this apparent shortcoming has a great potential for use in cross-national comparisons. For example, as a universal measure of effectiveness, CEA can be used to compare the success rates of life saving techniques and procedures in different health systems. Heidenheimer *et al.* (1983) used CEA explicitly to compare the relative efficiency of health systems. They ranked several developed countries, using as an input variable the level of health care expenditure measured as a percentage of the GNP. As a process variable they used patient access to specialists. For an outcome measure they calculated an average health status index based on 17 age- and sex-specific mortality rates. These specific rates are similar in that they all represent conditions of avoidable death. By contrasting countries for their relationship between the outcome measures and the input/process measures, the authors found a poor cost-effectiveness profile for the United States and West Germany and a much better one for Sweden. These findings should be considered carefully, because they are based on often unreliable and incomparable cost data, and because there is no international consensus on the benefits of medical treatment for the conditions cited above. These limitations may easily jeopardize the validity and conclusions of CEA.

Some of the limitations of the previous example may be overcome by narrowing the basis of comparisons. A comparison between 674 admissions to intensive care units in 5 tertiary care hospitals in the United States and 586 admissions to 7 similar hospitals in France suggests that the managerial efficiency in the United States' health system is greater than that of the French health system. The output measures, actual death rates and severity of illness, were extremely similar. However, though significantly younger than the US patients, the French patients remained twice as long in ICUs (Knaus *et al.* 1982).

A more recent method, called cost–benefit/utility analysis (Kaplan and Anderson 1988) is also useful for measuring managerial efficiency. This method combines classical cost–benefit analysis with an analysis of cost–utility which is the cost of producing a well-year of life, that is, a year with reasonably good health. So far, this method has been only used to select among community health programmes. It may potentially be useful in comparative studies focusing on similar or nearly similar health programmes in various regions or countries sharing common features like the Scandinavian countries.

Yet another method for estimating managerial efficiency is the evaluation of the establishment of control techniques in a health system. Control systems were developed for the appraisal of the performance of health systems in a number of countries including the UK and the US. In the UK, explicit performance indicators are used to assess hospital performance. These performance indicators include input levels of manpower, financial and estate management, process levels of service provision, lengths of hospital stay, waiting lists, and hospital outcomes (Birch and Maynard 1985). In addition to hospital-based indicators, district-based indicators were also developed. These indicators measure populations and their socio-economic characteristics plus their utilization levels (Harley 1988). In the US health system, managerial efficiency is measured more implicitly. For example, by using the Prospective Payment System (PPS) for Medicare patients. Because PPS is based on predetermined activity schedules for each type of episode of care, it is instrumental in constraining uncontrolled utilization and in improving the efficiency of the process of care.

Before we turn to our next topic, a word of caution is warranted. Due to the varying views on the nature of health benefits, efficiency is seen differently in various health systems. For instance, from the perspective of health care decision-makers, equity as a health benefit is often more important in the UK than in the US, causing the investments in similar health programmes to differ between these two countries. Clearly, such differences can reduce the validity of a comparative approach for studying efficiency (Culyer *et al.* 1982).

Indicators of efficiency

Because indicators for measuring efficiency are easy to operationalize, efficiency and its components are generally easier to measure than effectiveness. Here we present some basic methods for the computation of various types of efficiency.

Allocative efficiency

Allocative efficiency may be measured by the process of cost–benefit analysis which involves the measurement of costs and benefit expressed in the same monetary terms. Costs are divided into several components that may be evaluated concurrently. These components include: cost to the individual (generally not useful in cross-national comparisons); cost to the provider of care; cost to the Government; cost to society.

Costs can be evaluated by either market or non-market-based valuations. Market-based valuations can be either the price actually paid for services or goods, or the price equivalent of a time unit of human resources. This equivalent is generally expressed as the loss of time in hours or days. Values not explicitly expressed can be imputed like patients' leisure time or the value of housewives' production. Non-market valuations measure consumers' attitudes, and the views of providers, professionals, and policy-makers. Non-market valuations are more often used to evaluate benefits rather than costs. Furthermore, since it is unlikely that costs and benefits will all occur simultaneously, allowances must be made for a time lag in the allocation of these costs and benefits. Future costs and benefits must then be discounted to equivalent present values.

Also associated with future costs and benefits is the potential risk of failure. Probability models are more useful than deterministic solutions in dealing with uncertainty. In a typical probability model, the probability of attaining benefits at a certain given level is weighed and then multiplied by the monetary values of the benefits at that level. The 'expected value' of these benefits is the sum of these multiples.

A more elaborate description of cost–benefit analysis is beyond the scope of this book. Examples of practical implementation may be found in specific textbooks (Drummond 1980; Warner and Luce 1982).

Distributive efficiency

As suggested in an earlier section in this chapter, distributive efficiency can be measured by comparing longitudinal trends within systems. If two or more systems are compared, the dynamics of policy changes and their effects on the distribution of resources may be assessed. The analysis consists of the following steps:

1. Determine existing organizational arrangements in a system from several perspectives including hierarchic structures, centralization or decentralization, planning and budgeting, financial arrangements (reimbursement, funding), controlling and monitoring of costs, resources, and processes, and evaluation procedures.

The indicators to be used for determining these several perspectives of organizational arrangements were elaborated in Chapter 5 under the heading the 'Organization of the health system'.

2. Determine historical developments in each domain mentioned above, individually and overall.
3. Evaluate levels of improvement (or deterioration) in each domain and overall.
4. Based on the levels of improvement or deterioration, draw conclusions about individual systems and then compare these with systems cross-regionally or cross-nationally.

Distributive efficiency (equity based)

The indicators of equity described in Chapter 5 can be used to measure distributive efficiency and equity-based efficiency.

Dynamic efficiency

Cross-country comparisons are possible in two dimensions, static and dynamic.

Static comparisons When making static comparisons, we compare the 'prevalence' of a technology, that is the availability of a technology in a country, cross-sectionally. This can be done using one of two alternative variables:

1. the number of persons per technological unit;
2. the technological units per population.

Technological units include major equipment like computerized tomographs (CT), or specific procedures like bone marrow transplantation. Table 8.2

Table 8.2 Comparative availability of selected medical technologies

	Canada (1989)			Germany (1987)			United States (1987)		
	Number of units	Persons per unit (1,000)	Units per million persons	Number of units	Persons per unit (1,000)	Units per million persons	Number of units	Persons per unit (1,000)	Units per million persons
Open-heart surgery	32	813	1.23	45[a]	1355[a]	0.74[a]	793	307	3.26
Cardiac catheterization	39	667	1.50	161	379	2.64	1234	198	5.06
Organ transplantation	28	929	1.08	28[a]	2178[a]	0.46[a]	319	764	1.31
Radiation therapy	14	1857	0.54	191	319	3.13	967	252	3.97
Extracorporeal shock wave lithotripsy	4[a]	6500[a]	0.16[a]	21	2904	0.34	228	1069	0.94
Magnetic resonance imaging	12[a]	2167[a]	0.46[a]	57	1070	0.94	900	271	3.69

Sources: Canada: Canadian Hospital Association, Ottawa, Ontario; Canadian Association of Radiation Oncology, Vancouver, British Columbia; University Hospital, London, Ontario, and Canadian Medical Association, Ottawa, Ontario. Germany: Der Bundesminister für Jugend, Familie und Gesundheit, *Gesundheitswesens in der Bundesrepublik Deutschland* (Deutsche Krankenhaus Gesellschaft, 1988). United States: American Hospital Association, Division of Technology Assessment, *Hospital Statistics* (Chicago AHA, 1988).

[a]1988. Adapted from Rublee (1989).

provides an illustration of comparative data based on these two indicators (Rublee 1989).

Dynamic comparisons Rate of technological diffusion. The rates of technological diffusion are used to estimate the dynamics of introducing new technologies into a health system. Rates of technological diffusion may be compared in two ways:

1. Directly, by calculating the rate of diffusion per type of technology per population during a specified time period (e.g. How many CT scanners were installed in country X in a particular year per 100 000 population). Next, those rates can be compared across health systems.
2. Indirectly, by calculating rates of technological diffusion in a particular system during a specified period and then subsequently in following periods. Rates for several systems can then be compared for longitudinal trends. For example, the subsequent rates of installing CTs in the US may be computed for five years and the resulting curve compared with similar curves for Canada and the UK.

Managerial efficiency

Cost Effectiveness Analysis (CEA) can be used to measure managerial efficiency. In CEA, costs are measured as in CBA. However, unlike CBA, non-monetary benefits must be measured as changes in health states which can be variously measured. For life saving procedures, the extension of life is a useful measure of efficiency. In this case, the resulting outcome for the measurement of managerial efficiency would then be expressed in terms of 'cost per one year of life gained'. For situations not involving life-threatening conditions, other criteria may be sought. For example, when regimens of medical care are compared, their efficiency may be measured by the rate of complications per procedure, or by the rate of complications per unit of cost.

A detailed analysis of CEA and its potential applications can be found elsewhere (see for example Drummond 1980; Warner and Luce 1982).

Quality of care

Quality of care is a somewhat troublesome concept, particularly since we are concerned with comparisons at the system level. In this chapter, we focus on variations in the level of health caused by variables within the control of the health care system. Following this perspective, Donabedian's definition of quality can help us to focus on these variations. He addresses both the social and individual aspects of quality by suggesting that 'Given a specified quantity of resources devoted to medical care, the highest quality of care would be that which yields the highest net utility for the entire population' (Donabedian 1980). Unfortunately, this definition is insufficient for operationalizing the concept of quality. The following discussion is based on Vuori's elaboration of these issues (1982). He raised several questions:

1. Quality for whom?
2. How do we define quality?
3. Quality for what purpose?
4. What aspects of quality are we looking for?

With respect to the first question, health consumers, providers, administrators and decision-makers may all be interested in improved levels of quality. From a health system perspective, the attitudes of decision-makers and the consumers are the most relevant. However, the second question is particularly challenging because the operational definition of quality must address its several facets. Indeed, there have been international efforts to develop standard definitions and cross-country strategies for creating national quality assurance systems, expecially in the European region of the WHO (Vuori 1982; Euro WHO 1985). These efforts are also related to the third question, addressing the objectives and goals of quality assurance. Figure 8.3 illustrates a model in the form of a tridimensional matrix which shows the proposed targets for national quality assurance systems. This matrix expresses national quality assurance in terms of the content, which is the context of quality analysis; function, which is the timing of holding the activities; and level, that is the organizational level under study. Obviously, the development of operational definitions for

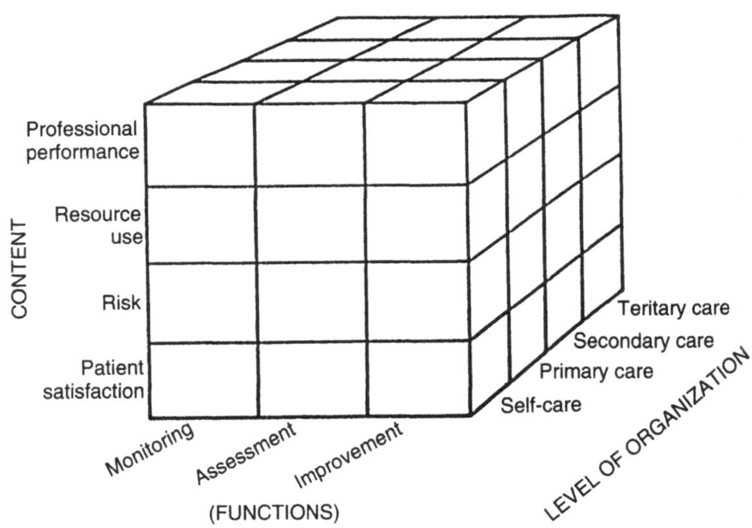

Fig. 8.3 Three-dimensional matrix illustrating the Components of an operational national quality assurance system. (From Euro WHO (1985).)

the concepts suggested in this model is a prerequisite for its implementation (Euro WHO 1985).

With respect to the fourth question, Donabedian's trichotomy of structure, process and outcome (Donabedian 1980), further elaborated by Vuori (1982) can be used to consider aspects of quality. For those interested in cross-comparisons this may be the most promising approach. Because with this approach, components of structure, process, and outcome can be clearly defined in operational terms, the approach can be used to evaluate quality straightforwardly. The structural elements in Donabedian's approach were discussed in Chapter 4, and the elements of process were discussed in Chapter 6.

In this chapter, we have focused on the quality of the outcomes of health care. This aspect is conceptually the most important form of quality assessment, because only by measuring outcome can quality be assessed to the final point of a given medical or health intervention. In the previous chapter we described the five Ds—death, disease, disability, dissatisfaction and discontent. In principle, the five Ds can be used to make a simple analysis of outcome and to evaluate its quality. However, these five Ds are generally too insensitive to the achievements of the health care system, and hardly specific enough to serve as true quality measures. Thus, methods more appropriate for measuring quality were developed. In these methods, to measure the general health status of a community, the health status of individuals are aggregated. For one such method the concept of Quality Adjusted Life Years (QALYs) is used. Bush and collegues (1973) first suggested QALY as a composite index when examining the cost effectiveness of screening for the congenital disorder phenylketonuria (PKU). QALYs are measured on an absolute scale of utilities ranging from zero to one where zero represents death and one represents perfect health. Health levels are assigned to individuals based on questionnaires in which respondents are asked to assign a utility level to their health status. The concept of QALY is discussed by Weinstein and Stason in an excellent article in the *New England Journal of Medicine* (1977). Stason and Weinstein (1977) also provide a practical application in which QALYs are used in a cost-effectiveness study of hypertension management. They show how varying degrees of hypertension affect the yearly cost of quality-adjusted life expectancy for American men and women. Theoretically, QALYs can be used in cross-country comparisons and also for the study of other diseases and conditions. However, their use can be hampered by the cost of large scale cross-comparisons, by uncertain validity, and by poor reliability of the responses from individuals representing different socio-cultural environments.

Rather than looking for a measure of general health outcome, we can instead, emphasize the explicit evaluation of disease-specific outcomes. As previously, this also requires outcome assessment at the individual level, which can then be aggregated to establish population-based levels as seen in the representative Rand Corporation Health Insurance Study (HIS) by Brook *et al.* (1979). One of the major goals of this multi-purpose study was to measure improvement or deterioration of health status caused by intervention in health care delivery. The effects of such intervention were measured by analysing the individual responses to several specific insurance plans. Since specific plans can be geographically allocated, the HIS approach can be used for cross-comparisons. But practically, such applications might be difficult because of the cost of data collection or the uncertain validity and reliability of the data collected.

The tracer method is a third approach first used by Kessner and colleagues (1973) for measuring the quality of health outcomes. In the tracer method, the health outcome for a specific process, generally a specific disease, is examined. Broad trends in the health system are then based on this specific analysis. This approach may be promising for cross-national evaluations since it overcomes some of the inherent difficulties of the previous approaches. Selecting a tracer condition for which information is readily available overcomes problems of insufficient data or the problems of validating various variables.

Kessner *et al.* (1973) considered a hypothetical health centre. Using actual figures, for each tracer, like otitis media or hypertension, they compared the number of clients actually cared-for with the expected number of clients. Expected numbers of clients consist of all those who would have been cared-for under the ideal conditions of complete needs assessment in a community, assuming the highest possible efficacy of care. The ratios between the figures for actual and ideal conditions were used to assess the quality of health care outcomes. Obviously, when reliable data can be generated, the tracer method can be used for cross-comparisons. However, except for research initiatives, the tracer method is unlikely to be applied in cross-regional or cross-national comparisons.

Indicators of quality-related outcomes

QALYs in cross-national comparisons

The use of QALYs to estimate outcome criteria is essentially a study of CEA for which the criteria for determining effectiveness are the gains in Quality Adjusted Life Years (QALYs). The application of QALYs is limited to situations where utilities can be assigned to specific health states as described in the previous section. These utility levels, ranging from zero to one, are determined by expert judgement based on individual responses by patients for each health condition. Useful examples with potential for cross-national comparisons include:

(1) a utility-based health classification system (Torrance *et al.* 1982) used in the measurement of the outcomes of neonatal intensive care units (Boyle *et al.* 1983);

(2) a rating scale technique for evaluation and policy analysis (Kaplan and Bush 1982).

For further details see for example Drummond *et al.* (1987).

Specific measures of quality—the tracer method

Quantitatively the tracer method can be formulated as follows:

$$S_i = \frac{T_i}{P_i} \quad \text{and} \quad S = \sum_{i=1}^{n} S_i$$

where: S_i = the success rate for the health condition that is tracer i;
T_i = the number appropriately treated for the condition (according to explicit standards of 'good medical practice') in a given population;
P_i = the number suffering from that condition in that population.

The ratio T_i/P_i expresses the percentage of the population at risk which has been 'successfully' treated for a given condition in a particular area. The calculation of S for several areas can be used to establish a comparative basis for such an analysis.

Equity

We discussed equity in Chapter 5 where we focused on equity in relation to the organization of a health system. That is, there we focused on the equity of both the structure and the process of a health system. Here we shall discuss the dimension of equity related to health outcomes. We shall assess the success of health care systems in implementing equitable care.

For example, in the Swedish health system there is remarkably equal access to health care across socio-economic levels (Swedish Ministry of Health and Social Affairs 1981). In spite of this, health outcomes were not equal (Stahl 1978). This can be plausibly explained in several ways. First, as shown in Chapter 7, health outcomes depend heavily on non-medical factors. Thus, suitable outcomes can be caused by health improvement resulting from changes in life style or in the environment even though the health care system itself may not be equitable. Second, most comparisons between inputs and outcomes are necessarily cross-sectional. However, the consequences of an inequitable distribution or of inappropriate processes of care may only be felt after the passage of time. Third, there is an inherent conflict of interest between equity and efficiency making it difficult to achieve equity as a health system outcome. In the case of equal allocation of resources to equals, called horizontal equity (West 1981), then equity and efficiency should converge. In such a perfect situation, only rarely encountered, the Gini index, discussed in Chapter 5, equals zero. In the usual case of vertical equity, when unequal subjects are treated unequally, equity and efficiency may conflict. For instance, organ transplants may save a few lives but only at the expense of the majority of the population whose basic services must thereby be reduced (Mooney 1986). Such problems have a strong ethical component that cannot be resolved by simply improving measurement instruments. Furthermore, the problems described here are not unique to the study of equity. These problems stem from the more fundamental problem of the definition of health. This is a delicate issue which has caused great concern in several health care systems. So long as we seek to measure health care outcomes, we must be concerned with the conflicting goals of equity and efficiency.

Indicators of equity

The same indicators proposed in Chapter 5 may be used to estimate equity from an outcome-oriented perspective. The only difference is in the use and the interpretation of the findings.

References

Altman, S. H. and Blendon, R. (1979). *Medical technology the culprit behind health care costs?* US Department of Health Education and Welfare, Publication No. (PHS) 79-3216. Washington DC.

Anderson, O. W. (1988). Introduction. Health care systems and the diffusion of technology. *International Journal of Technology Assessment in Medical Care*, **4**, (2), 169–70.

Babson, J. H. (1972). *Health care delivery systems a multinational survey*. Pitman Medical, London.

Banta, D. H. and Kemp, K. B. (1982). *The management of health care technology in nine countries*. Springer Publishing Company, New York.

Birch, S. and Maynard, A. (1985). Performance indicators and performance assessment in the UK National Health Service: implications for management and planning. *International Journal of Health Planning and Management*, **1**, 143–56.

Boyle, M.H., Torrance, G.W., Sinclair, J.C., and Horwood, S.P. (1983). Economic evaluation of neonatal intensive care of very low birth-weight infants. *New England Journal of Medicine*, **308**, 1330–7.

Brogren, E. O. and Brommels, M. (1990). Central and local control in Nordic health care: the public organization spectrum revised. *The International Journal of Health Planning and Management*, **5**, (1), 27–40.

Brook, R. H., Ware, J. E., Davies-Avery, A. *et al.* (1979). Overview of adult health status measures in Rand's Health Insurance Study. *Medical Care*, **17**, (7) (Suppl.), 1–131.

Bush, J. M. Chen, M. M., and Patrick, D. L. (1973). Health status index in cost effectiveness: analysis of PKU programme. In *Health status indexes* (ed. R. L. Berg). Hospital Research and Educational Trust, Chicago.

Ceresto, S. and Waitzkin, H. (1988). Economic development, political-economic system and physical quality of life. *Journal of Public Health Policy*, **9**, 104–20.

Charlton, J. R. W., Hartley, R. M., Silver, R., and Holland, W. W. (1983). Geographical variations in mortality from conditions amenable to medical intervention in England and Wales. *Lancet* **i**, 26 March, 691–6.

Cochrane, A. L., St Leger, A. S., and Moore, F. (1978). Health service 'input' and mortality 'output' in developed countries. *Journal of Epidemiology and Community Health*, **32**, 200–205.

Creese, A. (1983). The economic evaluation of immunization programmes. In *The economics of health in developing countries* (ed. K. Lee and A. Mills). Oxford University Press, Oxford.

Culyer, A. J., Maynard, A., and Williams, A. H. (1982). Alternative systems of health care provision: an essay on motes and beams. In *A new approach to the economics of health care*, (ed. M. Olson). American Enterprise Institute, Washington, D. C.

Deber, R. B., Thompson, G. G., and Leatt, P. (1988). Technology acquisition in Canada: control in a regulated market. *International Journal of Technology Assessment in Health Care*, **4**, (2), 185–206.

Donabedian, A. (1980). *Exploration in quality assessment and monitoring*, Vol. I. The definition of quality and approaches to its assessment. Health Administration Press, Ann Arbor, Michigan.

Drummond, M. F. (1980). *Principles of economic appraisal in health care*. Oxford University Press, Oxford.

Drummond, M. F., Stoddart, G. L., and Torrance, G. W. (1987). *Methods for the economic evaluation of health care programmes*. Oxford University Press, Oxford.

Ellencweig, A. Y. (1988). Development of medical care technology: the case of Israel. *International journal of Technology Assessment in Health Care*, **4**, (2), 255–67.

Euro WHO (1985). *The principles of quality assurance*, Euro Report No. 94. World Health Organization, Regional Office for Europe, Copenhagen.

Evans, R. G. (1984). *Strained mercy*. Butterworths, Toronto.

Fulop, T. and Reinke, W. A. (1981). Statistical analysis of the interdependence of country health resource variables, with special regard to manpower related ones. *Bulletin of the World Health Organization*, **59**, (1), 129–41.

Harley, M. J. (1988). Performance indicators in the management process. *Health Services Management Research*, **1**, (1), 29–42.

Heidenheimer, A. J., Heclo, H., and Teigh Adams, C. (1983). *Comparative public policy—the politics of social choice in Europe and America* (2nd edn.), Chapter 3. The Macmillan Press Ltd., London.

Holland, W. W. (1983). Concept and meaning in evaluation of health care. In *Evaluation of health care* (ed. W. W. Holland). Oxford University Press, Oxford.

Kaplan, R. M., and Anderson, J. P. (1988). A general health policy model: update and applications. *Health Services Research*, **23**, (2), 203–35.

Kaplan, R. M., and Bush, J. W. (1982). Health related quality of life measurement for evaluation research and policy analysis. *Health Psychology*, **1**, 61–80.

Kessner, D. M., Kalk, C. E., and Singer, J. (1973). Assessing health quality—the case for tracers. *New England Journal of Medicine*, **288**, 189–94.

Knaus, W. A., Le Gall, J. R., Wagner, D. P., Draper, E. A., Loirat, P., Campos,

R. A. *et al.* (1982). A comparison of intensive care in the USA and France. *Lancet* **ii**, 642–6.
Long, A. F. (1985). Effectiveness; definitions and approaches. In *Health services performance effectiveness and efficiency* (ed. A. F. Long and S. Harrison). Croom Helm, London.
McKeown, T. (1976). *The role of medicine: dream, mirage or nemesis*? The Nuffield Provincial Hospital trust, London.
Mooney, G. (1986). *Economics, medicine and health care*. Wheatsheaf Books, Sussex.
Rublee, D. (1989). Medical technology in Canada, Germany and the United States. *Health Affairs*, **8**, (3), 178–81.
Russell, L. B. and Sisk, J. E. (1988). Medical technology in the United States: the last decade. *International Journal of Technology Assessment in Health Care*, **4**, (2), 269–86.
Rutstein, D. D., Berenberg, W., Chalmers, T. C., Child, C. G., Fishman, A. P., and Perrin, E. B. (1976). Measuring the quality of medical care—a clinical method. *New England Journal of Medicine*, **294**, 582–8.
Shinn, R. L. (1986). Ethical issues. In *New options, new dilemmas. An interprofessional approach to life or death decisions* (ed. A.S. Allen). Lexington Books, Lexington.
Sorkin, A. L. (1976). *Helth economies in developing countries*, pp. 159–60. Lexington Books, Lexington.
Stahl, I. (1978). *Can we control health care costs?* Mimeographed report. Department of Economics, Lund University, Lund.
Stason, W.B. and Weinstein, M.C. (1977). Allocation of resources to manage hypertension. *New England Journal of Medicine*, **296**, 732–9.
Stocking, B. (1988). Medical technology in the United Kingdom. *International Journal of Technology Assessment in Health Care*, **4**, (2), 171–84.
Swedish Ministry of Health and Social Affairs (1981). *Starting points and guidelines*, HS-90. Stockholm.
Torrance, G. W., Boyle, M. H., and Horwood, S. P. (1982). Application of multiattribute utility theory to measure social preferences for health states. *Operations Research*, **30**, 1043–69.
Vuori, H. V. (1982). *Quality assurance of health services*, Public Health in Europe No. 16. World Health Organization, Regional Office for Europe, Copenhagen.
Warner, K. E. and Luce, B. R. (1982). *Cost benefit and cost effectiveness analysis in health care*. Health Administration Press, Ann Arbor, Michigan.
Weinstein, M.C. and Stason, W.B. (1977). Foundations of cost effectiveness analysis for health and medical practices. *New England Journal of Medicine*, **296**, 716–21.
West, P. A. (1981). Theoretical and practical equity in the National Health Service in England. *Social Science and Medicine*, **15c**, 117–22.

9. Limitations of cross-national and cross-regional comparisons of health systems

Until now, we have focused on presenting the various modules that make up a health system. After examining the conceptual basis for each module, we identified indicators for measuring the phenomena in each module and also examined how these phenomena change over time. Deliberately, we avoided the crucial question: did we choose and use indicators appropriately? This chapter is aimed at answering this question, and we shall do that in a two-stage process. First we shall examine it methodologically. We shall consider methodological problems and how they affect the use of the modular approach in cross-national comparisons. Then, by suggesting possible remedies, we shall attempt to solve these methodological problems.

The methodological perspective

Ecological fallacy

Cross-national and cross-regional comparisons are often problematic because they may be aggregate or ecological studies. Because data are generally available as averages or as population means, investigators are forced to use ecological models. Unfortunately, ecological studies are prone to ecological fallacy. As Michael and co-workers (1984) put it

> The ecological fallacy is a foxy, two-faced beast which lurks in the darkened corners of large population studies and tricks unwary readers into accepting unwarranted conclusions. This fellow can often be found infesting so called ecologic research when groups of people in selected geographic areas . . . are the units of study.

More formally, an ecological fallacy is a mistaken conclusion reached when characteristics of individuals are incorrectly assumed to be represented by the characteristics of a group. An ecological fallacy is often caused when the relationship between two or more given variables is affected by additional variables called confounding variables. These confounding variables may influence that relationship to some degree depending on which subgroups in a population are considered (Feinleib and Leaverton, 1984). There are many examples of ecological fallacy. For instance, merely comparing the levels of per capita GNP in two hypothetical systems can constitute an ecological fallacy. Because mean per capita GNP does not address equity, wealth may be differently distributed in the two countries even though their per capita GNPs are similar. Obviously, an even distribution of income, corresponding to a lower Gini coefficient, would contribute considerably more to a generally improved health status in a population than would a highly skewed distribution of wealth, corresponding to a higher Gini coefficient. Feinleib and Leaverton (1984) have offered an interesting example of how ecological fallacy can play a role in distorting relationships between variables. They analysed two similar comparisons of the relationship between fat consumption and mortality due to coronary heart disease (CHD) in 22 countries. The first comparison included total fat consumption and the second included dairy fats only. Within the larger context of the 22 countries, there was a significant correlation between fat consumption and CHD mortality in the results of both examples. However, as shown in Fig. 9.1, the correlation weakens for subsets of countries with similar characteristics, like English-speaking countries, or the Scandinavian countries. Moreover, in Fig. 9.2, we see that for each subset of countries the correlation of dairy fat consumption and CHD mortality is completely different from that for total fat consumption.

In addition to ecological fallacy, selective fallacy is also very important in cross-national studies. It occurs when data gathered in one specific area of a country are extrapolated to the whole country. Because a given specific area may not necessarily be representative of the whole country, conclusions for these areas may not be generalizable for the whole country. For example, in the international study on health care carried out by Kohn and White

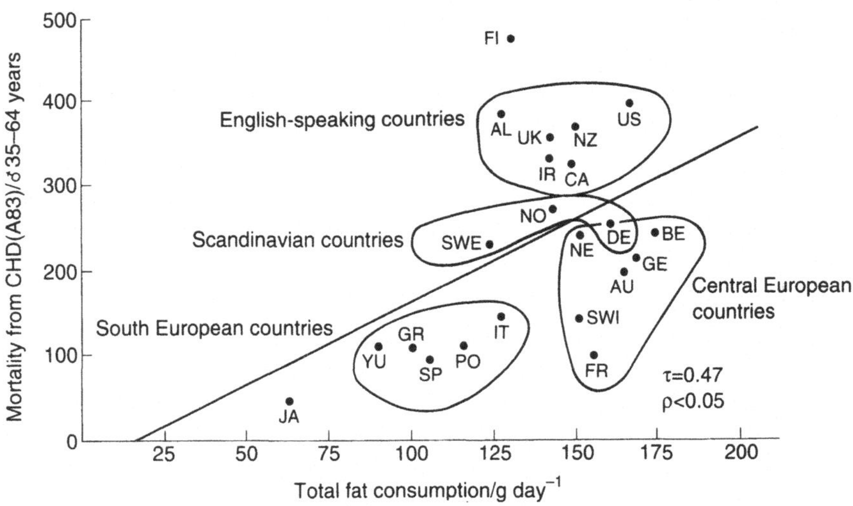

Fig. 9.1 Correlation between total fat consumption and mortality from Coronary Heart Disease (CHD). (From Turpeinen (1979), with permission.)

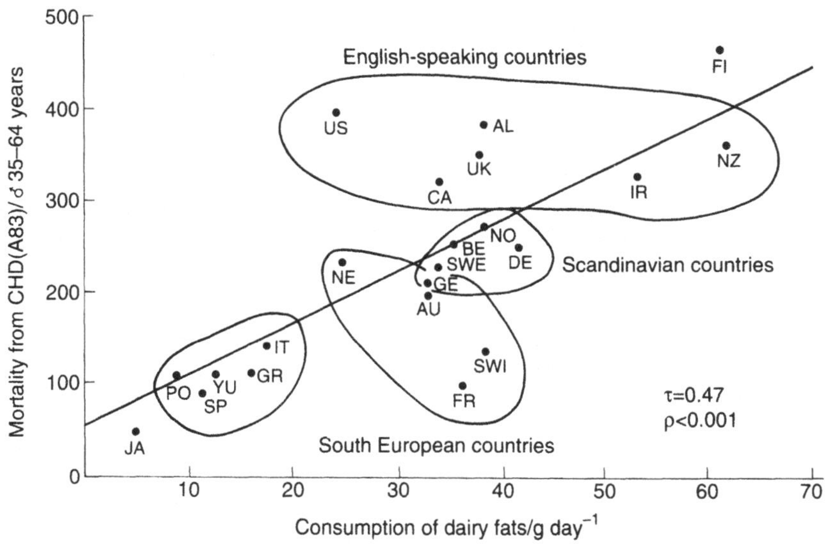

Fig. 9.2 Correlation between consumption of dairy fats and mortality from Coronary Heart Disease (CHD). (From Turpeinen (1979), with permission.)

(1976), the danger of ecological fallacy was eliminated because the information gathered was based exclusively on individual responses. However, these data were collected only in selected sites in countries studied, thus any attempt to generalize the findings at a country level would entail the danger of selective fallacy.

Though there is no complete remedy for ecological and selective fallacies, their ill effects can be reduced. Information gathered for an entire population can be validated by comparing it with data collected from individuals as did Kohn and White (1976) on a large scale. Alternatively, such information gathered on an ecological scale from one source can be tested against information gathered independently from another source. This may be rewarding for us because information for some of the variables in our model is routinely collected from different sources. For example, to estimate the validity of national statistics for cross-national comparisons, we can compare national data with available research findings collected independently in smaller areas within countries.

Problems of health indicators

Our perception of health indicators is also methodologically problematic for cross-comparative analyses. Health concepts and the indicators derived from them have been developed most often in the United States and sometimes in Western Europe. Applying these indicators in studies of countries with non-Western cultures may result in loss of indicator sensitivity, specificity, relevance or reliability. Their use may also be hindered by a lack of data. Consider, for example, general infant mortality (IMR) and infant mortality due to congenital malformations. In affluent Western societies, the IMRs for all births are 1 per cent or less, the overwhelming majority caused by congenital malformations. But in developing countries the IMRs are often as high as 10 per cent. Thus the great concern in wealthy countries over congenital defects must be overshadowed in developing countries by the concern to lower the general IMR. We can see that the indicator of infant mortality due to congenital malformations is far more relevant and sensitive in wealthy countries than in poor countries.

Non-transferability

Non-transferability is another central methodological problem. Non-transferability is an expression of systems dynamics: it demonstrates that a collection of separate components is not sufficient for the construction of a system. Even though sufficient information on several factors making up health systems may be gathered, merely comparing those factors does not constitute a valid framework for cross-comparative analysis. Because these components may interact in varying 'proportions' across systems, the picture is complicated and often distorted, and the validity of the conclusions and consequences reached in a particular health system must be questioned when other health systems are considered.

There are at least two elements alleviating the constraints imposed by the principle of non-transferability. One of these is the tendency of human societies towards achieving greater cohesiveness. Among other factors, the great improvements in automative information systems, the multiplication of communication channels, and the broad coverage by the mass media are responsible for these cohesive trends. The introduction of the same modern technologies in different countries and the growing standardization in professional education also contribute to these cohesive trends.

When different societies adopt similar medical technologies and professional approaches, they find a common denominator, thus permitting a more uniform base for the comparison of their health systems. This does not imply, however, that there will be convergence between either their health systems, as discussed in Chapter 2, or their societies. As a metaphor, consider language as a common denominator; for example, English is a common language in both Canada and in Nigeria, but neither their societies nor their health systems are similar.

The second element alleviating the constraints imposed by non-transferability is related to our method of analysis. With the modular approach, clusters of variables are assessed separately, thus reducing the likelihood of the misinterpretations associated with non-transferability. For example, suppose we want to compare the module of the quantitative issues on 'manpower' in several health systems. For most health systems, most of the quantitative variables in this module like rates of physicians per capita and rates of nurses per capita are easily available and fairly standardized. This permits analysts to establish a basis for comparison called 'quantitative aspects of health manpower'. However, it is quite difficult to analyse the companion module of qualitative comparisons on manpower. The qualitative components in this module include a complicated combination of professional orientation, professional socialization, and issues of professional prestige and status within the professional community and at large. Comparing such non-tangible assets is complex because it involves value-judgements based on the socio-cultural background of the evaluator. Even when comparisons are based on value-judgements, the modular approach is useful for determining, for each separate analysis, the limits of transferability. In operational terms, it can be used to determine the framework for cross-comparisons.

The association between phenomena and their measurement

The modular approach is based on a two-stage process, the definition of concepts and their operationalization by usage of indicators. A clear methodological problem arises with respect to the relationship between the measurement of a phenomenon and its concept. As with all measurements, the method of the measurement of health care indicators and the style of its use can interfere with the validity of the data. Suppose we wish to compare a given variable 'D' among several health systems. Galtung (1967) suggested a theoretical framework for the measurement of dependent variables. According to Galtung, 'D' will be a function of the following categories of variables.

$$D = f(I, N, I^*, R)$$

where: I = a set of independent variables;
N = national (or regional) characteristics;
I^* = a set of residual independent characteristics;
R = a set of variables introduced by the research methods.

While I and N relate directly to the concept, R reflects the interference caused by the research method and its effects on the measurement of D. Reducing the effects of R, the research methods, on D, the dependent variable, will increase the comparability among health systems.

Kohn and White (1976) suggested a less formal approach to this same problem. They identified several concepts and then translated each concept into a variable, measurable as an indicator. As shown in Table 9.1, a variable

Table 9.1 The hierarchy of measurement

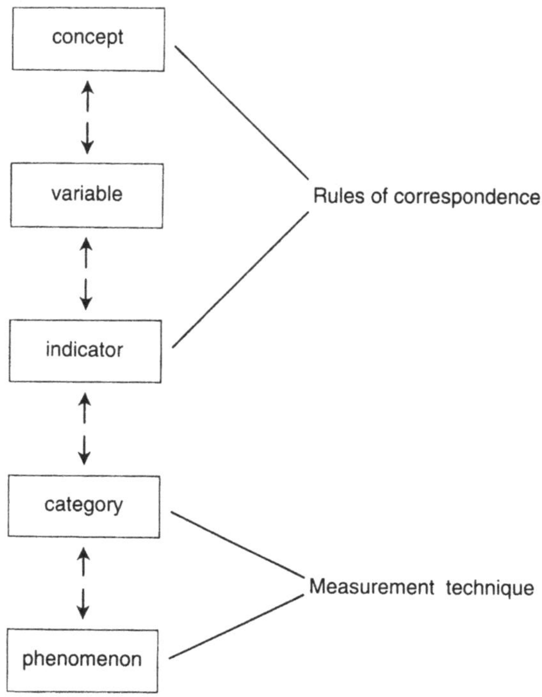

Source: Kohn and White (1976).

is operationally defined as an indicator and is divided into categories reflecting the size and characteristics of the actual phenomenon being measured. The process of the conceptualization of a phenomenon, and of defining an indicator for that concept, must follow rules that may be called 'rules of correspondence'. In this process there are two possibilities for error. First, poor operational definitions of concepts may result in poor indicators and reduced validity of comparisons. Second, unreliable measurement techniques can cause inaccurate results and loosely-associated phenomena and indicators. With respect to the first point, different socio-cultural environments can affect the rules of correspondence such that similar abstract concepts would be defined by dissimilar variables and indicators, thus affecting the construct validity of comparison.

Consider, for example, the concept of the 'physician–patient contact'. At the conceptual level, in some systems a simple telephone conversation between physician and patient is considered a physician–patient contact. In other systems, nothing less than a visit to a doctor can be counted as a 'contact'. Thus, at the indicator level, operational definitions for counting physician–patient contacts vary considerably.

The second problem, as Galtung (1967) described it, is the study of the effect of the chosen research method on the phenomenon under study. Research settings in different environments are dissimilar, and administrative and bureaucratic conditions vary, as do the resources available for carrying out data collection. These variations may increase the effects of the 'method' on 'results'.

Remedies for methodological problems

In the second part of this chapter, we focus on possible remedies for the methodological problems that may potentially affect the use of the modular approach. The discussion of remedies for the methodological difficulties in cross-comparisons coincides with the general requirements for the measurement of health-related phenomena. Following Dab and colleagues (1982), there are five major requirements for the measurement of phenomena in the health field:

(1) to have a reference concept;

(2) to relate to the phenomena covered by the indicator;

(3) to relate to appropriately constructed data;

(4) to be reliable, valid, and easily interpreted;

(5) to have possible uses.

Clearly, all of these criteria cannot always be implemented when making measurements. However, as shown in the next sections, they give a direction for the formulation of concepts and the selection of indicators.

Having a reference concept

Having a reference concept means that there is a logical relationship between a concept and the indicators proposed for operationally defining it. If such a reference frame is not easily identified for a given indicator, then that indicator must be carefully considered before it can be included in any analysis. Simple examples of the concepts of 'inputs' or 'resource use' like manpower facilities or financial indicators, will probably not be problematic. But as these concepts become more ambiguous, difficulties may arise, and relationships between the conceptual framework and the actual indicators used in analysis may be in doubt. A typical example is the relationship between the widely accepted set of indicators describing mortality, morbidity, and disability, and the reference concept of 'health outcome'. Unfortunately, these indicators do not measure 'health' but rather the state of 'bad health' or 'negative' health. In other words, the health outcome of a population is measured by considering its 'outliers', those who die, or those who develop disease or those who suffer from the consequences of illness during a certain period of time.

Phenomena covered by the indicator

This problem arises when an indicator is not completely relevant to the concept being studied. The most frequent inconsistency occurs when the indicator describes a topic or a concept incompletely. This problem persists even when indicators are carefully selected to reduce ambiguity in the definition of the reference frame. Selected indicators may be appropriate for representing a concept, but related data may not be available. When gathering data for a given indicator is problematic, other more easily obtained indicators seem more attractive. The danger for planners and decision-makers is that their reasoning may be affected by technical concerns rather than by problems of content. Their decisions may be based on available rather than essential data. This phenomenon may be called the 'information selection bias'. An illustration of an 'information selection bias' can be seen by examining the readily-available information on growth rates of elderly populations in several countries. Health policy-makers often use such information to substantiate their demands for more resources. In reality, using the indicator of growth rate in elderly populations is not really appropriate for health decision-makers. What truly counts in terms of resource use is whether the per capita expenditure on the elderly population is higher than that for the general population. Indeed, while higher per capita expenditure characterizes some groups of elderly persons at high risk, it is certainly not a valid observation for the entire aged population (Barer *et al.* 1987).

Appropriate construction of databases

It is common for policy-makers at different levels of the health care hierarchy to complain of poverty in the midst of plenty. Those policy-makers suggest that their data systems do not address the right questions. As this is common in individual systems, clearly cross-system comparisons may be similarly affected. For example, over the last two or three decades, some health statisticians have argued that death rates, the most commonly and systematically collected statistics on the health of communities and populations, are often inadequate to predict health outcomes. In developed countries, death rates in general, and infant deaths in particular, have declined to the level where it is hard to interpret small fluctuations in death rates as resulting from a health system impact (WHO Expert Committee on Health Statistics 1971).

This problem may be solved by categorizing health systems into subsets, each represented by a different set of appropriate indicators. Countries may be categorized into subsets according to a major health indicator, and then cross-comparisons will be made within these groups only. For instance, the WHO categorizes countries according to their infant mortality rates (e.g. high, 100 per 1000 live births; medium 20–100 per 1000 live births;

and low, less than 20 per 1000 live births) (UNICEF 1990). Consider infant mortality as an indicator: clearly one can use infant mortality data as an appropriate basis for comparison, only in countries with a high or a medium level of the indicator. On the other hand, mortality data in countries with low levels of infant mortality are not comparable because the variations in the indicator level are so small.

Another danger of an inappropriate use of information is related to the political implications of data collection. Deutsch (1963) identified the problem noting that 'information is power'. He argued that in a highly technological society control of the access to information is more important than physical control. In a democratic society, we assume that everyone has equal access to information. In reality, of course, access to information is highly uneven for many reasons even in democratic societies. The result is that certain types of information, readily available in some systems, will be strictly regulated in others. A notable example is the dissemination of information on infant mortality: easy to get in Western societies, but until recently hardly accessible in socialist countries like the USSR.

Reliablility, validity, and interpretation

Reliability

Reliability as shown in Chapter 1, is a measure of the stability and consistency of data. Reliability is of major importance in cross-national or cross-regional comparisons. When a phenomenon is measured in various environments, or more than once in a given single environment, it is crucial that similar information be comparable and reliable. Unfortunately, reliability and necessity are often inversely related. In industrialized countries, increased reliability is often associated with variables like total infant mortality or percentage of GNP as health expenditure. Because there is little variation in these indicators among industrialized countries, they are of little importance to health decision-makers. The problem with the more sensitive indicators is that they may be differently defined in different countries. For example, perinatal death is *generally*, but not *exclusively*, reported as occurring between 28 weeks of gestation and 1 week of age. Furthermore, the reliability of this indicator is reduced due to problems stemming from unstandardized procedures for perinatal death registration (Hunt *et al.* 1986).

In developing societies, on the other hand, basic mortality indicators are very useful for assessing the health of given populations. Unfortunately, data collection systems often collapse because of inaccurate measurement procedures and related technical problems. The unavoidable implication for both industrialized and developing countries is that inadequately supplied or missing crucial information interfere with making viable comparisons.

As Gilliand and Galland noted (1977), there are two possible responses to these problems:

(1) a conservative attitude, which leads to abandoning international comparisons while there is no correct reporting of data in accordance with the requirements of scientific analysis;

(2) . . . use the published data in spite of their imperfections . . .

Approach (1) precludes any international or interregional comparisons. In practice, we must use approach (2) and rely on imperfect information. Then, even inaccurate data can:

> . . . help to clarify understanding of economic, social and cultural phenomena and is preferable to ignorance, despite the bias that may be introduced through the use of imprecise and incomplete data.
>
> (Gilliand and Galland 1977)

Reliability is also affected when physicians do not accurately report all cases of diseases for which reporting requirements are established by law. In developed countries, the problem generally involves mild cases of communicable diseases for which hospital admission is not required. Paradoxically, in developing countries, inaccurately-reported cases are less of a problem: the problem is rather that the cases are not seen at all! Another threat to reliability is caused by the 'syndrome of outdated information'. This problem stems from the use of survey methodology to narrow the gaps in data when there is lack of regularly-reported information for several health and health-related variables. Properly performed surveys usually guarantee high levels of validity and reliability. However, such surveys are often based on outdated obsolete information. This happens when irregular, scarce surveys replace routine recording and data processing, as seen with population censuses. Though in some countries census surveys are carried out every five years, censuses have been traditionally surveyed every ten years, as in the US since 1790 and in Britain since 1801. Since censuses are by no means the best instrument to gather information on demographic, social, and economic trends in the population at large, the risk that census data will be used inappropriately is considerable. The main concern is not that data are unreliable, but that slow data processing and long intervals between consecutive censuses may force health decision-makers to rely on information which is ten or sometimes fifteen years old! In spite of this, there may be situations in which it is more effective to use survey methodology than documentary data, particularly if such surveys are performed on a limited rather than an entire population. This can be seen in the cross-national study comparing countries in which sentinel 'observation units' are used for the collection of a comprehensive set of integrated social and economic data (Scott 1978). These observation units were based on particular groups of the population representative of the entire population.

Validity

The concept of validity is closely related to the concept of reliability. As we have shown, reliability is the extent to which data actually reflect the characteristic under study. Clearly, low reliability reduces validity (if you don't hit close enough to the bull's eye you certainly can't win); but there are also other reasons to seek improved validity. When data is highly valid we are reassured that comparisons may be adequate and appropriate, and that the conclusions are worth noting. Unfortunately, in cross-comparisons of health systems, conditions for highly valid data are often missing. In reality, we have already shown that several concepts differ in their operational definitions across systems and across cultures so that there may be apparently different 'phenomena' covered by the same indicator. Even the simplest definitions may be subject to considerable controversy. For example, Bryant (1969) ask:

> What is a bed? It may be a rope stretched between the sides of a wooden frame, or it may be canvas with no sheets or blankets. It may have a mattress and sheets but may be attended only by auxiliary personnel; or doctors and nurses may be there, but a lack of equipment and materials may seriously limit the quality of service. These differences are seen between countries and within a country, and they may be the difference between the last century and this century in terms of medical care.

The problem of validity may be addressed in the study designs of comparative studies based on data from original research. The main problem in cross-comparisons, however, is the validity of comparing crude data from documentary sources. In this respect, standardizing terminology can be a powerful tool for bolstering the validity of data though it does not completely answer all the methodological difficulties. Over the last decades, the WHO made monumental efforts to standardize several resource variables including bed capacity and physician manpower, and process variables like hospital use and, particularly, mortality outcomes (WHO, *Statistics Annuals* publications). These efforts have substantially improved the power and usefulness of international comparisons.

These efforts of the WHO were based upon the recognition that there is no such thing as universal classification scales for variables used in international comparisons. Rather, such scales are chosen for comparative studies by their utility and adaptability. This may explain why international efforts have been concentrated on constructing and improving the International Classification of Diseases—9th Revision Clinical Modification (ICD-9CM) (Brown 1989). In fact, because ICD-9CM attracted so much attention, outcome data are the most natural to gather and the most convenient to collect. However, the use of ICD-9CM did not generally resolve the problems of acquiring and analysing information concerning the outcome of ambulatory care services. Designs for better classification systems for ambulatory care problems were thus sought (Hogarth 1978). These attempts resulted in the proposal of a specific scale, first submitted in 1975 and then revised in 1979, called the International Classification of Health Problems in Primary Care (World Organization of National Colleges and Academic Associations of General Practitioners/Family Physicians, WONCA 1979). Similarly, the proposed scale for chronic disease and disability has been effective in enhancing the validity of comparisons in the domains of disability and dysfunction (Wood 1983).

Both reliability and validity are also affected by the quality of data collection systems at the *micro* level which may vary across different hierarchies of any given *individual* health system. For instance, In Israel, within the *single administrative network* of the Ministry of Health, hospitals differ considerably in their reporting systems. While some hospitals enjoy an on-line computer system for processing medical charts and discharge forms, other hospitals still maintain a manual retrieval system that causes long delays in reporting and loss of some information due to problems in handling data. These differences result in information that may or may not be valid, accurate, and reliable at the *micro* level. Of course, this reduces the validity of aggregate data at the *macro* level too.

This same problem has been reported even when a rigorous survey methodology has been used. In the US, in practice, under-enumeration results in incomplete census coverage. Overall, under-enumeration rarely exceeds a very small percentage of the entire population, though for subgroups in the population, like Blacks in the US, it may be sizeable (Parsons 1972).

Possible uses and users of measurements

Using models of health systems is rather complicated when target audiences and the stated objectives of the model are not explicitly defined. To characterize information-use, Knox (1986) suggested three dimensions which he called taxonomies; these taxonomies include uses and users of information.

Uses of information

The first taxonomy includes routinely available information easily accessible to and usable by health planners and decision-makers. These include routine information about population needs, availability of resources, the determination of health standards, and health outcomes at large.

Knox's second taxonomy includes information meant to respond to a specific need. Though this second taxonomy can include routinely collected data, it more commonly includes data collected specially for a specific purpose. For cross-national studies, the special effort required to gather information responding to specific needs is expensive as is standardizing the responses and maintaining their validity. This is why easily collected and conveniently used information from the first taxonomy is generally used in cross-national comparisons. However, because routinely available information may be difficult to standardize and to validate, the likelihood of its potential use in comparative studies is definitely reduced. Kohn and White (1976) refer to this problem in their international study of health systems in 12 areas in various countries. When considering the feasibility of comparing physical access they note:

> Another question was how much information should be obtained on the transportation and communications networks of the study areas, when it is known that comparing the rates of motor vehicles and telephones per unit population cannot be used to explain travel time and distance to the nearest physician.

Users of information

Knox's third taxonomy includes the *users* of health information. In general, possible users of health information may be divided into the following groups:

(1) policy-makers at all levels;

(2) researchers and evaluators;

(3) the general public, either individuals or communities.

In a typical bureaucratic hierarchy, policy-makers may be divided into three separate levels, the local or community level, the regional or district level and the national level. For cross-national comparisons, a fourth additional level, the international level, is also relevant. The information needs of decision-makers are obviously different in both scope and depth at each level of hierarchy. This is why information satisfying the requirements at one level of care may not be sufficient for the needs of policy-makers in another level of care. A simple illustration can clarify this point. Average national figures on infant mortality may be sufficient for those interested in international comparisons and in ranking nations according to their overall health status. On the other hand, those figures will not generally satisfy the information needs of regional health planners. To comply with the differential needs for health services, regional planners require a more elaborate picture of the variations in mortality rates among districts and regions, and of the causes of these variations.

Researchers and evaluators are in the second group of potential users of cross-national and cross-regional comparisons. They generally need specific information often unavailable from documentary sources, so they tend to make extensive use of survey methodology in data collection. Unfortunately, it can be very expensive to survey a number of regions to discern inequalities in process or in outcomes. In addition, the validity of cross-national surveys can be affected by differences in the standardization of questionnaires or differences in responses due to socio-cultural factors.

Consider the findings of Kohn and White (1976) who conducted the largest cross-national survey of health systems. Their experience illustrates the problems encountered in validating questionnaires and comparing responses in cross-national surveys. They noted that there are instances when:

> . . . rather than attempt to impose specified sample designs on the study groups, a statement of sampling standards was drawn up that emphasized ends rather than means.

That is, in cross- national studies, final goals are more important than the methods for reaching them. Therefore, if at the end of a survey *construct validity* can be established, one can afford to make concessions in methodological design. The operationalization of this philosophy encouraged Kohn and White to select different sample frames for the different areas of their study. In some areas they used census lists for their sample frame, in other areas—tax lists, and in some areas they even used voter registration lists. Using these different sample frames did not really affect the outcome, which was a representative sample of the population in each area.

In addition to methodological concerns, there are other problems in cross-national research and its evaluation. For instance, when surveying a problem across a number of countries, questions must be presented to individuals in their own language. Quite apart from the cultural differences, translating the original survey instrument into different languages may be problematic. The variety of language structures and changes in emphasis in colloquial usage might easily transform the meaning of messages and reduce the validity of the responses. A possible remedy for this problem is to examine the verbal meanings of each item in the survey very carefully and to pre-test extensively the forms and the questionnaires.

Knox's third group of potential users of cross-national and cross-regional comparisons is the general public. Here we must define how the 'public' can function as a 'user'. The simplest approach is to define the public's need for information, which can be expressed through public opinion.

Hennessy (1981) pointed out that public opinion is '. . . the complex of preferences expressed by a significant number of persons on an issue of general importance.' This definition may be problematic for comparative studies. Clearly, a 'complex of preferences' may vary with culture and with social status. This issue has been reviewed by several authors. A typical example is the work of Almond and Verba (1963) who studied political culture across five nations. They noted that the '. . . political opinions of average citizens of any country will be heavily influenced by the culture of which they are a part.' From interviews of thousands of people in five countries they concluded that there are striking differences between the populations of different countries with respect to such criteria like knowledge and awareness of government and the policy-making process, political involvement, and understanding of political rights.

Furthermore, the expression of public concern is quite different in different societies. Western societies have a variety of means of expression, including voting power, the use of mass media, and the creation of lobbies for the promotion of issues and ideas. In non-democratic societies, however, the concept of public opinion has little or no meaning. Because of these problems in the application of Hennessy's definition, there is little chance that the general public will be a user of the comparative method. This is why the comparative method remains solely in the domain of the professional users, both policy-makers and researchers and evaluators.

There may be one exception to our conclusion. In some health systems, public participation has so increased that the public has acquired considerable power in the system itself (Bates 1983). Of course, only a few individuals participate actively in the health system, and these are not representative of the population at large. Nevertheless, these very active participants may be the only potential non-professional user-group for cross-comparisons of health systems. As Bates (1983) noted, consumers

> . . . are interested in easy access and quality of care at a low cost at the time of use. They want their particular needs met quickly and effectively no matter what the cost.

Along these lines there is of course ample opportunities for comparisons between attitudes and perceptions of consumers in different health systems.

References

Almond, G.A. and Verba, S. (1963). *The civic culture: political attitudes and democracy in five nations*. Princeton University Press, Princeton, New Jersey.

Barer, M.L., Evans, R.G., Hertzman, C., and Lomas, J.(1987). Ageing and health care utilization: new evidence on old fallacies. *Social Science and Medicine*, **24**, (10), 851–62.

Bates, E. (1983). *Health systems and public scrutiny*. Croom Helm, London.

Brown, F. (1989). *ICD-9CM Coding Handbook*. American Hospital Publishing, Revised Edition.

Bryant, J. (1969). *Health and the developing world*, p. 49. Cornell University Press, Ithaca.

Dab, W., Goldberg, M., Thebaud, A., and Gremy, F. (1982). Un outil multicritère d'analyse des indicateurs d'etat de santè d'une population. *Revue d'Epidemiologie et de Santè Publique*, **30**, 325–42.

Deutsch, K.W. (1963). *The nerves of government*. The Free Press of Glencoe, New York.

Feinleib, M. and Leaverton, P.E. (1984). Ecological fallacies in epidemiology. In *Health information systems* (ed. P.E. Leaverton and L. Masse). Praeger, New York.

Galtung, J. (1967). Some aspects of comparative research. *Polls*, **2**, (3), 1–19.

Gilliand, P. and Galland, R. (1977). Outline on International comparisons of public health, based on data collected by the World Health Organization. *World Health Statistics Report* **30**, 227–42.

Hennessy, B. (1981). *Public opinion*, (4th edn). Brooks/Cole Publishing Company, Monterey, California.

Hogarth, J. (1978). *Glossary of health care terminology*. WHO, Regional Office for Europe, Copenhagen.

Hunt, S.M., McEwen, J., and McKenna, S.P. (1986). *Measuring health status*. Croom Helm, London.

Kohn, R. and White, K.L. (1976). *Health care. An international study*. Oxford University Press, Oxford.

Knox, E.G. (1986). *Epidemiology in health care planning, a guide to the uses of a scientific method*. Oxford University Press, Oxford.

Michael, M., Boyce, W.T., and Wilcox, A.S. (1984). *Biomedical bestiary: an epidemiologic guide to flaws and fallacies in the medical literature*. Brown and Co., Boston.

Parsons, C.W. (ed.) (1972). *America's uncounted people: Report of the Advisory Committee on Census Enumeration*. National Academy Of Sciences, Washington, DC.

Scott, W. (1978). *Measurement and analysis of progress at the local level*, Vol. 1, An overview, UNRISD, 78.1. United Nations Research Institute For Social Development, Geneva.

Turpeinen, O. (1979). Effect of cholesterol-lowering diet on mortality from coronary heart disease and other causes. *Circulation*, **59**, (1), 1–7.

UNICEF (United Nations Children's Fund) (1990). *The state of the world's children*. UNICEF and Oxford University Press, Oxford.

WONCA (1979). *International classification of health problems in primary care*, ICHPPC-2 (revised edn). Oxford University Press, Oxford.

Wood, P.H.N. (1983). Prospects for control. In *Disability prevention: the global challenge* (ed. J. Wilson). Oxford University Press, Oxford.

WHO (World Health Organization) (1971). *Statistical indicators for the planning and evaluation of public health programmes*, 14th Report of the Expert Committee on Health Statistics. Technical Report Service, **472**, 18–19.

WHO (World Health Organization). *World Health Statistics Annual*. Geneva. (Various years.)

PART III

Applications

10. Cross-national comparisons—correlating input factors and determinants of process with outcomes

For cross-comparisons of a number of countries there are two main ways in which we can apply our modular approach. One, discussed in Chapter 11, is an in-depth comparison of some of the modules of the health system over a small number of countries. In the other, as discussed in this chapter, we can study the statistical associations among a few of the health system's modules for a larger number of countries. We can use these statistical associations to link health outcomes with their possible causes. This approach is very attractive because researchers and decision-makers are always intrigued by questions about how health outcomes may have been affected by a health system's inputs and processes. So, it is not surprising that cross-comparative studies of this kind have been made by researchers in many disciplines. These include historians, epidemiologists, demographers, economists, and health services researchers. All of these have attempted to test the hypothesis that there are significant relationships between the input and processes of health systems, on the one hand, and their outcomes on the other. From an historical perspective, McKeown (1976) examined several factors that can explain the decline in the mortality rate in developed societies, particularly in Britain, over the last two hundred years. After excluding several other factors, he concluded that nutritional levels were a major vehicle for improving the health outcomes of populations. Other factors outside of the health care system like water supply, sanitation, housing, and education, also played important roles in explaining the improvement in health status.

Because historical analysis is weak in using factual evidence, such analyses are likely to remain inconclusive. It is thus not surprising that instead of historical analysis, most recent studies have involved the application of quantitative analytic techniques for testing single hypotheses and complete models. We shall review a number of such studies here. We have divided these studies into two main groups according to whether their inputs or their processes are related to the health outcomes. Studies will then be classified according to the type of countries studied, developed or developing, and sometimes also according to their type of government: capitalist or socialist.

Finally, we shall compare among these groups. Each study also illustrates a different method of exploiting our basic approach. For each study, we shall address the variables from our special perspective. That is, as we have suggested in previous chapters of this book, we shall classify each variable into its respective modules. It should be recalled here that because various concepts presented in different modules can be operationalized by the same variable, that variables can be multi-modular.

Input-outcome comparisons

Cross-sectional correlation analyses

Cochrane and co-workers (1978) used cross-sectional design to compare several variables relating input characteristics to a health outcome indicator.

Table 10.1 Health system inputs

Modules	Variables
Manpower (quantitative):	- Doctors per unit population
	- Nurses per unit population
	- Paediatricians per live births
	- Obstetricians per live births
	- Midwives per live births
Facilities (quantitative):	- Acute hospital beds per unit population
Socio-economic development Direct effects:	- Percentage of GNP on health
Socio-economic development Indirect effects:	- GNP per capita
	- Percentage expenditure on health from public sources
	- Levels of education
	- Population per square kilometre area
Exogenous inputs Lifestyle:	- Cigarette consumption per capita per year
	- Alcohol consumption per capita per year
	- Calorie intake per capita per day
	- Sugar consumption per capita per day

Source: Cochrane *et al.* (1978)

For health outcome indicators they used several age-specific mortality rates. Inputs consisted of several variables (indicators) which, according to our model, we shall assign to the modules as shown in Table 10.1.

The restriction criteria for inclusion in the study, used by Cochrane and co-workers, were per capita GNP over $2 000 and population over 2 million. These very restricting criteria forced them to limit their study to only 18 countries. Findings were presented by the authors as correlations and regression analyses on their study variables. The associations between mortality and some of the input variables were not surprising, though some relationships between other inputs and outcomes were unexpected. For example, per capita GNP was strongly associated with mortality in both the youngest and the oldest age groups consistent with the notion that improved economic conditions affect the mortality levels at the extremes of the age range. Similarly, cigarette consumption was also positively correlated with mortality. On the other hand, the prevalence of doctors was positively associated with mortality in all age groups except for the 45 to 54 years group. This strong association was particularly marked for infant mortality which was so unexpected that it has been called in the literature 'Cochrane's Paradox' (Cumper 1984 p. 7).

In a critique of Cochrane's study, Cumper (1984) suggested that methodological deficiencies in Cochrane's approach can account for some of his unexpected results in correlating mortality to input variables. First, as we also suggested in Chapter 4, Cumper argues that purchasing-power parity rather than per capita income might be used as a standardizing criteria. Second, as Cochrane also notes, both the outcome of mortality rates and the input variables were used in the form of national averages. As we mentioned in Chapter 9, such averaging procedures may cause the serious problem of ecological fallacy.

Longitudinal correlation analyses

Preston (1975) was the first to report using Longitudinal Correlation Analysis in cross-comparative studies. His analysis of 30 countries was based on scatter diagrams each representing the relationship between a single input variable and a single outcome indicator. For his input variable he chose national income per capita measured in 1963 US dollars. For his outcome variable he chose average life expectancy at birth. To take account of longitudinal changes in these variables, he produced scatter diagrams for 1930 and for 1960. In each case, a logistic curve best fit the data. The explanation for the non-linear relationship between mortality and income is that eventually, further increases in income no longer decrease mortality so there are diminishing returns. Studying these logistic curves, Preston suggested the following conclusions:

1. The relationship between life expectancy and national income per capita has shifted upwards during the twentieth century.

Thus, in a country that attained a certain average life expectancy in 1960 there was a much lower income level than in a country that achieved the same mortality level in 1930.

2. Factors exogenous to a country's level of income probably account for 75–90 per cent of the growth in life expectancy in the twentieth century. Income *per se* accounts for only 10–25 per cent.

This observation is straightforward when considered by our modular approach. Since the inputs to health systems are represented by many modules, changes in a single module will normally affect any outcome measure only slightly.

3. Some of the observed scatter in cross-sectional relations is almost certainly caused by differences in national income distributions.

Because income distribution varied among the countries studied, Preston frankly admitted that his analysis may be biased. This is another example of a problem that we have discussed earlier. To avoid the danger of ecological fallacy, as here with respect to income, both *average income* and *income distribution* must be considered.

From Preston's work we see the need for further efforts in at least three directions. First, since changes in outcome measures cannot be adequately predicted from changes in income alone, a wider range of input variables must be considered. Second, the outcome of general health status must also be subdivided into specific components. This would permit a continuing analysis of changes in measures affecting particular health problems or specific population groups. Third, we must particularly emphasize the interplay between the effect on health status of two kinds of variables: variables in the economic input module reflecting economic growth factors, and variables in non-economic input modules including those reflecting the improvement in the qualitative aspects of physical resources, and those reflecting improvement in the organization of the health system. Technical change is an example of improvement in the qualitative aspects of physical resources. Attaining more equitable conditions, enhancing accountability, and increasing the appropriateness of health services are examples of improvement in restructuring the organization of a health system.

The WHO has initiated several attempts to expand analyses to the scope of these examples. Gilliand and Galland (1977) offer a methodological approach for using data collected by the WHO for international comparisons. They compared data for 68 countries selected mainly on the basis of data availability. As we see it, they used indicators reflecting four modules of our approach. Three indicators described input modules, and a single indicator, life expectancy, described the outcome module as follows:

(1) health manpower, quantitative, for which the indicator was
  - physicians per 100 000 population;
(2) indirect socio-economic effects, for which the indicator was
  - national per capita income (GNP per capita);
(3) physical resources, quantitative, for which the indicator was
  - hospital beds per 100 000 population;
(4) health outcomes, measured as life expectancy at birth.

These four basic indicators were intercorrelated twice for three distinct groups of countries. The countries were first divided according to per capita GNP, and second according to manpower availability. On the basis of these initial correlations Gilliand and Galland concluded that per capita GNP is a valid criterion for selecting countries for international analyses. Their further analyses were confined to a group comprising the twenty two countries with similar high levels of per capita GNP.

For those twenty two countries they considered four input variables of which, according to our analysis, three belonged to a single module which we call quantitative aspects of health manpower. These three variables were physicians per capita, dentists per capita, and nurses per capita. The fourth variable, beds per unit population, represents quantitative aspects of physical resources. After the four variables were selected, they were reduced into two factors by factor analysis. Factor analysis provides an overall picture for a given situation by projecting the observed values of the original variables for each country on a set of two newly constructed variables called factors or principal components. The observed values for each country are plotted in Fig. 10.1 where the axes represent these two factors.

As seen in Fig. 10.1, there was a 45 per cent and 30 per cent case dispersion explained by each of the two factors, respectively. The observed values for each country are plotted according to their projections on each of these two factors. In addition, the four original variables are plotted according to their correlation coefficients with these same two factors. In the figure we see four aggregates: first in the Nordic countries including Sweden, Norway, Finland, Denmark and Iceland. There are a high density of beds per unit population and a high proportion of dentists per capita. Second, in Eastern European countries there is a high density of physician staff per capita. Third, in the US and Canada there is a high density of physicians and nursing staff per capita. The fourth aggregate of Central European countries does not correspond to any original variable.

In summary, the Gilliand and Galland study provides yet another methodological approach for cross-national comparisons. However, it lacks the

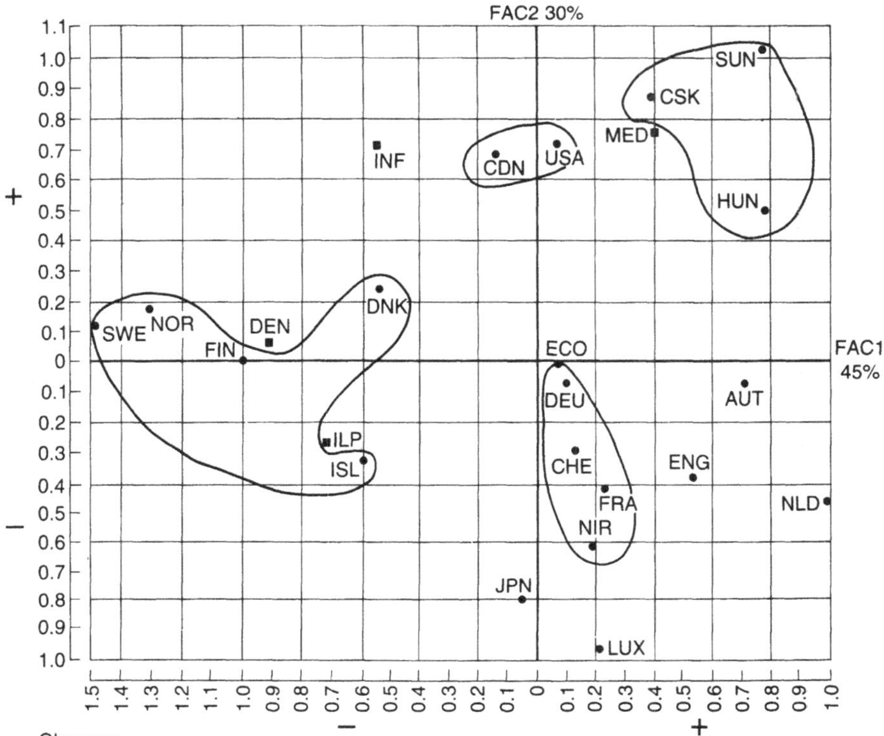

Glossary

AUT	Austria	INF	Density of nursing staff
CDN	Canada		
CHE	Switzerland	ISL	Iceland
CSK	Czechoslovakia	JPN	Japan
DEN	Density of dentists	LUX	Luxembourg
DEU	Germany, Federal Republic of	MED	Medical density
DNK	Denmark	NIR	Northern Ireland
ECO	Scotland	NLD	Netherlands
ENG	England	NOR	Norway
FIN	Finland	SUN	USSR
FRA	France	SWE	Sweden
HUN	Hungary	USA	United States of America
ILP	Bed/population ratio		

Fig. 10.1 Factor analysis—relationships between inputs and outcomes. (From Gilliand and Galland (1977), with permission.)

wide perspective needed for the comparison of rich and poor countries. In our view, the operational definitions of the variables chosen to represent the input modules in the study are not sufficiently standardized across countries. We previously referred to these problems in Chapter 9.

Longitudinal comparisons including developing countries

In an attempt to broaden the basis of comparisons and to provide useful characteristics pertaining to both developed and developing countries, Fulop and Reinke (1981) carried out an unusually comprehensive study including 131 countries. They wished to clarify the

> basic relationships at national level between socio-economic factors, health sector variables, and health status by quantitative as well as qualitative analysis.
>
> (Fulop and Reinke 1981)

Variables were selected on the basis of data availability and reliability. For the more than thirty measures considered, the twelve variables selected for further analysis are shown in Table 10.2 where they are arranged by modules according to our model.

Table 10.2 Twelve health variables according to modules

Name	Explanation	Name	Explanation
Module: indirect socio-economic development			
GNP	Per capita gross national product	TOFE	Ratio of percentage of total children in primary education to percentage of female children in primary education
PUTE	Pupil/teacher ratio in primary education		
PE	Percentage of children of primary school age in education		
Module: manpower – quantitative			
HLTH	Health employees per 10 000 population	DR	Physicians per 10 000 population
MD	Absolute number of physicians	NMW	Nurses, midwives per physician
Module: physical resources – quantitative			
BED	Hospital beds per physician		
Module: health outcomes			
LE	Life expectancy at birth	CBR	Crude birth rate
CHL	Percentage of population aged under 14 years		

Adapted from Fulop and Reinke (1981)

In addition to these twelve original variables, the authors defined change variables permitting the assessment of longitudinal trends. For instance, the change in the absolute number of physicians (DMD) was calculated as follows:

$$DMD = \frac{(MD_{75} - MD_{50})}{(MD_{50})} \times 100$$

Where: DMD = change in the number of physicians;
MD_{75} = number of physicians in 1975;
MD_{50} = number of physicians in 1950.

To determine the interdependence of health resource variables, regression analyses were performed. In the first stage, variables describing the socio-economic development module were analysed as a function of health resource variables. In the second stage, health status was analysed as a function of variables for both health resources and socio-economic development. The final regression equations are shown below, where the dependent variables are health status variables. The symbols for the variables are those defined in Table 10.2. T-values are given in parentheses under partial regression coefficients. The prefix I describes the initial value of the indicator—the 1950 value. The prefix D describes the difference between the current value of the indicator and its initial value.

$$\underset{(R^2 = 0.71)}{CBR} = 51.615 - \underset{(1.26)}{1.183}\ \text{LN}\ GNP + \underset{(2.55)}{0.178}\ PUTE - \underset{(1.56)}{0.050}\ \text{I}PE$$
$$- \underset{(4.02)}{4.366}\ \text{LN}\ \text{I}DR - \underset{(1.27)}{1.227}\ LN\ \text{I}BED + \underset{(0.06)}{0.001}\ \text{D}BED$$
$$- \underset{(1.09)}{0.986}\ \text{LN}\ HLTH - \underset{(2.04)}{1.467}\ \text{LN}\ NMW$$

$$\underset{(\text{R}^2 = 0.90)}{LE} = 64.741 - \underset{(0.13)}{0.078}\ \text{LN}\ GNP - \underset{(2.66)}{0.116}\ PUTE + \underset{(4.99)}{0.097}\ \text{I}PE$$
$$+ \underset{(4.66)}{3.275}\ \text{LN}\ \text{I}DR - \underset{(1.51)}{0.890}\ \text{LN}\ \text{I}BED - \underset{(3.44)}{0.027}\ \text{D}BED$$
$$- \underset{(0.45)}{0.251}\ \text{LN}\ HLTH - \underset{(0.22)}{0.097}\ \text{LN}\ NMW - \underset{(4.57)}{0.252}\ CBR$$

In accordance with earlier findings, more than 70 per cent of the variance of crude birth rates (*CBR*) as the dependent variable, could be explained by the three variables, per capita GNP, population per physician, and population per bed. When variables for life expectancy were the dependent variables, they were strongly associated with variables included in the module for indirect socio-economic development. This association explained more than 80 per cent of the variation in the dependent variable. When crude birth rate is included in the equation as an explanatory variable, and life expectancy is the dependent variable, this association may explain as much as 90 per cent of the variation. This last finding is not surprising and actually is not very relevant to our understanding of the causal relationship between health system inputs and health outcomes. As Fulop and Reinke (1981) put it:

> small improvement in R^2 for life expectancy is not as striking as the shift in importance from socio-economic factors to health resource variables as these are introduced into the equations.

They conclude that variables related to the indirect socio-economic modules explain a substantial share of the variations in health outcomes. Their conclusion is supported by Grosse (1980) who found that variations in infant mortality and life expectancy can be efficiently explained by levels of literacy and school enrollment. The inclusion of health resource variables in the analysis makes them more important than socio-economic factors in explaining variations in health status indices. The time factor in the analysis should also be considered. Fulop and Reinke suggest that there is a time lag in the response of health outcomes to the effect of health input variables. They concluded thus because, as they put it:

> the highest correlations are invariably observed between the current value [*i.e. the 1975 value*] of the dependent variable and the initial state of the independent variable [*i.e. the 1950 value*]
>
> (Fulop and Reinke 1981)

While Fulop and Reinke extended the scope of the countries studied in their analysis, they had a very limited choice variables. Fulop and Reinke operationalized only a few of the concepts of the inputs of health systems which we address in our modular approach. Cumper (1984), in a very comprehensive analysis published as a book, expanded the range of variables discussed in the cross-national analysis for a very large set of national health systems in 163 countries. Cumper defined four basic groups of variables of which each group corresponds to several of the modules in our model. While Cumper uses several input variables, for representing health outcomes he concentrates only on Infant Mortality Rate (*IMR*). In a very careful analysis, Cumper justifies the use of IMR for three reasons:

1. IMR is significantly correlated to other mortality indicators like age-specific death rates at older ages.
2. There is a similar correlation for the breakdown of infant and other mortality according to main causes of death.
3. Health interventions aimed at reducing infant mortality are also likely to affect mortality at older ages.

Cumper's analysis of the relationships between infant mortality rate and explanatory variables was conducted in two stages. In the first stage he selected four variables for which data sets were virtually complete. These variables were GNP per capita (*GNPN*), hospital beds (*BEDM*), physicians per capita (*PHYM*), and other health professionals per capita (*OHWM*). Regression analysis for these four variables accounted for 71 per cent of the variations in *IMR* in the data set. Logarithmic transformations were used because they best fit the data. The resulting equation for stage one is as follows:

$$\mathrm{L}\mathit{IMR} = 1.66 - 0.256\ \mathrm{L}\mathit{GNPN} - 0.202\ \mathrm{L}\mathit{BEDM} - 0.143\ \mathrm{L}\mathit{PHYM} - 0.055\ \mathrm{L}\mathit{OHWM}$$

where the prefix L stands for logarithmic transformations.

The results of this regression analysis are not surprising when one considers earlier evidence on the effects of per capita GNP on health outcomes (Cochrane *et al.* 1978; Fulop and Reinke, 1981). Chen and Lowenstein (1985) offer similar evidence for the role of the physician/population ratio in explaining the variations in infant mortality. For 60 countries, they also found a curvilinear relationship between infant mortality and the physician/population ratio. When this relation is linearized by logarithmic transformations, the physician/population ratio accounts for 53 per cent of the variance in infant mortality.

In the second stage of Cumper's analysis he used the results of the first stage to construct an intermediate variable consisting of the ratio of observed infant mortality to that predicted by the equation for L*IMR*. This intermediate variable was then used as the dependent variable in regression analysis with additional explanatory variables.

Having completed these two stages, Cumper was able to identify two sets of effects where:

(1) a health-promoting change is amplified by its indirect effects;

(2) a health-promoting change is offset by its indirect effects.

As an example of the first type, consider the effects of infant mortality on fertility. It was found that, after a time lag, a reduction in infant mortality led to a similar reduction in fertility. In the long-run, a reduction in fertility would lead to further reduction in infant mortality. However, such an amplifying effect is rare. More often, indirect effects cause a reduction of a health-promoting change. For example, a reduction in mortality can lead to increased population growth which would reduce the rate of the increase of per capita GNP. This would limit the resources available to the health system. Indeed, such conditions prevail in many developing countries. Also, deciding to allocate more resources to improve a single health outcome like infant mortality may cause a reduction in the allocation of resources for the improvement of other health outcomes. It could also cause a decrease in the allocation of resources to other sectors of society like education or welfare. In the long-run, the reallocation of resources to other areas of social interest could provoke adverse effects on the health status.

In his conclusion, Cumper attributes a massive weight to this phenomena of the indirect effects on health-promoting change:

> It appears that in the system of relationships determining national health levels, health-promoting activities are likely to generate indirect effects which offset, rather than reinforcing their primary effects.
>
> (Cumper 1984, p. 109)

Only if better health leads to increased economic production could we weaken this strongly pessimistic assertion. While not rejecting the feasibility of such options, Cumper admits that he is not able to demonstrate it either.

Concentrating only on developing countries, Grosse (1980) also addressed the relationship between several input variables and health outcome represented by life expectancy. We have assigned these input variables to modules as shown in Table 10.3.

Table 10.3 Modules for input variables for developing countries

Variable	Module
Sanitation	Exogenous outcomes—physical environment
Health expenditure	Direct socio-economic development
Health personnel	Quantitative aspects of manpower
Health facilities	Quantitative aspects of physical resources
GNP per capita, literacy rate, etc.	Indirect socio-economic development
Income distribution	Organization of health care—equity

Adapted from Grosse (1980)

Grosse found that the variations in life expectancy could be best explained by the use of two variables. These two variables were literacy rates, which we assign to the module of indirect socio-economic development, and the distribution of sanitary installations, which we assign to the module of exogenous outcomes. However, he did not find any correlation between income and the change in life expectancy over time. He arrived at the very important conclusion that the effects of economic performance on health outcome become less visible over time. That is, whenever some level of economic development has already been achieved, the level of economic production in a nation is not associated with changes in life expectancy.

In a major comprehensive study focusing on developing countries, Carrin (1984) concluded similarly. He explains:

> Economic progress cannot buy continuous improvement in life expectancy. Around the age of seventy the marginal effect of GNP becomes rather small. Countries with a high life expectancy can then only hope that economic progress will contribute to lower morbidity rates.
>
> (Carin 1984, p. 4)

In his study, Carrin proposes a theoretical framework in a path model for linking health outcomes and economic development. He used regression analysis on national data, at the ecological level, for 51 developing countries. In Table 10.4 we show regression coefficient estimates for variables explaining the variations found for a series of health outcomes. The results of Carrin's study suggest very similar correlations to those shown in other studies cited above. Here, too, GNP per capita and literacy levels seem to be decisive factors in determining health outcomes.

Grosse (1980) and Carrin (1984) showed that the effects of the explanatory variables on the changes in outcome levels over time were ambiguous. This ambiguity prompted other investigators to examine the relationship between socio-economic development and the decline in mortality in developing countries. Pendleton and Yang (1985), for example, hypothesized that a decline in mortality in developing countries is related solely to the rate of transfer of health and medical technologies from the developed nations. If this hypothesis were correct, then indirect socio-economic development would hardly affect the decline in mortality. To test the hypothesis, they separated developing nations into two categories:

(1) those in early transition (i.e. the poorer countries, N = 44);

(2) the more developed countries, later called transition nations (N = 48).

A path model linking socio-economic and health variables to mortality was developed and tested separately for each of the two groups of countries. In applying their model, Pendleton and Yang found that the impact of the independent variables was different for each group of countries. For the poorer countries there was a strong impact of health services on changes in life expectancy, infant mortality and crude mortality. For the more developed countries, there was a much lower effect of the health services on variations in mortality rates, while variables representing socio-economic development were more important in explaining these variations.

Pendleton and Yang's results support Gwatkin's (1980) contention that the direct impact of medical care declines with advanced economic development. It explains why in studies described previously in this chapter in which several groups of countries were examined simultaneously, there was no relationship found between health resource modules (beds and manpower)

Table 10.4 Coefficient estimates of the basic needs model

Number of equation	Dependent variables	Explanatory variables							R^2
		Doctors per 100 000 people (1970)	Calorie consumption (1970)	Protein consumption (1970)	Access to water (1970)	GNP (1970)	Primary school enrolment (1970)	Population growth (1960–1970)	
(1)	Life expectancy (1970)					0.68^{++} (65.6)		-0.33^{++} (15.3)	0.41
(2)	Infant mortality (1970)					-0.59^{++} (34.5)		0.21^{+} (4.2)	0.31
(3)	Deaths due to infectious diseases (1970)					-0.68^{++} (25.0)		0.72^{++} (28.3)	0.64
(4)	Life expectancy (1970)					0.34^{++} (16.4)	0.48^{++} (33.3)		0.50
(5)	Infant mortality (1970)					-0.23^{++} (7.3)	-0.63^{++} (53.8)		0.53
(6)	Deaths due to infectious diseases (1970)					−0.21 (1.0)	-0.48^{++} (5.3)		0.36
(7)	Life expectancy (1970)	0.72^{++} (30.2)	0.18 (2.1)	0.19 (2.5)	0.13 (1.6)	0.01 (0.00)			0.67
(8)	Infant mortality (1970)	-0.41^{+} (4.8)	−0.41 (0.62)	−0.18 (1.0)	−0.14 (1.5)	−0.41 (0.92)			0.43

Source : Carrin (1984) p. 144

Note:
- F values in parentheses ($^{+}$ = significance at 5 %, $^{++}$ = significant at 1 %);
- all equations are linear;
- regression coefficients are beta weights (equal to the coefficient times the standard deviation of the corresponding variable divided by the standard deviation of the dependent variable).

and changes in health outcomes. In conclusion, Pendleton and Yang's results were congruent with their hypothesis for only the least developed nations where the impact of technological diffusion outweighs the effects of the indirect socio-economic variables.

The previous findings were confirmed in a cross-sectional study in which 73 countries were divided into 4 groups according to their per capita income (Pegels 1989). Within each group, regression analyses were performed to evaluate several effects on health outcomes. In the poorer countries, both educational status and daily calorie intake per capita significantly affected health outcome as measured by life expectancy. In the wealthier countries, life expectancy was inversely related to per capita daily calorie intake and positively correlated to the rate of population per nurse. When infant mortality was considered as the health outcome in low income countries, the most important determinants were lack of education and the variables of manpower resources (both physicians and nurses per capita). In the upper income countries, lower education and higher calorie intake explained most of the variations in infant mortality.

In most studies of health systems cited above, the relationships between input variables and health outcomes were investigated. In a departure from this usual pattern, Ceresto and Waitzkin (1988) studied the effects of various political-economic systems on health outcomes. They examined the 123 countries having a population of over one million. As in Pegels's study, countries were classified into 5 categories by their level of economic development. However, Ceresto and Waitzkin introduced a new measure which can be linked to our module of 'system structure' as presented in Chapter 4 of this book. Their measure designates the type of political-economic system in the country under study. These political-economic systems were 'capitalist' (market economy), 'socialist' (centrally-planned economy), and 'recent post-revolutionary'. This third category includes countries like China which through a process of social revolution have reoriented their political-economic systems to a more centrally planned economy. For each of the 5 groups of economic development, the countries were then classified as 'capitalist', 'socialist' and 'post revolutionary'. However, only 'capitalist' countries were found in the upper level of economic development. Other input measures used by Ceresto and Waitzkin, like literacy rate, secondary education rate, and daily per capita calorie intake, had already been used in previous studies. However, their outcome measure, the Physical Quality of Life Index (PQLI) differed from outcome measures in other studies. Rather than a set of separate indicators for outcome, it is a single index. In an empirical formula, PQLI combines life expectancy, and infant mortality and literacy rates. As seen in previously mentioned studies, multivariate analysis showed that the level of economic development is a strong predictor of the PQLI. Turning to the effects of the political-economic system on health outcomes, Ceresto and Waitzkin reached the surprising conclusion that when controlling for income levels, socialist countries as a group have achieved a more favourable level of PQLI than have capitalist countries. These findings can be explained on the basis of Ceresto's earlier work (1982) in which he found more equitable distributions of incomes in socialist countries than in capitalist countries. Through the elimination of confounding effects in a procedure that is similar to the Elling's (1980) 'case-contrasting approach' which we discussed in Chapter 2, Ceresto and Waitzkin suggested that income distribution is a plausible explanatory variable for variations in PQLI. However, we found a great deal of evidence contradicting their assertion that 'socialist' countries have an advantageous status. First, from data on infant mortality (Szymanski 1982) and on mortality due to cardiovascular disease (Cooper 1981) we see that mortality rates in 'socialist' countries are higher than in the corresponding 'capitalist' countries. Second, defining the two groups of countries solely on the basis of per capita income is insufficient. This classification places the wealthiest 15 high income 'capitalist' countries in a group in which there are no comparable 'socialist' countries at all. The 'socialist' countries can be compared with 'capitalist' countries only at a lower level of income. But at that level, Ceresto and Waitzkin's comparisons are less valid since they compare the 'wealthiest' socialist countries with capitalist countries of only intermediate wealth.

Ceresto and Waitzkin presented their health outcome variables in very broad categories like overall infant mortality and general life expectancy. Because of this, their evidence on the effects of the input variables on health care outcomes is incomplete. We have attempted to carry out a more refined analysis. In our analysis (Nagbe and Ellencweig 1987) we asked: is there any association between cause-specific infant mortality rates and investment in health resources? Can changes in health care resources significantly reduce cause-specific infant mortality rates? The rationale of our study was that the effects of input variables on outcomes would be more tangible if we were to select only cause-specific outcomes amenable to intervention by the health care system. We had two study objectives:

(1) to evaluate the effects of various health care investment inputs on cause-specific infant mortality rates in an ecological model;

(2) to evaluate the effects of changes in health inputs on the differences seen for the health status in terms of cause-specific infant mortality rates.

Our data consisted of cause-specific infant mortality rates for the population of 40 countries that reported infant mortality data to the WHO; this size of our sample of countries depended on data availability. We included only countries reporting at least once in each of the two periods 1970–73 and 1980–83. Cause-specific infant mortality rates included the following specific causes:

- infectious diseases (all types);
- pneumonia;
- meningitis;
- complications at birth (all types);
- accidents (all).

In all, we studied 20 developed and 20 developing countries. Countries were classified into one of these two groups according to per capita income as determined by the World Bank (World Bank 1984). We classified high income or high middle income countries as developed and low middle or low income countries as developing. As stated above, we were interested in the specific outcome indicators and in the effects of the input variables that can be related to the manpower and physical resource module. Therefore, in our analysis we only used input indicators showing such direct relationships. The list of variables that we used in this analysis is given in Table 10.5.

To respond to our two study objectives we used both cross-sectional and time-dependent analyses. The cross-sectional analysis included Pearson correlations and multivariate regression analysis. It yielded several statistically significant associations generally in agreement with earlier findings. Here we report only the findings of the regression analysis. Findings are

Table 10.5 Variables used in cross-national comparisons

Label	Variables
Outcome Variables	
INFD X[a]	Infant mortality rate per 10 000 population per year from all types of infectious diseases.
PNEU X[a]	Infant mortality rate per 10 000 per year from pneumonia.
MENGT X[a]	Infant mortality rate per 10 000 per year from meningitis.
BIRCOM X[a]	Infant mortality rate per 10 000 per year from all types of complications at birth.
ACCDNT X[a]	Infant mortality rate per 10 000 per year from all types of accidents.
Input Variables	
DOC X[a]	Physician rate per 1000 population
NURSP X[a]	Registered and practical nurses rate per 1000
MID X[a]	Rate per 1000—midwives
MDT X[a]	Rate per 1000—medical technicians (laboratory, X-ray etc.)
PHAR X[a]	Rate per 1000—pharmacists
BED X[a]	Bed rate per 1000 population

[a] X = 70 For the early seventies, X = 80 for the early eighties.

reported separately for the two time periods, for the early 1970s and the early 1980s and the statistical analyses are shown in Table 10.6. We see that the incidence rate of health conditions amenable to health interventions and the levels of health resources are inversely related. The module of physical resources affects outcomes the most: in 5 of the 10 equations, bed availability and health outcomes were inversely related. With regard to manpower resources, the incidence rates of pneumonia and meningitis were inversely related to the availability of pharmacists and medical technologists, but not to the rates of doctors and nurses per capita. Perhaps the availability of ancillary services like the distribution of pharmaceutical or medical laboratory services is especially sensitive to variations in specific health outcomes. This may happen because for these services, greater differences are expected between developed and developing countries.

The next step of our analyses included a time component. Our primary effort was to carry out a multivariate regression analysis in which the

Table 10.6 Regression analyses for the association between outcomes and inputs

Dependent variable		Equation[a] (sig t)[b]	F_s[c]	R^2[d]
INFD 70	=	−0.605 *BED* 70 (0.0002)	0.0002	0.366
PNEU 70	=	−0.415 *PHAR* 70 (0.018)	0.0018	0.172
MENGT 70	=	−0.432 *BED* 70 (0.013)	0.013	0.187
BIRCOM 70		None		
ACCDN 70		None		
INFD 80	=	−0.542 *BED* 80 (0.016)	0.016	0.294
PNEU 80	=	−0.407 *BED* 80 (0.022)	0.022	0.166
MENGT 80	=	−0.373 *MDT* 80 (0.04)	0.04	0.140
BIRCOM 80	=	−0.378 *BED* 80	0.035	0.143
ACCDN 80		None		

Notes:
[a] Standardized coefficients
[b] Significance of the t-statistic
[c] F_s Significance of F-statistic
[d] Adjusted R-square of equation

dependent variables reflect changes in cause-specific health outcomes over time, and the explanatory variables reflect changes in input variables through the same time period. These comparisons did not reveal significant correlations as other authors found using a similar rationale (see for example, Grosse (1980) and Carrin (1984) whose findings we reported earlier in this chapter). As an alternative, we have chosen to assess longitudinal trends in the Pearson correlation coefficients. Our rationale is that a trend was strengthened over time if the positive (or negative) Pearson correlation coefficient for two given variables was more significant in the 1980s than in the 1970s. Because trends for developing countries may differ from those for developed countries, we assessed trends for all the countries studied in our analysis together and then separately for developed and developing countries. The results of the Pearson correlations and their trends over time for all the countries are listed in Table 10.7(a). The separate correlations for developed countries are in Table 10.7(b) and those for developing countries are in Table 10.7(c).

Table 10.7(a) shows that except for complications at birth, we found that trends in cause-specific outcomes were not strengthened over time. In fact, over time, we found either a weakened effect or no effect of inputs at all. This result means that the association between the cause-specific outcomes and the several input measures were statistically more significant in the 1970s than in the 1980s. If statistical trends reflect reality, then we can conclude that when levels of resources were lower, as was the case in the 1970s,

Table 10.7(a) Pearson correlation coefficients: all countries (N = 40)

	BED X[a]	*DOC* X	*NUR* X
INFD X	−0.568 (0.00) −0.661 (0.00) NC[b]	−0.554 (0.00) −0.661 (0.00) NC	−0.328 (0.022) −0.340 (0.018) W
MENGT X	−0.336 (0.020) −0.403 (0.006) W	−0.282 (0.043) −0.393 (0.007) W	−0.553 (0.00) −0.302 (0.033) S
PNEU X	−0.154 (N.S.) −0.308 (0.030) W	−0.274 (0.048) −0.330 (0.022) W	−0.322 (0.025) −0.339 (0.019) W
BIRCOM X	−0.358 (0.014) −0.030 (NS) S	−0.289 (0.039) 0.042 (NS) S	−0.359 (0.014) −0.118 (NS) S

Notes: [a]Upper line value for the 80s.
Bottom line value for the 70s
Values in parentheses are respective p-values for correlations
[b]Trend value over time; stronger (S), weaker (W) or no change over time (NC)
[c]NS = not significant

Table 10.7(b) Pearson correlation coefficients: developed countries (N = 20)

	BED X	*DOC* X	*NUR* X
INFD X	−0.244 (N.S.) −0.394 (0.028) W	−0.187 (N.S.) −0.276 (0.09) W	−0.451 (0.013) −0.637 (0.00) W
MENGT X	0.037 (N.S.) 0.029 (N.S.)	0.047 (N.S.) −0.107 (N.S.)	−0.308 (0.072) −0.397 (0.027) W
PNEU X	0.091 (N.S.) 0.010 (N.S.)	−0.147 (N.S.) −0.114 (N.S.)	−0.286 (0.080) −0.323 (0.061) W
BIRCOM X	0.108 (N.S.) 0.098 (N.S.)	0.050 (N.S.) 0.002 (N.S.)	−0.316 (0.065) 0.203 (N.S) S

Notes: see Table 10.7(a)

Table 10.7(c) Pearson correlation coefficients: developing countries (N = 20)

	BED X	*DOC* X	*NUR* X
INFD X	−0.449 (0.035) −0.443 (0.056) S	N.S.	−0.544 (0.022) −0.553 (0.020) NC
MENGT X	0.107 (N.S.) 0.498 (N.S.)	N.S.	−0.103 (N.S.) −0.254 (N.S.)
PNEU X	−0.389 (0.08) −0.217 (N.S.) S	N.S.	−0.458 (0.05) −0.293 (N.S.) S
BIRCOM X	−0.145 (N.S.) 0.176 (N.S.)	N.S.	−0.215 (N.S.) 0.074 (N.S)

Notes: see Table 10.7(a)

the adverse effects of input variables on specific outcomes were more pronounced. This conclusion supports the earlier findings of Grosse (1980) and Carrin (1984) for the effects of input variables on broad outcomes like infant mortality and life expectancy. They also found that changes occurring at lower levels of resources have stronger effects on the outcome variables than the same changes occurring at a higher level of resources. We can attribute this effect to the decreasing marginal effect of inputs on outcomes as shown by the Rand Curve discussed in Chapter 4. As the level of resources increases, the improving effect of each of them on outcomes becomes less marked.

Time-trends analysed separately for developed and developing countries are dissimilar. While the trends in developed countries were similar to the trends for the entire group of countries studied, for developing countries we found an opposite trend. For those countries, over time, the association between resources and outcomes becomes stronger. This phenomenon may be caused by the effects of the early developmental stages of health systems in many developing countries. In these countries, better organization of care and better deployment of resources could help in diagnosing new cases of disease that had previously not been noticed, thus apparently increasing the incidence rates for cause-specific mortality.

The only exception to this pattern is for neonatal death caused by complications at birth. For this cause of death, the trends over time are strengthened for all the input variables. Due to improved technology, the negative association between health input variables and the neo-natal mortality rate becomes more significant during the 1980s. That is, higher levels of resources invested in the health care system resulted in a decrease in infant mortality caused by birth complications.

Process–outcome comparisons

Health care organization and outcomes

Departing from the study of inputs *per se*, we shall now address the relationship between the variables used to describe the organization of a health system and the variables describing its outcomes. Comparisons of this kind

Table 10.8 Cross-national rankings of health care expenditures and measures of health status, 1975

	Health care expenditure as percentage of GNP	RANK	Patient access to specialists	Health status based on 17 mortality rates	RANK
West Germany	9.4	1	Uncontrolled	1.23	6
United States	8.7	2	Uncontrolled	1.17	5
Sweden	8.5	3	Uncontrolled	0.73	1
France	7.9	4	Uncontrolled	1.10	4
Netherlands	7.9	4	Referral only	0.79	2
Britain	6.1	6	Referral only	0.93	3

Note: The index employed in the health status column reflects how the average of that country's rates for 17 age- and sex-specific mortality rates relate to the mean of the above 6 countries plus 4 others (Australia, Canada, Italy and Switzerland).

Source: Maxwell, R.J. (1981). *Health and Wealth*, pp. 52, 90. Lexington Books, Lexington, Mass.

are less common because it is more difficult to define operationally and to measure organizational elements at a systems' level than to make straightforward comparisons of inputs and outcomes. The work of Heidenheimer and colleagues (1983), as described in Chapter 8, is a remarkable example of an assessment of this kind of relationship. The authors ranked health status, defined as an index based on 17 mortality rates, and then related it to 2 explanatory variables:

(1) the percentage expenditure on health from GNP, an input variable;

(2) the patient access to a specialist.

This latter variable is related to the organizational arrangements in a health system. The results of their comparisons for 6 countries are shown in Table 10.8. However, because of the difficulties in operationalization of other variables describing health care organization, Heidenheimer and colleagues used patient access to a specialist as a single variable of its kind. Because of this, their qualitative conclusions can serve only as suggestive hints for health policy-makers.

Associations involving the process of care

There are only a few reports linking process to outcomes in an international context. Goodman, for example, (1986) examined the relationship between the use of medical technologies and mortality rates at the ages of 25–34 and over 75 years for 8 developed countries. He used the US mortality rates as reference values for the entire group. He found that relative to the US mortality rates, on the average, countries whose mortality rates rise with age use medical technologies less than does the US. Because sophisticated technologies are relatively lacking in these countries, Goodman concluded that

> the fewer the medical resources that are available, the lower the likelihood that an elderly patient will have access to them, relative to a younger patient.

The relative lack of studies on international comparisons of the process of health care prompted us to carry out some illustrative comparisons of our own. First, we concentrated on the effects on the process of variables representing structural modules. We studied 25 developed countries using the OECD (1985) as our data source, plus information from local Ministries of Health for certain countries like Israel. We used only the most recent figures. For most countries, we found most recent data for the years 1980 to 1983. The variables used in our analysis are shown in Table 10.9. Because utilization depends heavily on age structures, we calculated age-adjusted rates for the variables describing process modules. We selected 3 age categories for the adjustment procedure: 0–14, 15–64, and over 65 years. We

Table 10.9 Structure/process comparisons – variables and their definitions

ADM	–	Admission rate to acute care hospitals per 1000 population (AADM – adjusted admission rates)
ALOS	–	Average length of stay in acute care hospitals (AALOS – age adjusted ALOS)
CONT	–	Number of contacts with physicians (excluding dentists) in a year (ACONT – age adjusted CONT)
STAF	–	Staff per hospital bed
PHYS	–	Physician rate per 1000 population
BED	–	Bed rate per 1000 population

performed statistical analyses for both the crude and the adjusted rates. These included Pearson correlations and regression analysis. In Table 10.10, the results of the regression analysis are shown for these adjusted rates.

Table 10.10 also shows that adjusted admission rates to hospitals were positively associated with the availability of manpower resources. This finding corresponds to Roemer's (1961) early observation, well known as the 'Roemer postulate'. The postulate is based on the empirical observation that the utilization of hospital beds depends on their availability.

Our results suggest that Roemer's postulate is true internationally. When the adjusted average length of hospital stay (AALOS) is the dependent variable, regression analysis shows that it is positively associated with the volume of beds per capita. AALOS is also correlated to the volume of contacts with physicians in the community. This also indirectly reflects resource availability, since one would expect more contacts with more physicians per capita. Finally, adjusted length of stay and adjusted admission rates are negatively associated. This may simply be a result of the constraints imposed on hospital bed availability. With higher admission rates, the

Table 10.10 Regression analysis process and input variables

Dependent Variable		Equation[a] (sig t)[b]	Fs[c]	R^2
AADM	=	0.609 STAF (0.002)	0.0020	0.345
AALOS	=	0.663 BED − 0.537 AADM + 0.349 ACONT (0.015) (0.025) (0.033)	<0.0001	0.798

[a] Standardized coefficients [b] Significance of the t-value
[c] Significance of the F-value

burden on hospital bed availability becomes greater, causing a drop in average length stay.

We carried out a second series of international comparisons relating structure and process modules to health outcomes. For greater sensitivity, we chose infant mortality due to congenital disorders as a tracer condition. Here we focused on the relationships between age- and cause-specific mortality rates and a number of structure and process variables for 20 developing countries. Our data sources for congenital mortality were the *WHO Statistics Annual* (1980, 1982). Data sources for other variables were taken from the OECD (1985). The dependent variable used in our analysis was congenital mortality (*CONMOR*), and the explanatory variables were health personnel per bed (*STAF*), nursing personnel per bed (*NURSTAF*), and the average length of stay for children aged 0–4 years in acute care hospitals (*ALOS*).

We hypothesized that because congenital malformations may be amenable to medical intervention, an increase in health personnel per bed would cause a decrease in mortality. We also anticipated that a more intensive treatment pattern in hospitals, reflected by longer stays, would cause a decrease in mortality rates due to congenital disorders. Our analysis confirmed our hypotheses and yielded the following equation:

$$CONMOR = \underset{(0.026)^{b}}{0.603^{a}\,STAF} - \underset{(0.008)^{b}}{0.764^{a}\,ALOS}$$

$$R^2 = 0.350$$

[a] Standard coefficients [b] Significance of t

Conclusion

In this chapter we wished to analyse a broad spectrum of associations between health outcomes and their underlying causal factors. Significant relationships reported by many authors show that on the ecological level, it is possible to show relevant associations between many inputs and health outcomes. Using our terminology, these inputs are modules containing indicators for manpower, physical resources, and both direct and indirect socio-economic development. Less frequently, there are similar associations for modules representing the organization of health systems or the process of health care delivery.

The extensive use of such comparisons indicates that it is possible and useful for researchers and decision-makers to use this type of cross-comparisons. Indeed, such comparisons can crudely indicate differences in the effectiveness of health care systems. However, one should not underestimate the inherent dangers of this approach. Such dangers include ecological fallacy, lack of standard definitions for variables across countries, problems in data collection, and data reliability. While these problems have already been fully addressed in Chapter 9, it is appropriate to recall here that application of cross-national comparisons inevitably results in a similar 'application' of some of these problems. Therefore, it is always recommended to weigh the benefits of these ecological comparisons in explaining *macro* characteristics of health systems in countries and regions against the danger that methodological problems can strongly affect the validity of such conclusions.

References

Carrin, G. (1984). *Economic evaluation of health care in developing countries—theory and applications*. Croom Helm, London.

Ceresto, S. J. (1982). Socialism, capitalism and inequality. *Insurgent Sociologist*, **11**, 5-29.

Ceresto, S. J. and Waitzkin, H. (1988). Economic development, political economic system, and the physical quality of life. *Journal of Public Health Policy*, **9**, 104-20.

Chen, M.K. and Lowenstein, F. (1985). The physician population ratio as a proxy measure of the adequacy of health care. *International Journal of Epidemiology*, **14**, (2), 300-4.

Cochrane, A.L., St Leger, A.S., and Moore, F. (1978). Health service 'input' and mortality 'output' in developed countries. *Journal of Epidemiology and Community Health*, **32**, 200-5.

Cooper, R. (1981). Rising death rates in the Soviet Union: the impact of coronary heart disease. *New England Journal of Medicine*, **304**, 1259-65.

Cumper, G.E. (1984). *Determinants of health levels in developing countries*. Research Studies Press, Letchworth, England.

Elling, R.H. (1980). *Cross-national study of health systems—political economics and health care*. Transaction Books, New Brunswick.

Fulop, T. and Reinke, W.A. (1981). Statistical analysis of the interdependence of country health resource variables, with special regard to manpower-related ones. *Bulletin of the World Health Organization*, **59**, (1), 129-41.

Gilliand, P. and Galland, R. (1977). Outline on international comparison of public health, based on data collected by the World Health Organization. *World Health Statistics Report* **30**, 227-38.

Goodman, J.C. (1986). Rationing health care: an international perspective. In *Policies and prescriptions. Current directions in health policy* (ed. C.M. Lindsay). The Centre for Independent Studies, St Leonards, Australia.

Grosse, R.N. (1980). Interrelation between health and population: observations derived from field experiences. *Social Science and Medicine*, **14c**, 99-120.

Gwatkin, D.R. (1980). Indicators of change in developing country mortality trends: the end of an era. *Population Development Review*, **6**, 615-44.

Heidenheimer, A.J., Heclo, H., and Teich Adams, C. (1983). *Comparative public policy*, (2nd edn). Macmillan, London.

McKeown, T. (1976). *The modern rise of populations*. Edward Arnold, London.

Nagbe, C. (1987). A study of the impact of health resources on cause-specific infant mortality rate. MPH Thesis, supervised by A.Y. Ellencweig, School of Public Health and Community Medicine, Hebrew University, Jerusalem.

OECD (Organization of Economic Co-operation and Development) (1985). *Measuring health care 1960–1983*, Social Policy Study, No. 2. Paris.

Pegels, C.C. (1989). A cross-national country group study of three health level outcomes and four potential causes. *International Journal of Health Planning and Management*, **4**, 107–16.

Pendleton, B.F. and Yang, Shu-O. W. (1985). Socio-economic and health effects on mortality declines in developing countries. *Social Science and Medicine*, **20**, (5), 453–60.

Preston, S.H. (1975). The changing relation between mortality and level of economic development. *Population Studies*, **29**, (2), 231–48.

Roemer, M.I. (1961). Bed supply and hospital utilization—a 'natural' experiment. *Hospitals*, **35**, 36–42.

Szymanski, A. (1982). On the uses of disinformation to legitimize the revival of the cold war: health in the USSR. *International Journal of Health Services*, **12**, (3), 481–96.

WHO (World Health Organization) (1980, 1982). *World Health Statistics Annual*. WHO, Geneva.

World Bank (1984). *World Development Report* (1984). Oxford University Press, New York.

11. Integration of modules into a comprehensive model—a three-country example

In Chapter 10 we applied our model to multi-country comparisons using a small number of modules. Alternatively, we can compare a few countries on a broad basis using a larger number of modules. In Chapter 11, we shall explore the potential for the comparability over a broad range among three different representative health systems. We have chosen the Canadian health system as an example of a fully developed national health system. The Israeli health system is an example of a developed national health system which in some areas faces the problems of developing nations. The Nigerian health system is an example of the health system of a developing nation.

As described in Part I of this book, we begin our comparison with modules representing the resources available to the health systems. We continue the analysis with the comparison of health resources, and with the description of the process of care. Finally, we consider the outcomes of the health system and also general health outcomes.

Manpower aspects

Canada

Trends in health manpower in Canada show a gradual decrease over time in the rate of population per physician. The population per physician decreased from 636 in 1972 to 510 in 1983 and to only 467 in 1987. However, there are wide variations among Canadian provinces: in 1987, the rate ranged from 433: 1 in Quebec to 736: 1 in New Brunswick (Statistics Canada 1990). The causes for the growth of the physician population in Canada are due both to local graduation and to the immigration of physicians who graduated in foreign countries of which only a small proportion are Canadians (Barer *et al.* 1989). The balance between the supply of local and foreign graduates has changed over time. For example, in the middle 1970s, each year only 60 per cent of newly graduated physicians matriculated from local Canadian medical schools; by the middle 1980s, local schools accounted for 85 per cent of physician supply. In the future, this decrease in the proportion of immigrant physicians within the Canadian medical community may result in a more homegeneous health care in Canada. Because more physicians are likely to be Canadian graduates, a more uniform professional socialization is probable. In the age distribution of physicians in Canada, the relatively young are strongly represented with 50 per cent of the physicians younger than age 45. At the same time, 11 per cent of active physicians are beyond the retirement age of 65 (Woodward and Adams 1985). On the other hand, medicine is still a masculine profession in Canada, with only about 16 per cent female physicians.

In Canada, professional socialization still encourages physicians to retain community-based offices in the traditional model of family practitioners. It is thus not surprising that the ratio between generalists and specialists is relatively high. Canada has maintained roughly equal numbers of generalists and specialists and this ratio has not changed much over the recent years (Lomas and Barer 1986).

Nurses represent about two thirds of all human health resources in Canada. Nurses share a similar growth trend with the doctors. The population per nurse rate decreased between 1972 and 1983 from 129:1 to 114:1 and the figure for 1987 dropped to 107:1. However, unlike the trend for doctors, a shortage of nurses is still common in Canada, especially because one third of the nurses work part time (Statistics Canada 1990). Besides this, there are considerable geographical variations in nurse manpower availability: the rate is 123:1 in Newfoundland, and only 97:1 in Ontario. When considering health professionals other than physicians and nurses, the most remarkable change in resource availability is seen for dentists. Table 11.1 (p. 264) shows that between 1975 and 1983, there was a striking 23 per cent decrease in the rate of population per dentist. No comparable growth was recorded for any other health profession during such a short period.

Israel

According to the Israeli Ministry of Health (MOH 1990), between 1972 and 1983, Israel's manpower supply in the various health professions grew considerably. Table 11.1 shows that over that period, the population per physician decreased from 513:1 to 356:1. Generally, sources for an increase in physician manpower are the domestic production of physicians, the return of Israelis trained abroad, and emigration from Eastern Europe, and—to a lesser extent—from the American continents. While all these sources together contributed a net increase of some 500 physicians per year, the picture has been dramatically changed by the massive immigration of Soviet Jewry to Israel. Beginning in 1990, this wave of immigration brought with it a very high proportion of physicians. As Israel is already over supplied with physicians, the effects may be harsh.

Because a high percentage of physicians have been educated abroad, the professional background of physicians in Israel is extremely heterogeneous. Not only do immigrant physicians differ from locally-trained physicians

Table 11.1 Rates of per capita health manpower

	Canada[a]	Israel[b]	Nigeria[c,d]
Physicians	1:585 (1975)	1:513 (1972)	1:22 000 (1973)
	1:510 (1983)	1:356 (1983)	1:7700 (1982)
Dentists	1:2610 (1975)	1:2325 (1972)	1:10 500 (1985)
	1:2000 (1983)	1:1695 (1983)	
Nurses (all)	1:129 (1975)	1:403 (1972)	-
	1:114 (1983)	1:275 (1983)	1:1055 (1985)
Pharmacists		1:1820 (1972)	-
	1:1680 (1983)	1:1610 (1983)	1:19 000 (1985)

Sources: [a] Statistics Canada (1980)
[b] Ministry of Health, Israel (MOH 1990)
[c] Chuke (1988)
[d] Itayavyar (1988)

in their general and professional socialization, but their age structure is also different. Immigrant physicians are frequently older than local graduates (Ellencweig 1983). In general, physicians in Israel are relatively young with 53 per cent younger than age 45, and only 10 per cent are aged 65 or over. Physician manpower in Israel is also characterized by the relatively large proportion of female doctors, about one third (Central Bureau of Statistics 1987).

Israeli physicians are also characterized by a large proportion of specialist doctors. The desire of young Israeli physicians to become specialists comes from the professional socialization process in Israel. In this process is emphasized the superiority of the hospital-based specialists, over community-based doctors, as the most prestigious post in the medical hierarchy.

Nursing is a predominately female profession, and in Israel about 90 per cent of practicing nurses are women. The profession is also characterized by a relatively young age structure, with over 70 per cent of active nursing manpower below the age of 45. 55 per cent of the nurses in Israel are qualified registered nurses while 45 per cent are practical licensed nurses.

Like physician manpower, nursing manpower shows a similar trend of a nominal increase. For all types of nurses, including registered nurses, licensed practical nurses, and midwives, the rate of population per nurse decreased from 403:1 in 1972 to 275:1 in 1983. Despite this relative decrease in nursing manpower, the shortage of nurses remains a major issue on the national agenda. As a result of the heavy demands of modern hospitals, a substantial percentage of nursing manpower quit the profession. Other nurses who continue to work prefer to be in only part-time employment.

In Israel, the biggest jump in manpower availability is seen for dentists. Between 1972 and 1983 the rate of population per dentists decreased by 27 per cent. The dental profession may be so attractive, because unlike their peers in medicine and general surgery, dental surgeons benefit from a nearly free-market system in dental care.

Nigeria

The absolute number of health care professionals in Nigeria is far below that needed to provide appropriate health care for the population. Even so, in Nigeria there has also been a decrease in the rate of population per physician. The major vehicle of physician production in Nigeria is local medical schools. According to one source, the increase in the number of local medical schools, to 12 in 1985, reduced the population per physician rate from 22 000:1 in 1973 to 12 550:1 in 1980 (Chuke 1988). Other sources report a rate of 8330:1 population per physician in 1980 (Pearson 1986), and 7700:1 for 1982 (WHO 1988). Even so, about 35 per cent of Nigeria's physicians are foreigners. (Ityavyar, 1988).

Nursing personnel is scarce too. In 1980 the population per nurse rate was 3000:1 and the population per midwife was 3600:1. Dentists were even scarcer: 10 500 population to one dentist in 1985 (Chuke 1988). In general, manpower figures for Nigeria are typical for other developing countries also. In addition to the scarcity of manpower resources, inadequate collection of data makes basic indicators like the quantitative indicators on manpower unreliable and figures change from one source to another.

Cross-country comparisons

When we compare the health manpower module among these three countries, Canada and Israel are seen to be in a very similar condition. Over the last two decades there was a nominal increase in the manpower of all the medical professions in both countries, and there are signs of an oversupply in physician manpower. On the other hand, Nigeria lags far behind with an unacceptably low availability of health manpower. The trends across time, however, are reassuring (Table 11.1). Paradoxically, an increasing annual output of doctors from Nigerian medical schools in the early 1980s could not be met by an economic capacity to employ them. This caused the annual enrollment in local medical schools to drop again (Chuke 1988). On the other hand, as Benjamini *et al.* (1986) and Barer *et al.* (1989) note, both Canada and Israel are committed to full employment of physician manpower. Also, as will be shown later, in both countries the amount of public incomes available for physician reimbursement remains relatively constant. The immediate implication of these trends in employment and funding is that the steady increase in manpower must result in a decreasing per capita investment in each unit of manpower resource like physicians or nurses. In Israel, this development inevitably leads to labour unrest (Ellencweig 1987); in Canada, such labour unrest occurs less frequently, but may become more common in the future (Barer *et al.* 1989). In Israel the consequences are that the limited public resources force physicians to search for alternatives to supplement their income. One popular escape has been the development of a black market in medical care, recently described by the State Inquiry Commision on the Performance of the Health Sector as a 'widespread and dangerous phenomenon' (State of Israel 1990). Of course, because it is available to only a few, income from supplementary sources is unevenly distributed among physicians. The majority of physicians remain increasingly dissatisfied. This dangerous situation may also be found in Canada if the decreasing income per active physician will force some physicians to adopt black market strategies in the future. This would probably take the form of extra-billing, that is, the billing of patients by the doctor at his own discretion.

Before the enactment of the 1984 Canada Health Act, extra-billing was common. Physicians can no longer bill their patients because fees are now exclusively covered by the Government (Taylor 1986). However, as federal sources dwindle, some commentators believe that extra-billing is about to return (Law, personal communication). In fact, a new formula for the transfer of funds from the federal government to the provinces has reduced the federal contribution from 44.6 per cent of the total spent by provincial governments on health care in 1980 to only 36.7 per cent in 1990 (Iglehart 1990).

In Nigeria, where medical manpower is grossly undersupplied, the already scarce health personnel prefer to practice in the lucrative medical centres located in major cities (Federal Ministry of Economic Development 1975). This problematic trend exacerbates the imbalance within the health system. To solve the problem of this lack of adequate medical service in many areas, alternative health personnel, generally regarded as 'healers' are recruited. While these healers are involved in indigenous medicine, the WHO is attempting to train them to perform basic modern accepted medical techniques (Pearson 1986).

The only dissimilarities between Canada and Israel with respect to the personal characteristics of physicians are gender-related. At least in these two countries women physicians tend to carry lower work loads than male physicians (Barer and Ellencweig 1988). Thus, to some extent, the higher rate of females in medicine in Israel may offset the problem of the oversupply of physicians since an equal number of female doctors would fill fewer full-time equivalent positions than would their male colleagues.

Finally, quality assurance in manpower resources is most emphasized in Canada and least emphasized in Nigeria. In Canada, formal licensure to practice medicine is granted by the individual provinces but specialization is overseen by professional medical associations. However, the impetus for monitoring quality is provided by the by-laws of admission privileges. Because most doctors in Canada work as private practitioners, their access to hospital practice is determined by admission privileges. The specific rules and restrictions of these privileges create a positive and long lasting incentive for quality assurance. In Israel, licensure to practice by the Ministry of Health is mandatory. Specialty certification is issued by the Scientific Council of the Israel Medical Association upon successful completion of examinations. In spite of these two requirements, there is no follow-up procedure for ascertaining quality. Until 1988, even these two restricting measures were not in effect for the large mass of immigrant physicians who were automatically granted a license to practice medicine. As of April 1988, immigrant physicians have been required to pass qualifying examinations in order to practice medicine in Israel (MOH 1990). Nigeria has also set licensure mechanisms for several medical professions. Some of these mechanisms are regulated by federal law like the Medical and Dental Practitioners Act and the Nursing and Midwifery Registration Act (Chuke 1988). In addition, doctors trained overseas must pass an assessment examination. However, many other professions are not covered by this regulation, and currently there are no follow-up procedures to monitor the quality of health professionals already in practice.

Physical resources

Canada

In Canada, hospital services are provided by more than 1200 hospitals. In these hospitals there are some 176 000 beds which comes to about seven beds per 1000 population (Statistics Canada 1990). Nearly half of these are short-term medical and surgical beds, while about one quarter are designated for extended care. Beds in mental care facilities account for nine per cent of all beds. While an increase in the absolute number of beds is constantly reported, over the years the rate of bed per population has been kept relatively constant (WHO, 1983). The impetus for the maintenance of quality in the Canadian hospital system is due to a national voluntary accreditation agency.

Ambulatory services in Canada are generally provided by solo practitioners, and some of these also provide ancillary services like laboratory or X-ray services. On the other hand, except for the elderly and patients with chronic disease, pharmaceuticals are almost entirely distributed privately, through commercial pharmacies.

Israel

The total bed to population rate in Israel is about 6.15 beds per 1000 population. About 44 per cent of total beds are in the short-stay general sector. Long-term beds, including beds for extended care and rehabilitation, account for almost 30 per cent of the total, while beds for mental care account for 26 per cent. Over the years, there was a steady decline in the use of short-term general beds for which the rate declined from 3.3 per 1000 population in 1975 to some 2.7 per 1000 population in 1988 (MOH 1990). Primary care is provided mainly in health clinics, though there are also independent physician practices. Because operational definitions differ among health care providers, it is difficult to assess the exact number of community clinics. However, Kupat Holim, the largest provider/insurer in Israel, operates 1600 clinics which are located in nearly every settlement throughout the country. A special institutional feature in the Israeli health system is the specialized preventive family health centre. In 1988, there were nearly 1000 centres providing well child, pre- and post-natal care, and other kinds of personal preventive care (MOH 1990).

Nigeria

Hospitals in Nigeria are divided into two categories: tertiary care and secondary care institutions. The tertiary care institutions are generally university teaching hospitals and are located in several capitals of the 19 Nigerian states. In 1980, there were 9 such institutions with a total of 5700 beds. Secondary care hospitals including general, maternity, and armed forces hospitals, had an additional 67 800 beds, while specialized hospitals like mental, ophthalmic and orthopaedic hospitals had 4600 more beds (Pearson 1986). Their total bed per 1000 population rate was about 0.9 per 1000, of which, the overwhelming majority were short-term general beds. By international standards, the bed to population rate in Nigeria is still very low.

Primary care in Nigeria is based on health clinics and dispensaries. In 1980, there were approximately 3400 institutions of this kind in Nigeria (Pearson 1986). A significant amount of primary care is also provided by private practitioners.

Cross-comparisons of the physical resources module

In Chapter 4, we described the Rand Model for the qualitative aspects of physical resources. We then suggested that based on this model, health systems may be divided into four Regions. Considering the three countries described in this chapter, there is no doubt that the quality of physical resources in both Canada and Israel is adequate while Nigeria lags far behind. Over the last decade, the Israeli system was able to cut the number of short-term beds by almost 20 per cent. This suggests that some beds in some hospital services are frequently unnecessary, corresponding to Region IV of the Rand Model. Alternatively, it is possible that in particular services, some of the beds are only marginally used, corresponding to Region III of the Rand Model. We can draw the same conclusion for Canada where there are still about 20 per cent more short-term beds per capita than in

Israel. In both Israel and Canada there are standards for building hospitals and for capital investment in the health system. However, apart from construction, the Israeli Ministry of Health has no standardized procedures for assessing present or prospective technologies. Neither does it have sufficient financial leverage to effect decisions on the purchase of medical equipment (Ellencweig 1988).

In Canada, since hospitals are not reimbursed for capital investment, the acquisition of major medical equipment is constrained. Capital funds are available from the provincial governments which can decide whether or not to permit hospital expansion. Following our suggestion in Chapter 4, Canada can be ranked as a country for which there is adequate control over construction and the acquisition of medical equipment in the health sector. Nigeria, with a beds to population rate of less than 1 per 1000 is undoubtedly in Region I of the Rand model. In Region I, the increase in health status is linearly related to the acquisition of new equipment and technologies. The Nigerian health system still suffers from too few facilities and installations in both the hospital and the primary care sectors. There are varying levels of control over physical resources in Nigeria, such as better controls in the privileged tertiary hospital sector. For these academic institutions, taken over by the Federal Government, there are satisfactory policies for the planning of construction and for acquisition; for other hospitals and facilities the situation is more ambiguous. As a typical example of the lack of any appropriate control on the purchase of equipment we quote the Nigerian Minister of Health (Ransome-Kuti 1990) who describes the condition in recent years:

> Enormous quantities of sophisticated equipment were purchased, contrary to the principle of self-reliance and the concept of appropriate technology. Dental chairs, theatre equipment, and X-ray machines were supplied to health centres but could not be used.

Direct and indirect socio-economic development

In considering the socio-economic development for each of the three countries under study, we shall first examine the broader indirect effects and then turn to the more specific direct effects.

Canada

As shown in Table 11.2 (p. 271), Canada's demographic profile reflects the pattern of a developed country. Life expectancy at birth is 73.0 for males and 79.8 for females; the birth rate is 15.0 per 1000 population; and the infant mortality rate is 7.9 per 1000 live births. The population is predominantly urban. Individual achievement in Canada is high too: there is virtually no illiteracy, and unemployment is low. Canada is among the wealthiest countries in the world: in 1987 the per capita gross domestic product (GDP) was $US 17 200. In spite of this glowing report, Canada's wealth is inequitably distributed. In 1981, the highest 20 per cent of the households shared 40 per cent of the income, while the lowest 20 per cent shared only 5.3 per cent (World Bank 1988). These figures, almost identical to the US figures, place Canada in an unfavourable position among the industrial countries: France, Australia, and New Zealand are the only three countries which have a more inequitable income distribution.

In 1987, the share of health expenditure of the Canadian GDP was 8.6 per cent, significantly higher than the corresponding figure of 7.3 per cent for 1975 (OECD 1989). However, the rise in health expenditures was slower in Canada than in the US (Evans *et al.* 1989). When this information is translated into per capita expenditure through the use of purchasing-power parities, the 1987 level of per capita expenditures was increased to nearly $US 1500. For developed countries, this level of per capita expenditure on health is second only to that of the US. While health expenditure has grown, in the late 1980s its structure remained relatively similar to that of the 1960s. Institutional services account for 53 per cent of the health expenditure of which above 40 per cent is spent on hospitals. Professional services take 22 per cent of the total while pharmaceuticals account for another 12 per cent of the health expenditure. That the ratio of hospital costs to total health costs in Canada has remained stable over time is due to the strict controls imposed by provincial governments on hospitals. These controls encompass two dimensions:

(1) the approval and funding of hospital operative budgets;
(2) as previously mentioned, the lack of private capital markets for hospitals which depend exclusively on provincial agencies to support expansion or the replacement of major equipment.

A similar phenomenon prevails with respect to physicians' income. In Canada, physicians are practically all reimbursed by provincial governments on a fee-for-service schedule. Unlike physicians in the US, Canadian physicians were unable to raise their fees because the Government managed to constrain the fee schedules. In Canada, complex negotiations between the provincial ministries of health and the medical associations are held to regulate physicians' fees. This process provides the Government with enough leverage to affect considerably the demand for raises in the fee schedules (Evans *et al.* 1989).

According to the indicator of organizational development described in Chapter 5, the health sector structure in Canada can be defined as organized and developed. Its organization is based on a national health insurance programme provided separately by each province but similarly designed for all the provinces. The Provincial Ministries of Health assume full responsibility for the provision of health care and for the reimbursement of health care providers. Nearly all hospitals are public non-profit organizations, while as an autonomous group, physicians often enjoy an entrepreneurial position which maintains a collective agreement with the Government. Such collective agreements are subject to a uniform fee schedule, as mentioned above. In Chapter 4, we suggested that the percentage of total health expenditure spent by the public sector could be used as a proxy measure for the extent that a society values health. Using this proxy measure, we see that the public sector in Canada spends as much as 76 per cent of the total expenditure on health, indicating that the value placed by Canadian society on health is relatively high.

Israel

According to the demographic characteristics listed in Table 11.2, to a great extent, Israel can be considered a developed country. However, in 1987 for

Table 11.2 Characteristics of socio-economic development

Indirect	Canada[a,b]	Israel[a,c]	Nigeria[a,d]
Population (1987/8) (000's)	25652	4477	103 000
Annual population growth (1980–86)	1.1	1.7	3.3
Life expectancy (mid 1980s) (at age 0)			
Males	73.0	72.5	52
Females	79.8	75.5	52
Birth rate (1988) per 1000 population	15.0	22.6	45
GNP per capita (1986)	15 100	6200	370
GDP per capita	17 200	-	-
Health expenditure (percentage of public expenditure)	76	50	-
Adult literacy rate (1985) >14 years	99	94	43
Percentage of urbanization	77	90	30
Health expenditure (percentage of GNP)	9.7	7.7	-
Health expenditure per capita $US (1987)	1470	442	-

Sources: [a]World Bank Development Report (1988) Oxford University Press
[b]Statistics Canada
[c]Central Bureau of Statistics, Israel
[d]Chuke (1988)

example, the per capita GNP in Israel was only $US 6 800. This and its other economic characteristics place Israel in the World Bank's middle income category (World Bank 1988). In 1980, the income distribution in Israel was almost identical to that in Canada: the highest 20 per cent of Israeli households shared 39.9 per cent of the income, while the lowest 20 per cent shared only 6 per cent. Such a profile shows Canada to have one of the least equitable income distributions for high income countries (see above); but for the middle income category the distribution in Israel is among the most equitable (World Bank 1988).

According to our health structure indicator, the health care structure in Israel can be defined as intermediate to highly organized and developed. There are two reasons why Israel's health system is not classified as fully organized:

1. Israel's health system is based on membership in prepaid sick funds called 'Kupot Holim'; however, membership is not mandatory and both the enrollment and the extent of coverage are subject to restrictions imposed by the management of each individual sick fund.
2. Though some 96 per cent of the population are members of sick funds, insufficient coverage and sometimes unsatisfactory standards of care encouraged the development of a parallel system of private and semi-private medicine.

It is thus not surprising that only 50 per cent of the health expenditures in Israel is funded by the public sector. However, this does not mean that the private sector, *per se*, consumes the other half of the national health expenditure, because private funding also includes the costs of membership fees incurred by households and the costs incurred by employers for the health care of their employees.

Nigeria

Nigeria is the most populated country in Africa and is typical of a developing country. In 1988, as UNICEF (1990) reports, Nigeria's low life-expectancy was about 50, its very high infant mortality was about 105 per 1000 births, and birth rate was high (45 per 1000!). While currently the annual population growth is nearly 3.3 per cent in the first half of the 1980s the per capita increase in the GNP was only 1.9 per cent. When compared with that of other developing countries, this annual increase rate in GNP appears relatively high because Nigeria is a major oil exporter. However, the benefits of the economic growth were offset by the more rapid growth in population. This trend causes an actual decrease in GNP per capita, a phenomenon observed in many other countries of the developing world. (see also Chapter 10)

Nigeria is undergoing rapid social and economic changes. Over the last decades, the structure of the economy has been considerably altered with the emergence of industrial centres, especially in the oil industry. Urbanization is extremely rapid and the creation of a new proletariat in metropolitan areas has been accompanied by increasing urban unemployment (Bienen 1985).

The issue of income distribution in Nigeria is not as salient as it is in developed economies. This is because economic growth is more important to Nigerian society than distributional problems. This is partly due to the fact that inequity is not a class-based phenomenon in Nigeria, but it is rather based on geographical location and on ethnic traditions. The rural and the impoverished sectors are still relatively ignored and the existing wealth is highly divided among elites which are formed according to ethnic affiliations (Bienen 1985).

The health sector in Nigeria is decentralized with separate local ministries of health in each of the 19 states. These local ministries are responsible for both public health and for general hospitals. Federal responsibility is limited to the administration of tertiary care hospitals and to the implementation of national programmes in prevention and health education. Along with the public sector, there is a large private sector run by large companies for the health of their employees, by missionary organizations, or by independent practitioners. Thus, the system can be conveniently categorized as developing, with an intermediate level of organization. Note that the health care system in Nigeria also includes a strong indigenous component. In several areas, particularly the rural areas, traditional healers and village midwives take care of most health problems (Pearce 1986).

Cross-comparisons of the socio-economic development modules

According to both the direct and the indirect socio-economic development modules, Canada is more developed than Israel or Nigeria. Israel follows closely, while Nigeria is a typical example of a developing nation. The general societal indicators from both demographic and the socio-economic perspectives are very similar for Canada and Israel. However, an examination of the direct financial attributes and the structure of the health sectors reveals differences in terms of the per capita GNP: investment in health in Canada is nearly four times higher than in Israel. Obviously this difference does not entirely reflect the *real* investments in health, because labour and goods are presumably less expensive in Israel than in Canada. However, there is still no doubt that the real level of expenditure in Canada is far greater than that in Israel. The full extent of the gap between the two countries can be explained by more abundant resources in Canada, as already seen in the case of physical resources, or as will be described later, by higher accessibility to, and better quality of, care. An analysis of the full extent of the differences in the structure of the health sectors is also offered in the next section, where we discuss organizational issues of the health system.

Nigeria has neither the wealth of the two other countries nor their socio-economic status. In this developing country, the very existence of a modern health care system is still at stake. Not only does the health system face difficulties, but from the British colonial administration it also inherited the philosophy that the hospital, and not the rural and community health centres, is the cornerstone of the health system (Pearce 1986). Even supplying additional funds and transforming the structure of the health sector would not necessarily lead to the full westernization of the Nigerian health system. Instead, the Nigerian health system will probably develop in such a way that indigenous medicine will also play a major role (Pearce 1986).

The configuration and organization of the health system

Here we shall consider the organization of the health system (see Chapter 5). We shall examine only those elements of the organization and configuration which are comparable between Canada, Israel, and Nigeria.

Canada

In Canada, control in the health care system is seen in the federal–provincial system of hospital and medical insurance. By substantially contributing to each of the provincial governments, the Federal Government can influence the provincial health care systems. Nevertheless, the province is still the main vehicle for the provision of health care. The control of the health system by the provincial governments is also primarily financial, that is by hospital funding and collective reimbursement of physicians' fees.

Planning in the Canadian health care services is mainly decentralized and is a provincial concern. The planning process can be defined as 'partnership planning' as we described in Chapter 5. Partnership is reached through an equilibrium among the Federal Government, the provinces, and the health care providers. The major issues are public administration, comprehensiveness, universality, and accessibility. For these issues, the role of the Federal Government was never challenged by the provinces, but they always maintained their right to interpret federal guidelines (Evans 1988). Partnership planning between provinces and health care providers is reached by a complex process of collective bargaining including physicians and hospitals. Provincial governments have generally been more effective in using their financial leverage to implement their strategy in hospital expansion and capital investment than in controlling the physician market. Nevertheless, some degree of control has been exercised through negotiations on the structure of physicians' fee schedules. The control by provincial governments depends on regional parameters within provinces (Palley 1987). For example, the provincial government in Quebec has generally been more successful in controlling the physicians' demands than that in Ontario (Vayda and Deber 1984; Barer *et al.* 1988).

In summary, financially Canada's health system is fully supported while provincial governments control the reimbursement function but not the delivery of care. Canada's health system is thus a public health insurance system and not a public health service. Structurally it is fully decentralized. Because of this, and because the index of democratization, as defined in Chapter 5, is also very high, in Canada's health system, power is truly decentralized.

The next dimension of the organization of a health system which we shall consider is co-ordination and continuity. In many cases the inherent structure of the Canadian health care system guarantees vertical co-ordination. This kind of co-ordination is secured by the manner in which physicians may share an ambulatory practice and hospital privileges. Vertical co-ordination also implies that there is a fair degree of continuity within the system. Because a number of preventive activities like general medical screening, care in pregnancy, and immunization are performed by general practitioners, it is likely that there will also be horizontal co-ordination.

Regarding the next dimension, the organization of the work teams, the financial incentives for entrepreneurial practice, lead to the preponderance of solo practices. It is interesting that, though the ratio of physicians per capita is steadily increasing, there does not appear to be any competition to attract patients. Instead, physicians deal with the 'patient shortage' by sharing the patients among themselves. This is a feasible solution in Canada; a second opinion is always welcomed there, because specialists can see patients only upon referral from GPs, and because there is even a separate fee item for second opinions on the fee schedule (Evans *et al.* 1989).

We now turn to the dimension of appropriateness of care for which Canada's health system is well known. This can be shown by the full coverage of the population and by the well-balanced professional distribution of physicians in Canada where there are almost equal numbers of generalists and specialists. Finally, Canada's health system has a very sophisticated structural accountability in that all medical procedures are fully reported to the provincial ministries of health. Thus, at the provincial level, Canada has outstanding information systems based largely on the information collected for billing purposes. Consequently, Canada is internationally considered one of the top ranking countries with respect to the dissemination of information on its health care system. However, this rosy view is darker when regarding the quality of care. Though procedures are fully reported, their content remains unmonitored (Terris 1990).

Israel

In Israel the health system is controlled by the voluntary 'sick funds', by the Government, and by a variety of public non-profit institutions providing hospital care. Practically, the MOH has long been considered weak, exercising only a limited influence on the health system beyond the services that it owns outright (Ellencweig 1987). Thus, the sick funds enjoy considerable autonomy in deciding the extent of coverage and how individual providers will be financed and reimbursed. So it is not surprising that there is a plethora of methods for the reimbursement of individual providers in the health care system: salary, capitation, and even fee-for-service. In any case, most health employees are salaried, and wages are subject to an uneasy collective bargaining process between the health care providers and professional associations. Cost-containment policies dictated by the powerful Treasury impinge on the health labour force since the growing supply of health manpower in Israel cannot be complemented by a similar increase in financial resources. The clear consequences of this situation are seen in the continuous and serious unrest in labour relationships (Barer *et al.* 1989; Ellencweig 1987). In the light of these comments, it is not surprising that health care planning in Israel usually takes the form of 'partnership planning' in which all the principal actors in the health system participate: the Government, the sick funds, and the professional organizations.

The Israeli health care system is well known for its centralized structure. The headquarters of both the MOH and the sick funds assume major responsibilities in the decision-making process (Ellencweig 1983). Recently, however, it has been proposed that the system be restructured (State of Israel 1990). If this proposal is accepted, there may be extensive decentralization of responsibility and authority into five or six health regions.

For co-ordination and continuity of care, the picture is gloomy. In fact, there are two systems of medical care in Israel: ambulatory care and hospital-based care. These two systems are found side by side but they are not generally amalgamated. Hospital-based physicians are not only separated from their ambulatory care counterparts, but they also tend to ignore information conveyed to them by community-based practitioners (Ellencweig 1983; Barer *et al.* 1989). This lack of vertical co-ordination impinges on the continuity of care, as does the lack of horizontal co-ordination. Horizontal co-ordination is lacking both at the ambulatory level, where preventive and curative care are separate, and at the hospital level, where the flow of information among the various networks of hospitals is inadequate (Ellencweig 1983).

The Israeli health care system has a positive pattern for the dimension of the appropriateness of care. This is so because nearly all the population (96 per cent) is covered by the sick funds, and also, as seen in Table 11.1, (p. 264), because the ratio of health personnel per capita is appropriate by international standards. On the other hand, the issue of equity of care is questionable because the geographic distribution of health resources across the country is uneven. There may be differences of up to 30 per cent in the ratio of resources per capita for both manpower and facilities between the wealthier and the less privileged regions (Ellencweig and Grafstein 1989).

Accountability in the Israeli health care system is also unsatisfactory.

There is no viable information system for ambulatory care. Reporting on hospital care is adequate, but it is still very sluggish and uneven. When detailed reporting on hospital procedures is processed, as required by the Central Bureau of Statistics, the various hospitals report at different times. A clear example of this sluggish reporting is that the report on the details of hospital activity in 1983, including diagnoses, was published only in 1989 (Central Bureau of Statistics 1989).

Nigeria

The Nigerian health system may be classified as a model of partial intervention in the health care system by the federal or state governments. While public services are provided to a minority of the population, the majority remains beyond the reach of the public health system. This large sector of the population may be served by a parallel private system of care, by traditional care, or may be left to its own destiny (Pearson 1986). This lack of care is what Nigerian officials praise as 'self reliance' (Ransome-Kuti 1990).

Within a relatively narrow scope, the Federal Government has some financial and administrative leverage in determining the extent of employment in health care, and in making decisions on the construction of hospitals and the acquisition of medical equipment. In the non-government systems, physicians are largely reimbursed by the fee for service method. Fees are paid either by individuals or by large employers. Institutional reimbursement for private institutions is similar. For the large sector of voluntary institutions, particularly those registered with the Christian Health Association of Nigeria (CHAN), donations are an important source of funding.

In Nigeria there are a variety of planning styles. In 'central' or 'system' planning, principles are laid out by federal or state governments. These authorities issue general plans for predetermined time periods. More often 'individual' or 'no planning' situations prevail in which individuals or organized groups of employees must assume total responsibility for their own health. Central planning of health care by the Federal Government was included in the several national development plans in Nigeria launched since 1945. Only the third plan in 1975 seriously addressed the lack of infrastructure in primary health care. However, practically, the process of restructuring the system has been hindered by political and tribal rivalry between the federal and the state governments (Ransome-Kuti 1990). While efforts to carry out the central planning function were recently resumed, it is very doubtful whether co-operation between the federal and the state governments is possible given the array of fragile ethnic and state relationships in Nigeria. We can ask the same question about decentralization. While the health care system is formally decentralized, it is doubtful if the communication channels between federal and state authorities are effective. There is evidence that the Federal Government allocated more resources to areas in which it has a higher level of political support (Pearce 1986). Therefore, though the decentralization of the health system is formally accepted, practically, the Federal Government possesses both power and control (Jarmon 1988).

The plethora of health care agencies operating in Nigeria, the lack of insurance mechanisms, and the scarcity of data collection all impinge on the co-ordination within the system, on the appropriateness of care, and on the system's accountability. It is hard to achieve co-ordination because the Federal Government is neither able nor willing to supervise the provision of modern health care. In addition, Government certainly has little or no effect on traditional medicine. Appropriateness of care is undoubtedly insufficient, as seen by the low proportion of the population covered by modern health services, and the very low ratios of health professionals per capita. Appropriateness of care is also hampered by the focus on curative rather than preventive services in Nigeria (Chuke 1988). This trend impinges on the balance between the hospital sector and the community care sector. In Nigeria, where all health services are scarce, people still cry out for hospitals (Pearson 1985). Accountability, as perceived in developed countries, is simply nonexistent. In fact, health status indices are not reported to the WHO or to other international agencies. The only form of reliable information is based on occasional research or on surveys. As the Nigerian Minister of Health (Ransome-Kuti 1990) admits:

> Although Nigeria has no accurate data, publications from Nigerian Universities and surveys conducted by various government agencies provide a good picture of the state of people's health.

Finally, equity is seldom achieved while continuing and profound geographical disparities in health resources prevail. For instance, 44 per cent of the Nigerian population in northern Nigeria had only 27 per cent of hospital beds in 1980. The remaining 9 southern states had 73 per cent of hospital beds (Ityavyar 1988). In addition, urban–rural inequalities are considerable as the Federal Government admits (Federal Government of Nigeria 1982).

> . . . the distribution of health establishments is lopsided in favor of urban centers with just 20 % of the population and to the neglect of the rural areas where 80 % of the population resides. Even where in some cases dispensaries and maternity clinics are located in rural areas, services were unreliable as a result of shortage of drugs and personnel to run them regularly. An aspect of the access problem is that even in the areas supposedly covered, available health establishments for first level curative care are sometimes too far away from target population.

Cross-comparison of the configurational and organizational aspects

Canada and Israel may be regarded as welfare states. In both, Government assumes the responsibility for the provision of health care; but, also in the two countries, Government does not generally provide health care directly to the population. In both Canada and Israel, the principle of non-profit health insurance prevails. In both societies it is accepted that all its members should participate in the cost of health care, though only a few may benefit from it extensively. At this point, the similarity between the two countries ends. By and large, Canada has adopted a strategy of financing without organization. This strategy involves heavy regulation on the supply side but little involvement in the organization of care, which at least for the physician market is a fully entrepreneurial domain (Rodwin 1989). On the other hand, Israel has instituted complex bureaucratic structures for the organization of health care institutions owned by the Government or by the sick funds. These structures are highly centralized and permit little autonomy to local managements in regions or medical centres. By receiving substantial support from the Government, sick funds have managed to preserve their 'quotas' of health care. Thus, until recently, the pluralism of Israeli health care agencies did not impinge on the growth in competition. The ageing of the population and the rise in the standard of living have increased the demand for more health services of higher quality. This and the reductions in government support for health insurers have changed the picture, there is now more competition among providers as well as a booming private market in Israel.

This could also happen in Canada, if federal support to the provinces continues to shrink. There might be an impetus to reinstate some kind of private market, at least in the form of extra-billing (Law personal communication).

With regard to decentralization, both Canada and Nigeria are typical examples of a decentralized system. This can be objectively explained. Canada, the second largest country in the world, is so vast that it cannot be centrally governed. Nigeria is also large, and its population of over a hundred million include more than 250 different ethnic groups. These factors alone make it feasible to call them decentralized health systems. Above all, Canada and Nigeria are constitutional federations so that their health systems are primarily based on the full decentralization of administrative and legal functions. Decentralization by itself is not a recipe for success; sometimes decentralization can endanger co-ordination as is found in Nigeria, where there are no strong control mechanisms to offset conflicting local interests in the system. This did not happen in Canada because federal laws have helped to preserve a similar, though not identical, character for all provincial health insurance systems. This legislation, which took the form of a 'stick and carrot' policy, succeeded in providing the provinces with positive financial incentives to keep track of the principles laid by the Federal Government.

To conclude: in Canada, the level of health resources per capita is high, and there is no separation between the hospital and ambulatory sectors. This explains why Canada enjoys the most favourable conditions among the three countries. It is more difficult to judge whether Canadians or Israelis enjoy a more equitable level of health care. In both countries incomes are similarly and relatively inequitably distributed. In spite of this, in both countries there are health insurance schemes that formally dissociate the provision of health services from income levels. This alone does not guarantee equity because of the uneven distribution of health resources and there are considerable deficiencies both in the Canadian north or in the Israeli periphery.

Aspects of health care delivery

Canada

In Canada, the utilization of primary care services is within the acceptable range of utilization for developed countries. In 1987, it was 6.6 visits per capita per year. In 1973, it was 4.4 visits per capita per year (Statistics Canada, 1990), so there has been a considerable increase over 15 years. The ageing of the population and improved accessibility under national health insurance may explain part of this increment. It may also have been caused by the method of physician reimbursement, because fee-for-service offers physicians incentives to increase their patient loads. In any case, the average utilization figures for the entire population are misleading. Though the elderly are the highest users of health services, about 10 per cent of them do not see a doctor in any given full year (Ellencweig *et al.* 1990). In addition, because relatively few clients consume a substantial share of health care services, utilization is very skewed (Shapiro and Roos 1986). Considering the incentives to the physicians to increase the volume of medical procedures, the overall rate of utilization in Canada is actually relatively low.

Trends are less conclusive for the hospital sector where the admission rate to hospitals is 145 per 1000 population per year and has been nearly constant for several years (OECD 1989). In 1987, the total average length of stay for all kinds of health care institutions was 13.2 days per person per year – nearly similar to the rate a decade earlier (OECD 1989). However, variations occur in the average length of stay for specific disease categories. For example, the average length of stay for diseases of the circulatory system decreased from 24.5 days per person per year in 1980 to only 20.7 days per person per year in 1984 (OECD 1989). There are also many examples of the extensive use of medical procedures where no real need is apparent. For instance, rates of tonsillectomies in British Columbia and in Ontario were between ten and twenty times higher than the corresponding rates in Sweden and England where physicians are reimbursed by other methods than fee for service (Terris 1990).

Evaluated by the proxy measure of resources per capita, physical accessibility is high as also seen by focusing on the gatekeeping function of a primary care physician. Economic accessibility based on full coverage is high too, though comprehensiveness of care is incomplete. Neither dental care nor pharmaceuticals are covered by the regular health insurance plans. Social accessibility reflected by disputes over ethical issues have constantly shaken the Canadian health care system. For example, the issue of abortion is often brought before the public. In court cases, libertarian groups have frequently challenged the generally conservative stand of Canadian provincial and federal legislatures about free abortions (Goldberg and Mercer 1986, Chapter 3).

An overview of the indirect attributes of utilization in Canada shows that the rationing of utilization is common. In the hospital system, rationing is achieved by following a 'cash-limited' formula according to which negotiated budgets are set on the principle of cost plus. There is, however, an important qualification in this arrangement. Hospitals frequently run deficits which the Government covers for political reasons (Evans 1984) thus limiting the applicability of the 'cash-limit' formula. Through negotiations on the structure of the fee schedule physician reimbursement is also somewhat rationed, somewhat affecting their professional autonomy (Barer *et al.* 1988). Surprisingly, controls on expenditures do not include quality assessment, and the Canadian programme fails to monitor the quality of the process of care (Terris 1990).

Israel

According to an Israeli national health survey, in 1981 there were 12 visits to physicians per capita per year, a very high rate by international standards (Central Bureau of Statistics 1983). To understand the process of ambulatory health care delivery in Israel, we must consider the effect of large groups of immigrants, of which the most recent large wave is from the USSR. Frequent visits to physicians are encouraged by easy access to the physician's services, his role in social guidance, and his controlling influence over immigrant society (Ellencweig 1982).

Hospital care utilization in Israel shows patterns typical of industrialized countries. In 1988, there were 160 hospital admissions per capita per year, similar to the admission rates of a decade ago. The average length of stay in general hospitals was relatively short. In acute care hospitals, the average length of stay was 5.1 days per person per year in 1988, a decrease from 8.9 days per person per year in 1970. The decline in the average stay, as well as in total hospital days, can be explained by massive reduction in hospital beds which increased the pressures on physicians for early discharges.

We can summarize that there are opposite trends in physical accessibility in Israel. The excess physicians per capita makes ambulatory services highly accessible for frequent visits; however, the decline in the rate of general hospital beds, plus the relative scarcity of beds in the long-term, and rehabilitation wards, produce long waiting-queues for elective surgery and chronic care.

Economic accessibility is fairly good because except for dental care and long-term care the voluntary health care insurance plans marketed by the sick funds are comprehensive. Long-term care is covered by the Government following the Nursing Act Legislation of 1987, though a substantial share of the financial burden is still carried by individual households. Cost-containment policies in Israel were traditionally carried out on the supply side by the Government cutting resources. Programmes for the quality assurance of the process of care and serious efforts to control utilization are both rare. (Ellencweig 1988).

Nigeria

Little can be said about the quantitative utilization of health services in Nigeria. Because data is very scarce accessibility can only be evaluated crudely. With modern health care accessible to only one third of the population, economic accessibility is unsatisfactory. Physical accessibility is also minimal. As shown in Table 11.1 (p. 264), even for those enjoying a certain accessibility to health care, coverage is often limited to care by semi-professionals. For example, in northern Nigeria, the scarcity of nurses makes it necessary for Community Health Officers (CHOs) and Community Health Assistants (CHAs) to perform medical duties inappropriate to their training. In villages and other small communities, where even CHOs and CHAs are unavailable, other types of health workers predominate. These are primary health workers who are local residents who have received only a minimal training in basic health functions (Pearce 1986). Even in public hospital care, there is often limited accessibility to prescriptions, and patients would have to buy them privately (Ityavyar 1988). Social accessibility to health services in Nigeria, as measured by the acceptability by the population of health service usage, is also controversial. Many people would like to be treated by modern physicians, but they maintain the same expectations for the European trained doctor as they had for the traditional healer. Because they expect the physician to discover their problems by himself, they are unwilling to discuss their problems and complaints with him (Osuntokun 1985).

Cross-comparisons of delivery of care

While the demand for health services stems from unmet needs, the utilization of health services can be seen as satisfying this demand (Holland 1983). We have found that Canada, Israel, and Nigeria differ with respect to each of these components. We found that the highest level of perceived needs by the population is in Israel. This causes a high volume of initial physician contacts, because this is nearly the only process in the health care system for which the patients' choices have a role in creating demand. In Canada, the volume of initial contacts is lower, but it is rapidly increasing over time. This increase may be due to a 'physician-induced demand' where, to increase their incomes, Canadian physicians could transfer patients among themselves. This is particularly true since 1984 when extra-billing was legally abolished by the Canada Health Act. In Nigeria, there may be demand, or need, for modern medical services, but because resources are scarce and unevenly distributed, modern health care utilization is unlikely.

We turn now to the indirect modules of utilization. Canadian 'privileged' physicians enjoy the highest level of physician autonomy. Surprisingly, in this sense, Israel and Nigeria are quite similar. In the health system hierarchies of both countries, departmental divisions prevail in hospitals, and physicians are overworked. These structural patterns impinging on physician's autonomy is rooted in the British colonial tradition to which both these countries were exposed in their pre-independence days.

In all three countries, ethical and moral issues play a role in health system dynamics. In each of them, these issues are couched in a context specific to the country itself. In Canada and in Israel, ethical issues are subject to continuous public debate. Thus, the opinions of religious groups or those expressed through the mass media may substantially influence policy-makers' decisions. Issues like abortion, euthanasia, and autopsy have been discussed nationally for years. The solution to these problems must represent a delicate balance between the conservative and religious circles on the one hand, and the liberal circles on the other. In Israel, the Orthodox Jewish establishment is directly represented in parliament. This Orthodox block has traditionally had a powerful role in supporting the narrow coalition governments centred around either the left- or the right-wing parties (Yishai 1980). In Canada, there is a high proportion of Catholics, so the ethical issues of health care, as they impinge on religious problems, are of major concern to many people. Abortion in particular has become a divisive social issue. In several cities, attempts to open abortion clinics have sparked fierce controversy and legal action (Goldberg and Mercer 1986, Chapter 3). In Nigeria there is a military government and public opinion plays a minor role in any decision-making. In Nigeria, issues of ethics and morals are discussed only in relation to the process of the allocation of the scarce resources. In theory, 'the Government is determined to set in motion the process that will ensure that every Nigerian obtains the health services he or she needs, when and where they are needed . . .' (Ransome-Kuti 1990). In practice, past experience has shown that the tribal structure in Nigeria dictates that the areas best represented at the government level will receive most of the resources (Pearce 1986). This ensures that the rural sector continues to be relatively ignored (Bienen 1985).

Outcomes

Canada

As shown in Table 11.3, the mortality pattern in Canada is characterized by longevity, a low infant mortality rate, and the predominance of ischaemic heart disease. Malignant neoplasms and cerebrovascular disease are also leading causes of death. The improvement in overall health status in Canada has primarily been due to the drop in infant mortality rates which declined about 71 per cent between 1960 and 1985. A study of the changes in the rates of the leading causes of death over this period shows a slight increase in the effects of malignant neoplasms and a slight decrease in the incidence rates of circulatory diseases. The most dramatic increase was in female death rates due to lung cancer which nearly doubled between 1976 and 1986. The greatest decrease occurred for the death rate for cerebrovascular disease, which dropped by a third over the same period (Statistics Canada 1990). By international standards, the rates of notifiable infectious diseases in

Table 11.3 Comparison of health outcomes

	Canada	Israel	Nigeria
Infant Mortality rate (per 1000 live births)			
1960	27.3	27.2[a] (50.3)[b]	190
1985	7.9	7.7 (16.3)	120
Crude death rate (per 1000)			
1960	8	6	24
1985	7	7	15
Mortality rates per 100 000 Various causes (1986)			
Circulatory disease	314.0	300.0	
Cancer	187.4	142.0	
Pneumonia	23.8	17.7	
Infective and parasitic disease	4.2	14.0	
Accidents all	35.5	37.0	

[a] Jewish population [b] Non Jewish population

Sources: 1. Statistics Canada (1990) 2. *Health and Health Services in Israel* (MOH 1990) 3. *World Health Statistics Annual* (1988) 4. UNICEF (1990)

Canada are generally low. For example, the rate for tuberculosis declined from 21.2 cases per 100 000 population in 1971 to 7.7 cases per 100 000 population in 1987. Similarly, measles, pertussis, and polio, for which there are also effective immunization programmes, have nearly been eliminated. Of the sexually transmitted diseases, the rate of reported cases of gonococcal infection declined. However, the incidence of Acquired Immune Deficiency Syndrome (AIDS) has risen rapidly. By October 1988, there were 2118 cases reported in Canada (Statistics Canada 1990). Disability in Canada for the years 1983–84 was extensively studied in a nationwide survey (Statistics Canada 1986). Among individuals 15 years and older, 12.8 per cent reported some level of disability; this rate increased to 38.6 per cent for those aged 65 years or over.

In 1974, the Canadian Minister of Health, Marc Lalonde, issued a document in support of well-being (Lalonde 1974). Since then, Canada has been an international leader in promoting well-being. Lalonde argued that immediate action was necessary to improve environmental conditions and to change negative life styles. However, no major implementation programme by the Federal Government followed Lalonde's recommendation. In a second initiative in 1986, the Minister of National Health and Welfare recommended that Canada's health policy should emphasize disease prevention, self-care, and more equitable health services (Epp 1986). As yet, no major additional funding has been provided for supporting this recommendation (Spasoff 1990).

Regardless of policy options, the quantitative indicators show that the levels of well-being in Canada are satisfactory. For example, deaths caused by accidents are relatively low by Western standards. The daily per capita calorie supply is 129 per cent of that required. Cigarette smoking is declining: in the Canadian province of Alberta, for example, smokers in various age groups range only between 25 and 30 per cent of the population (*WHO Statistics Annual* 1989). However, alcohol-related problems are still a major social and health issue which contributes almost 1 per cent of hospital days throughout the country. On the other hand, public opinion in Canada is among the most alerted to environmental issues in the world, so the conservation of the physical environment is high on their agenda. The state of the psychological environment measured by suicide rates is also within acceptable range. Suicide rates are more unfavourable for males than for females. According to WHO (1989), in 1986, there were 22.1 deaths per 100 000 males while the corresponding figure for females was 6.2 per 100 000. These rates are nearly similar to the rates in the UK and the US and are lower than the corresponding rates in Scandinavia (44.6 deaths per 100 000 males in Finland) or in Eastern Europe (58.1 deaths per 100 000 males in Hungary!)

Israel

Mortality statistics in Israel follow the general trend for industrialized societies (MOH 1990). The major cause of death is ischaemic heart disease, but the leading causes of years of life lost are malignancies and accidents. Overall longevity is high. In 1986, life expectancy at birth was approximately 73 for males and 77 for females. From 1950 to 1954, the years of massive immigration from North Africa and Asia, mortality due to infectious diseases was very high, at 31 per 100 000 population. Massive preventive programmes in immunization and health education, and improved care in the community have been effective in lowering these rates so that by 1986 they were only 1 per 100 000 population (MOH 1990).

While the mortality patterns in Israel are similar to those of other industrialized countries, the incidence of morbidity due to infectious disease is still high. In particular, enteric infectious disease is a major problem in Israel. Bacillary dysentery, food poisoning, and viral hepatitis are still a great concern (MOH 1990). However, the incidence of infectious disease is unevenly spread among the population: the highest incidence rates are found for lower socio-economic classes in settlements inhabited mostly by immigrants from Asia–Africa and their descendants, and within the rural Arab minority (Ellencweig and Slater 1986). Immunization rates of children are satisfactory with a coverage rate approaching 90 per cent for measles, polio and, diptheria–pertussis–tetanus (DPT). These diseases have practically been eliminated by the policy of global immunization. A noteworthy exception is the 1988 outbreak of poliomyelitis in one district of central Israel. This outbreak resulted in 15 confirmed cases of polio and led to the unprecedented decision of the MOH to immunize the entire population of Israel under the age of 40 (Ellencweig 1989).

Data on disability among the Israeli population is provided by a recent survey by the Central Bureau of Statistics (1988). The results of this survey show that only 34 per cent of the population over the age of 65 are in need of additional help and only 10 per cent are restricted in their activities of daily living (ADL).

In Israel, there are opposing trends for indicators of well-being. Longevity, as a general standard for well-being, is high but the scores for lifestyle indicators are far less satisfactory. Though smoking rates in the population declined from 42 per cent in 1970 to only 30 per cent in 1987, smoking rates for females are still rising (Ministry of Health 1987). In 1987/8 casualties, including deaths, due to motor vehicle accidents were 514 per 100 000 population. This was an increase over the casualties rate of a decade earlier. But death rates themselves due to road accidents decreased from 18 per 100 000 population in 1970–79 to 12 per 100 000 population in 1987/8 (MOH 1990). On the other hand, alcohol and drug consumption in Israel are relatively low and are only a secondary problem for public health. Among the sexually transmitted diseases, AIDS is increasing, but its incidence is still far lower than in many other countries. By May 1989, a surprisingly low total of 79 cases had been recorded, of whom 50 have died (MOH 1990).

Nigeria

Like many other countries, Nigeria does not report mortality data regularly. In the absence of reliable detailed data on mortality, only crude figures are available. The estimate for infant mortality rate is 120 per 1000 live births, and the general crude death rate is 15 per 1000 population. Mortality data for Lagos, the federal capital, show that pneumonia and gastroenteritis are the leading causes of death (Chuke 1988). Morbidity figures are similarly scarce, but the frequent prevalence of several diseases is recognized. Tuberculosis is widespread in both rural areas and the urban slums, onchocerciasis is common in the north, and leprosy is found in some areas particularly in the eastern regions of the country (Pearson 1986). Government reports on the incidence rates of the top twenty major infectious diseases places malaria first followed by dysentery, measles, and pneumonia (Basic Health Service Programme 1976). Apart from the changes in the rates of infectious diseases, changing dietary habits and lifestyles have resulted in an increased prevalence of hypertension and diabetes. Another major problem in Nigeria is both childhood and adult anaemia. Childhood anaemia is caused by overall insufficient dietary intake and by genetic disorders. Adult anaemia, particularly in rural areas, is primarily due to widespread hookworm infestation.

Well-being indicators in Nigeria are low. Overall life expectancy at birth does not exceed 50 years. The daily calorie intake is only 90 per cent of the recommended standards (UNICEF 1990). There has been an increase in the use of alcohol and drugs (Obot 1990). Particularly in rural and semiurban areas, the water supply is inadequate and many dwellings have no modern sanitation facilities (Ityavyar 1988). Road traffic accidents are of special concern, and Nigeria leads the list of accident rates in the world. This peculiar situation for a developing country is the result of a combination of dangerous driving, an increase in car ownership, and poor vehicle maintenance (Pearson 1986).

Cross-comparisons of outcomes

When mortality is used as a basis for cross-comparisons, the health outcomes of both Canada and Israel are similar. When morbidity is used, the health outcomes of these two countries differ to some extent. When well-being indicators are examined, the two countries appear very different. Health outcomes in Nigeria, however, differ greatly from those in Canada and Israel no matter which indicator is used. This is not surprising because very poor health outcomes are the most striking characteristic of the health system in most developing countries.

The differences in the health outcomes in Canada and Israel enable us to divide health outcomes into two levels, 'traditional' and 'positive'. Each level corresponds to conditions prevailing in the two countries. 'Traditional' outcomes include the rates for mortality, morbidity, and disability. 'Positive' outcomes include well-being indicators relating to improvements in lifestyle and in the environment. We can divide health outcomes in this way because even though health systems in individual countries may have similar 'traditional' outcomes, they may still have different 'positive' outcomes. This is the case for Canada and Israel where the 'traditional' outcomes are nearly similar but where the 'positive' outcomes are not. These 'positive' outcomes can be divided into lifestyle indicators, like cessation of cigarette smoking, decrease in road accidents, and awareness of physical fitness, and into environmental indicators, like awareness of the levels of water and air pollution. Indicators for both lifestyle and environmental indicators score higher in Canada than in Israel. Because it is impossible actually to measure the overall effects of well-being, we cannot make quantitative cross-comparisons of this concept. Nevertheless, the division of health outcomes into 'traditional' and 'positive' health outcomes is still useful since it makes comparisons of health outcomes more sensitive to the differences between developed countries.

Issues of effectiveness, efficiency, and outcome-related quality

While, as already outlined in Chapter 8, it is hard to measure overall effectiveness of a health system, we can comment on the relative efficiency within each of the three health systems studied.

Canada

First we shall address the issue of allocative efficiency in Canada. In the late 1980s, the total cost of health care to the Canadian society was set at 9 per cent of the GNP. Of this sum, the public share was 76 per cent (Schieber and Poullier 1989). This level of the public expenditure in health care is much higher than that of the US (41 per cent) but lower than that of the UK and the Scandinavian countries (85–90 per cent). The public expenditure in Canada is lower than in the UK and in the Scandinavian countries mainly because in Canada generally neither dental care nor pharmaceuticals are publicly funded. While the cost component in the Canadian health system is clear, it is more difficult to assess its benefits. It would be easier to see if there are incentives to the health providers in the system to investigate alternative methods of care so as to improve health outcomes. Some commentators suggest that there are no such incentives in the 'financing without organization' health system of Canada. They suggest that instead, the system favours a 'status quo' in which providers are seeking to maximize their own profits under constraints imposed by the 'rules of the game' (Stoddard 1985; Rodwin 1989).

The dynamic efficiency of the health care system in Canada can be assessed by studying technology diffusion. For example, in a comparison of technology diffusion in Canada and the US, Rublee (1989) suggests that in the US there is an excess of innovative technology. Rublee reports that in the US there are nearly eight times more Magnetic Resonance Imaging (MRI) units and radiation therapy units per capita and six times more lithotripters than in Canada. Even so, an excess of health care technology may also be found in Canada. The electronic fetal monitor, for instance, is widely used for detecting fetal distress *in utero*, and a positive alarm is understood as a signal that birth by Caesarian section is necessary (Banta and Thacker 1979). However, the repeated incidence of false positive alarms has increased the use of Caesarian section, resulting in an increase in obstetricians' incomes (Evans 1984, Chapter 10). Surely, here there were no incentives for physicians to change their style of practice so as to use technologies more efficiently (Rodwin 1989).

Another issue in technology diffusion is the locus of care. With respect to the percentage of procedures until recently conducted in hospitals, Canada has a long way to go. In Ontario, for example, recent legislation has provided funding and regulation for diagnostic and treatment facilities located within the community (Fried 1990). This legislation can thus encourage patient care outside of hospitals.

Finally, we shall discuss managerial efficiency based on cost-effectiveness analysis. As mentioned previously, it is difficult to make a systems' analysis of effectiveness. Instead, we can measure effectiveness by using a 'tracer' condition like life expectancy at birth. On the one hand, as measured by this proxy condition, Canada has a high level of 'effectiveness' because life expectancy at birth is among the longest in developed countries. On the other hand, from a perspective of the costs of health care to society, Canada is in an intermediate position among the industrialized countries. Consequently, managerial efficiency in Canada is not too high because its high 'effectiveness' is achieved at a relatively high level of cost of health care.

Israel

In Israel, health care expenditure is less than 7.5 per cent of the national GNP – among the lowest for developed countries. The public expenditure on health care is not more than 50 per cent, also relatively low by Western standards. This relatively low level of public expenditure in the Israeli health system may be explained by a number of factors. These include:

1. Individual households contribute substantially to the cost of health care by paying membership fees in sick funds and health care co-payments.
2. There is a massive contribution by employers for employees' benefits.
3. An increasing share of health care is provided by the private market (Rosen 1989).

Dynamic efficiency in Israel is characterized by the inability of the MOH to control the proliferation of modern technology. The MOH has no standardized procedures for assessing prospective or existing technologies. Also, the MOH has only limited influence on the allocation of capital investment in health care. This limits the role of government in improving the efficiency of the health care process (Ellencweig 1988).

We can use life expectancy at birth as a tracer condition for the effectiveness of the health care delivery system. Because in Israel life expectancy at birth scores high and the cost of health care to society is relatively low, the resulting level of managerial efficiency is among the highest in industrialized countries. However, since there is no appropriate system for monitoring the quality of health outcomes in Israel, perhaps this high level of managerial efficiency is negated by an inadequate quality of health outcomes.

Nigeria

The lack of relevant data precludes a serious analysis of the effectiveness and efficiency of the health system in Nigeria.

Cross-comparisons of effectiveness and efficiency

Managerial efficiency is better in Israel than in Canada. For nearly similar health outcomes Israel's financial input in the health system is much lower. However, this explanation appears too simplistic when we consider the quality of health outcomes in our definition of effectiveness. While it is not possible to quantify the outcome-related quality component, there are signs that the quality of the health system outcomes in Canada is better than in Israel. These signs are seen for both 'traditional' and 'positive' indicators. Particularly with respect to communicable and infectious diseases, in Canada there are better outcomes for morbidity indicators than in Israel. The outcomes for well-being indicators are also higher in Canada as shown above. Satisfaction with the health system is another important dimension in the evaluation of the health system outcomes. The extent of public support for the health system in Canada is high, as seen in a recent comparative study of satisfaction with the health systems of Canada, the UK, and the US, as we will discuss later in chapter 12 (Blendon and Taylor 1989). In Israel, satisfaction with the health care system is much lower, especially in reference to the performance of the major health insurers (Pizam and Newman 1975).

Conclusion

The aim of the analysis presented in this chapter is twofold:

(1) to provide a thorough analysis of the health systems in Canada, Israel, and Nigeria;

(2) to illustrate the application of the modular approach.

In this chapter we showed that the modular approach can be used to compare individual health systems. The structured analysis used here provides a plausible framework for the analysis of three countries whose health systems differ to a large extent. Comparing modules separately enabled us to concentrate on relevant issues within and between countries. This also reduced the danger of diverting the discussion when several issues are compared simultaneously. Another benefit of the modular approach for this type of comparison is that lack of information need not hamper our cross-comparisons. When data on a certain indicator within a given module is missing, data on other indicators within the same module can be used in their place, thus compensating for the lack of information.

References

Banta, H.D. and Thacker, S.B. (1979). *Costs and benefits of electronic fetal monitoring: a review of the literature*, National Centre for Health Services Research, PHS 79-3245. Department of Health Education and Welfare, Washington, DC.

Barer, M.L. and Ellencweig, A.Y. (1988). Physician workload and their life cycle. Unpublished results.

Barer, M.L., Evans, R.G., and Labelle, R.J. (1988). Fee controls as cost controls: tales from the frozen north. *The Milbank Quarterly*, **61**, (1), 1-64.

Barer, M.L., Gafni, A., and Lomas, J. (1989). Accommodating rapid growth in physician supply: lessons from Israel, warnings for Canada. *International Journal of Health Services*, **19**, (1), 95-115.

Basic Health Service Programme of the Federal Republic of Nigeria (1976). *Report of the Project Formulation Team*. Federal Ministry of Health, Lagos.

Benjamini, Y.A., Gafni, A., and Blankett, J. (1986). The Israeli physician's strike: an inevitable outcome of the structure of Israel's health care system. *Journal of Collective Negotiations in the Public Sector*, **15**, (3), 211-22.

Bienen, H. (1985). *Political conflict and economic change in Nigeria*. Frank Cass, London.

Blendon, R.J. and Taylor, H. (1989). Views of health care: public opinion in three nations. *Health Affairs*, **8**, 149-57.

Central Bureau of Statistics (CBS) (1983). *Use of health services survey 1981*, Special Series No. 717. Jerusalem.

Central Bureau of Statistics, CBS (1987). *Labour force – data from sample emuneration, 1983 Census of Population*, Publication No. 13. Jerusalem.

Central Bureau of Statistics (CBS) (1988). *Selected characteristics of persons aged 60 and over*, Special Series No. 840. Jerusalem.

Central Bureau of Statistics (CBS) (1989). *Hospitalizations, 1983*, Special Publications Series No. 867. Jerusalem.

Chuke, P. O. (1988). Nigeria. In *The International Handbook of health care systems* (ed. R. B. Saltman). Greenwood Press, New York.

Ellencweig, A. Y. (1982). Patterns of utilization of medical services in Israel in comparison to other countries: physician-patient contacts. *Social Security*, **23**, 90–9 (Hebrew; summary in English).

Ellencweig, A. Y. (1983). The new Israeli health care reform: an analysis of a national need. *Journal of Health Politics, Policy and Law*, **8**, (2), 366–86.

Ellencweig, A. Y. (1987). Modern dilemmas in health care – an analysis of the Israeli doctors' strike. *Industrial Relations Journal*, **15**, 117–29.

Ellencweig, A. Y. (1988). Development of medical care technology, the case of Israel. *International Journal of Technology Assessment in Health Care*, **4**, 255–67.

Ellencweig, A. Y. (1989). The polio epidemic in Israel: an analysis and consequences. *Health Policy*, **13**, 177–88.

Ellencweig, A. Y. and Grafstein, O. (1989). Inequities in health – the case of Israel. *Israel Journal of Medical Sciences*, **25**, 27–32.

Ellencweig, A. Y. and Slater, P. E. (1986). Factors affecting hospitalization for selected diseases in Israel. *Israel Journal of Medical Sciences*, **22**, 417–25.

Ellencweig, A. Y., Stark, A. J., Pagllicia, N., McCashin, B. and Tourigny, A. (1990). The effect of admission to long-term care program on utilization of health services by the elderly in British Columbia. *European Journal of Epidemiology*, **6**, (2), 175–83.

Epp, J. (1986). *Achieving health for all: a framework for health promotion*. Ministry of Supply and Service, Ottawa.

Evans, R. G. (1984). *Strained mercy, the economics of Canadian health care*. Butterworths, Toronto.

Evans, R. G. (1988). We'll take care of it for you: health care in the Canadian community. *Daedalus*, **117**, (4), 155–89.

Evans, R. G., Lomas, J. L., Barer, M. L., Labelle, R. J., Fooks, C., Stoddart, G. L. *et al.* (1989). Controlling health expenditures – the Canadian reality. *New England Journal of Medicine*, **320**, (9), 571–7.

Federal Government of Nigeria (1982). *The Fourth National Development Plan*, p. 276. Federal Government, Lagos.

Federal Ministry of Economic Development (1975). *Nigeria – Third National Development Plan 1975–1980*, p. 263. Federal Government, Lagos.

Fried, B. J. (1990). *Finding a course for Canada's health services system*; Presentation at the Conference on 'Public Sector in Turbulence', December. Jerusalem, Israel.

Goldberg, M. A. and Mercer, J. (1986). *The Myth of the North American City*, Chapter 3. UBC Press, Vancouver.

Holland, W. W. (1983). *Evaluation of health care*, Chapter 1. Oxford University Press, Oxford.

Iglehart, J. K. (1990). Canada's health system faces its problems. *New England Journal of Medicine*, **322**, 562–8.

Ityavyar, D. A. (1988). Health service inequalities in Nigeria. *Social Science and Medicine*, **27**, (11), 1223–35.

Jarmon, C. (1988). Nigeria – *reorganization and development since the mid Twentieth Century*, Chapter 1. E. J. Brill, Leiden.

Lalonde, M. (1974). *A new perspective on the health of Canadians*. Government of Canada, Ottawa.

Law, M.M. (1990). Formerly deputy Minister of Health of Canada, Personal communication.

Lomas, J. and Barer, M.L. (1986). And who shall represent the public interest? The legacy of Canadian health manpower policy. In *Medicare at maturity* (ed. R.G. Evans and G.L. Stoddart). Management Studies Program, the Banff Centre, Banff, Alberta.

MOH (Ministry of Health) (1987). *Aspects of cigarette smoking*. Department of Health Education, Jerusalem.

MOH (Ministry of Health) (1990). *Health and health services in Israel 1990*. State of Israel, Jerusalem.

Obot, I.S. (1990). Substance abuse, health and social welfare in Africa: an analysis of the Nigerian experience. *Social Science and Medicine*, **31**, (6), 699–704.

OECD (Organization for Economic Co-operation and Development) Secretariat (1989). Health care expenditure and other data. *Health Care Financing Review*, Annual Supplement, pp. 111–94.

Osuntokun, B.O. (1985). Traditional beliefs in Africa and their interaction with modern ideas and beliefs: implications for health policies. In *Health policy, ethics and human values* (ed. J. Bankowski and J.H. Bryant). CIOMS, Geneva.

Palley, H.A. (1987). Canadian federalism and the Canadian health care program: a comparison of Ontario and Quebec. *International Journal of Health Services*, **17**, (9), 596–616.

Pearce, T.O. (1986). Social change and the modernization of the medical sector. In *Social change in Nigeria* (ed. S. Afonja and T.O. Pearce). Longman, Essex.

Pearson, C.A. (1985). The role of hospitals in community health. In *Principles and practice of community health in Africa* (ed. G.O. Sofolune and F.J. Bennett). University Press Limited, Ibadan.

Pearson, C.H. (1986). Nigeria. In *Primary health care 2000*. (ed. J. Fry and J.C. Hasler). Churchill Livingstone, Edinburgh.

Pizam, A. and Newman, Y. (1975). Measurement of satisfaction with ambulatory medical service in Israel. *Business Economics Quarterly*, **2**, 41–52.

Ransome-Kuti, O. (1990). Nigeria: developing the primary health care system. In *Achieving health for all by the year 2000. Midway reports of country experiences* (ed. E. Tarimo and A. Creese). World Health Organization, Geneva.

Rodwin, V.G. (1989). New ideas for health policy in France, Canada and Britain. In *Success and crisis in national health systems: a comparative approach* (ed. M. Field). Chapter 9. Routledge, New York.

Rosen, B. (1989). *The public-private mix in the Israeli health care*, RR-13-89. Brookdale Institute of Gerontology and Adult Human Development, Jerusalem.

Rublee, D.A. (1989). Medical technology in Canada, Germany and the United States. *Health Affairs*, **8**, (3), 178–81.

Schieber, G.J. and Poullier, J.P. (1989). International health care expenditure trends 1987. *Health Affairs*, **8**, (3), 169–77.

Shapiro, E. and Roos, N.P. (1986). High users of hospital days. *Canadian Journal on Aging*, **5**, 165–74.

Spasoff, R.A. (1990). Current trends in Canadian health care: disease prevention and health promotion. *Journal of Public Health Policy*, **11**, (2), 161–8.

State of Israel (1990). Report: *The majority view. The State Committee on the Operation and the Effectiveness of the Israeli Health Care System*. Government Printing House, Jerusalem (Hebrew).

Statistics Canada (1986). *Report of the Canadian Health and Disability Survey, 1983–4*, Catalogue 82-555, Ottawa.

Statistics Canada (1990). Health. *Canada Year Book 1990*, Chapter 3. Ottawa.

Stoddard, G. (1985). Rationalizing health care. In *Ottawa and the provinces: the distribution of money and power* (ed. T. Courchene, D. Conklin and G. Cook). Ontario Economic Council Conference, Toronto.

Taylor, M. G. (1986). The Canadian health system 1974–1984. In *Medicine at maturity* (ed. R. G. Evans and G. L. Stoddart). Management Studies Program, The Banff Centre, Banff.

Terris, M. (1990). Lessons from Canada's health program. *Journal of Public Health Policy*, **11**, (2), 151–60.

UNICEF (United Nations Children's Fund) (1990). *The state of the world's children 1990*. Oxford University Press, Oxford.

Vayda, E. and Deber, R. B. (1984). The Canadian health care system: an overview. *Social Science and Medicine*, **18**, (3), 191–7.

Woodward, C. and Adams, O. (1985). Physician resource databank: numbers, distribution and activities of Canada's physicians. *Canadian Medical Association Journal*, **132**, 1175–86.

World Bank (1988). *World Development Report* 1988. Oxford University Press, New York.

WHO (World Health Organization) (1983, 1988). *World Health Statistics Annual*. WHO, Geneva.

World Health Statistics Annual (1989). *The WHO Monica Project, a world wide monitoring system for cardiovascular diseases*. WHO, Geneva.

Yishai, Y. (1980). Health policy and religion: conflict and accommodation in Israeli politics. *Journal of Health Politics, Policy and Law*, **5**, 431–46.

12. A modular approach to competitive reform in health systems

David Chinitz*

Introduction

In Chapters 10 and 11 we used the modular approach to compare health systems in two ways. In one, we dealt with countries which are similar over several modules while diverging widely in one module. In the other, we based our comparison on a larger array of modules, attempting to characterize health systems more completely. For both approaches, we assumed that each module shares the same content validity across various countries.

In this chapter, we shall weigh the usefulness of the modular approach in cases where we cannot be certain that a given module has the same meaning across different systems. We shall focus on change in health systems, in particular on the introduction of increased competition in health care finance and delivery. We hypothesize that within each module the phrase 'increased reliance on competition', varies in its meaning across systems.

One of the most far-reaching changes that can take place in a health system is, of course, reform. Reform is the conscious effort on the part of a country or government to change the basic nature of its health system. The impetus for reform usually comes from significant dissatisfaction on the part of policy-makers, providers, and especially the public, with the performance of the system in processing inputs and producing outputs. Understanding health system reform demands simultaneous attention to changes taking place in several input, process, and output modules.

Today, many countries are considering health system reform. A common theme is the introduction of competitive markets as the primary mode of health system organization. Perhaps this is due to the fact that, aside from the the health system in the US, most health systems in developed countries are based on social solidarity and collective provision of care. In such countries, health care is not a good mediated in the so-called free market. Instead, governments dominate the planning and sometimes even the operation of the health care system, seeking to ensure that access is based on need and

*Research Associate and Instructor, Hebrew University School of Public Health, and Senior Researcher, JDC-Brookdale Institute, Jerusalem, Israel.

not on one's ability to pay. In recent years, many welfare states have come under financial pressure resulting in reductions in funding for social programmes including health. But, as medical technology provides a never-ending stream of new and expensive treatments and diagnostic techniques, such public systems are also subject to the pressure of increasing demands from patients and, perhaps even more so, from their physicians. Privatization, competition, and reliance on market forces are sometimes seen as having the potential to increase efficiency of health systems, to obtain additional revenues from private sources, or both (Maynard 1986).

For example, the health care systems in the Netherlands, Sweden, and the UK are all highly socialized (van de Ven 1988; HMSO 1989; Saltman and von Otter 1990; Ham *et al.* 1990). In all three countries, the Governments are considering introducing competition as a way of making the health systems more efficient and responsive to consumer demands. Even the Canadian health care system is subject to such pressures. By eliminating the rights of physicians to bill patients in addition to receiving public reimbursement, Canada has made an explicit policy out of limiting the extent of the private health care sector. But in some of the Canadian provinces there is talk of reintroducing private medicine (Iglehart 1990). In the US the directors of public programmes like Medicare are experimenting with the use of competition, carefully managed and regulated by the Government, as a framework for supplying health care services to their target populations.

A common by-product of health system reform is the tendency to look outside the system for ideas and solutions. Indeed, this is one of the most important reasons for engaging in the type of international comparisons we have been discussing in this book. The US health system is widely perceived as highly competitive. Health administrators and policy analysts in several countries including Israel and the UK have consulted the literature and experts in the US on the do's and don'ts of competitive health care (Bevan and Brazier 1987; Enthoven 1987; State of Israel 1990).

This is where our modular approach comes into play. Though many health policy analysts and decision-makers acknowledge the difficulties and dangers of simply adopting aspects of health systems from one country into another, they seldom act on this awareness systematically. By evaluating the introduction of competition in the context of each of the modules, we can better assess the implications of its introduction into any given health system. Using the modular approach may also help us to explain why an idea which seems so compelling to individuals in one country is unacceptable in another.

After briefly introducing the notion of competition, we shall consider the role competition plays, or could play, with regard to several of the modules in various health systems. We shall deal with:

(1) health care inputs (physician manpower and the professional attributes of physicians);
(2) 'needs' (expectations from the health system and the problem of the adverse selection of health insurance clients);
(3) organization of the health system (market structure);
(4) systems outputs (consumer satisfaction and the percentage of the GNP devoted to health care).

We shall close with some concluding remarks.

What is competition?

Especially in countries accustomed to socialized health systems, speaking about competition in health care evokes strong, sometimes emotional, responses. Competition is often confused with privatization, which conjures up the image of expensive private health services available only to the rich and powerful.

Perhaps the best definition of competition in health care, or in any field, is the decentralization of decision-making through the use of a price system (Hayek 1945). The price system is essentially a set of signals which consumers and producers can use for making decisions. Prices transmit information about the relative supply of, and demand for, different goods and services.

Economists often speak about competition in the context of different types of ideal markets. In a perfectly competitive market, economic agents are price-takers, none is large enough to determine prices on his own. In addition, all agents have equal and complete information about prices and the quality of all goods and services. In such a situation, no supplier is able to sell his goods above the market price. Moreover, the fear of losing customers through competition from existing competitors, or of losing to new ones who are free to enter the market, drives prices down and encourages producers to produce efficiently. Producers seek to keep the costs of production at or below market prices.

Economists recognize that these conditions for a perfectly competitive market are usually lacking. Information flow is not always smooth and not all the economic agents possess the same amounts of information for any given transaction. Prices do not always reflect the minimum costs of production. Some markets have relatively few agents, consumers, or producers, and this violates the 'price taking' assumptions of the perfectly competitive market.

Non-perfectly competitive markets are still more decentralized decision-making mechanisms than, say, government control and central planning. For example, a government may rely on political or legislative processes to decide what its contribution to the health system will be. The Government can implement that decision by allocating its financial contribution through a centrally planned government-owned organization like a national health service. Or, alternatively, it can distribute its contribution to consumers who can then use the monies to purchase health care services in the market. The health care providers may be private for-profit enterprises, non-profit organizations, or government-owned institutions.

Even including the US, no health system is based only on competition in the market place without any government intervention. Market-mediated health care transactions are problematic due to the asymmetry of information among the providers, consumers, and financers of medical care. If it is in their interest to do so, physicians can convince patients to undergo treatment which may be unnecessary (Arrow 1963). Insurance companies are interested in avoiding clients who constitute bad risks. Governments can restrain competition by monitoring the utilization of physicians, imposing limits on the purchase of medical technologies, controlling capital investment in health care facilities, licensing of medical manpower, and limiting physician pay scales.

Applying our modular approach is useful for understanding and evaluating the current and possible mix of market vs. centrally-planned government mechanisms for health service delivery in any given country. A separate analysis of each module can illuminate aspects of health care competition sometimes overlooked and usually not addressed systematically by health care analysts.

Competition and the resources at the system's command: physician manpower and professional attributes ('I never met a physician I didn't like!')

Frequently, manpower supply is not the central focus of pro-competitive health policy analysts (Enthoven and Kronick 1989; Iglehart 1990). This may be because the proponents of competition assume that the supply and behaviour of physicians and other health personnel will somehow respond predictably to the rigour of market forces. But the manpower available and the personal and professional attributes of physician manpower in a health system can heavily influence any attempt to introduce competition.

In Chapter 4 we discussed the issues involved in making cross-national comparisons of the manpower at the disposal of health systems. For example, comparing the rates of physicians per unit population across several countries gives only a very rudimentary assessment of where a given country stands on this most basic of health system inputs. To give an idea of how the health manpower resources of one system really compare with those of others, the basic rate of physicians per unit population must be supplemented with information on geographical dispersion, income levels, backgrounds and personal attributes. We shall apply this comparative approach to the problem of competition in health care delivery.

The implications of competition in the delivery of health care services vary for countries with different levels of manpower resources. Consider a system with a large number of physicians per capita: we might expect that, according to the law of supply and demand, an increase in competition would cause the reduction of the relative income level of physicians. Over time, perhaps even the absolute number of physicians might be reduced because fewer individuals would be willing to work for the lower wage determined by the market.

This picture is too simple. Health is not the typical economic good of the competitive model discussed above. What is special about health is that the supplier, in this case the physician, has a strong influence over the demand for his services. This is one explanation for the phenomenon of the simultaneous increases in the rate of physicians per population and the average physician workload. For example, Canadian health economists have documented the increases in physician contacts per capita population as the number of physicians rises. In Canada, strict controls of physician fees have been implemented to contain the increased expenditures resulting from the increase in physician contacts per capita (Barer *et al.* 1988).

Past government policies, like those pursued in the US during the first part of this century (Starr 1982), were intended to increase the availability and geographical dispersion of physicians: such policies limit the power of the market to ration the number of physicians and their income. Firmly-established university medical schools and other medical education programmes do not simply disappear just because physicians seem to be numerous. In Israel we see a good example of the problem of constraining the supply of physician manpower. Israel has one of the highest physician per unit population rates in the world. It also has a very high rate of medical schools per unit population. In addition, as we have mentioned in Chapter 11, to exacerbate the situation there has been an influx of thousands of physicians arriving in the recent wave of immigration from the Soviet Union: in the first wave of 100 000 immigrants there were estimated to be about 2900 physicians (Haaretz 1990)! Early arrivals in the present wave of immigration were all offered a free course to prepare them for the state medical licensing exam. It is difficult to deny them licensure. And there is no explicit government policy limiting the number of licensed physicians in the country. In any event, it seems clear that many Soviet immigrant physicians may be forced out of the profession. How an increasingly market-oriented system will affect this problem of physician oversupply in Israel remains to be seen.

In the US, health maintenance organizations (HMOs) and other managed health care organizations have apparently had enough of an impact on the level of physicians' incomes and on their working conditions to cause a downward trend in the number of applicants to medical schools (Altman and Rosenthal 1990). There are still enough applicants for medical schools to fill all of the available slots, but the number of applicants for each position has dropped (Greenberg 1990). It seems that physicians believe that managed health care will result in lowered physician incomes and reduced professional autonomy (Schulz *et al.* 1990). In Canada, on the other hand, despite government control over health budgets, the supply of physicians has remained constant. As we have mentioned, this may be because until now physicians practicing in the autonomous fee-for-service framework of Canadian Medicare have been able to maintain their relative income position (Evans *et al.* 1989; Iglehart 1990).

Physician oversupply does not always have a positive impact on indicators like availability of service, queues for elective procedures, or adequacy of the process of care. In Israel, for example, the rate of physicians per unit population is high, but physician availability and access are still problematic. Hospital budgets are not sufficient to permit the use of operating theatres for more than one shift daily. Physician wage agreements stipulate that official hospital and clinic working hours be terminated in the early afternoon. There are long queues for many elective procedures in Israel. Some physicians engage in various forms of private practice in the afternoon, which provides additional access only to those who can pay the price (State of Israel 1990). Thus, though physicians are numerous, the health system behaves as though they are scarce. In Chapter 4 we discussed the Rand curve which is a graphical representation of the returns, in terms of health outcomes, to varying levels of health inputs. The curve is divided into four areas:

I increasing returns;

II diminishing returns;

III a state of no further positive returns;

IV negative returns.

In Israel, it seems that the relationship between the physician manpower as an input and health outcomes has reached area III, or perhaps even IV, of the Rand curve. In terms of the Rand curve, the level of physician input has therefore risen beyond the point of diminishing returns, to the area of zero or negative returns.

Whether or not an oversupply of physicians can be made advantageous by introducing competition depends on the organization of the rest of a given health system and on the professional attributes of the physicians in it. Regarding the organization of care, for example, if there is third party insurance and neither the physician nor the patient bears most of the cost of medical care, an oversupply of physicians will not necessarily lead to increased physician access or to lower physician wages. Physicians who are not cost-conscious will, *ceteris paribus*, expend greater amounts of resources on each patient treated, thereby reducing access for others. Physicians can also increase their wages by creating demand and increasing service levels.

Similarly, the attitude of physicians toward their profession is likely to impinge on the introduction of competition in health care. Are physicians willing to take financial responsibility under conditions of budgetary constraints? Are they trained in preventive care, case management, and medical management? Perhaps because of the underlying cultural milieu, physicians in the US have begun to adapt themselves to the rise of large medical corporations and to the conversion of medicine into a business (Freedman 1985). Physicians working in a variety of HMOs are learning to accept financial constraints and even some intervention in the professional aspects of their work. Sometimes physician reimbursement is linked to performance measures, creating an incentive for physicians to conform to norms determined by HMOs. But it should not be forgotten that before such incentive schemes were implemented, physicians in the US could largely control their own incomes without sacrificing any professional autonomy. Increasingly, physicians in the US are abandoning the model of solo independent practice and accepting positions as salaried employees of health organizations (Fay 1987; Altman and Rosenthal 1990; Ku and Fisher 1990). In addition, the role of the 'physician leader' is emerging. Physician leaders are a cadre of doctors who mediate between health care managers and practising physicians. Physician leaders also facilitate the introduction of new management techniques aimed at controlling cost and quality in health organizations (Goldfield and Nash 1989).

The situation is different in other countries like the UK and Israel. In Israel most physicians are employees who perceive their salaries as low. This is despite the fact that their average wages are two and one-fifth times the national average wage. Israeli physicians may see their wages as low because they compare them with the wages of physicians in Canada and the US. In those countries, the average physician's wages are four to five times higher than the national average wages there (State of Israel 1990). Whatever the source of this perception, it is manifested in frequent strikes for higher wages (Modan 1985; Yishai 1990). However, most Israeli physicians have not yet accepted the notion of linking increased wages to increased responsibility for the overall cost of care, or tolerating interference in medical decision making. Though a cadre of family practice doctors has been trained to promote preventive and holistic care, they are not expected to be responsible for limiting the costs of health care.

In England, the new National Health Service (NHS) reform included transferring greater budgetary responsibility and financial risk sharing to family practitioners. The White Paper (HMSO 1989) on reforming the NHS proposes 'practice budgets' for general practitioners (GPs) with practices of a certain minimum size. GPs would be responsible for negotiating the purchase of both out-patient and in-patient services for those patients registered in their practice. The GPs would then pay for these services out of their practice budgets; any savings could be 'ploughed back' into the practice. Physicians in the UK are only now beginning to respond to this proposal (Glasman 1990; Henwood 1990; King 1990).

Competition and needs; expectations and adverse selection ('If you want it, catch it if you can!')

In our discussion of the needs module (above, and see Chapter 3) we offered various approaches for comparative needs assessment. The perception, and perhaps the actual fact, of unmet needs is one of the central reasons for reforming health systems. When public or centrally planned systems are, or appear to be, failing to meet needs, privatization and competition are solutions touted to match or align consumer needs with overall system capabilities. This appears to be the case in both the UK and in Israel (Maynard 1986; State of Israel, 1990).

It is interesting that in the US the perceived inadequacies of health care in *both* the public and private sectors has led to proposals for increased competition in health care. Some of these proposals emphasize the need for substantially refining competition as it is found presently. Thus, in his outline of his competitive health plan Enthoven (1987; Enthoven and Kronick 1989) spoke of national health insurance in the context of managed competition in the delivery of health services. One of the purposes of the proposed reform is to make the health system more equitable by providing universal insurance coverage. On the other hand, Enthoven sought the elimination of the over-utilization of health services. This over-utilization is a result of the structure of competition in health delivery in the US which, until a decade ago, was dominated by what he calls the 'guild free choice' of the medical profession. According to Enthoven, while that system allowed physicians to prescribe treatment without considering cost, it offered no real freedom of choice to the mainly uninformed and disorganized consumers of health care (Enthoven 1986, 1987).

Health needs and demands seem to be ever increasing. The successful treatment of diseases and the development of new technologies create more demand for health services. We might want to separate demand based on true needs from illegitimate demand, as we did in Chapter 3. But this is not always easy! For the same level of 'objective need', one society may perceive its unmet health needs as great while another society may feel that its needs are mainly met. Since most Israelis, for example, seem to have high expectations of their medical system, they often feel that many of their health needs are unmet (State of Israel 1990).

An example of such differences in perspectives on health needs is seen in the results of a recent study of the Israeli health care system by the State Commission of Inquiry (State of Israel 1990). The Commission published both majority and minority reports. One of the differences between the two reports is seen in their opposing interpretations of the success of the Israeli health system in meeting the health needs of the country. The majority and the minority used the same basic health indicators to compare the Israeli health system with several European systems. The majority concluded that

Israel's unmet needs are large and growing. The minority concluded that Israel's health system is relatively successful. Both the majority and the minority recommended increasing competition in the delivery of health care as we describe below in the section on process. In addition, the minority recommended only relatively minor adjustments to the existing competition among Israel's sick funds. The majority, on the other hand, sought to retain competition but also to strengthen the Government's control and planning of the health system. In some countries the perception of great unmet needs encourages an increase in centralization of health systems. In other countries like the US where there is a strong tradition of competition, even in the face of perceived unmet needs the Government's role may be limited at least in the actual planning and delivery of health services.

Societies differ in their determination of legitimate demands. This is reflected in the decisions made by governments about which health services and technologies will be covered by public insurance. In the UK, the NHS made certain explicit age-related decisions about the allocation of kidney dialysis equipment (Aaron and Schwartz 1984). In Israel, dialysis is available to everyone suffering renal failure, but crowding in dialysis facilities in public hospitals is beginning to be felt.* In the US, legislators and administrators of public programmes have considered excluding high cost services like organ transplantation from public insurance coverage but public pressure sometimes results in a reversal of such initiatives (Welch and Larson 1988).

Decisions about what services will be included in public insurance programmes must be made as a result of administrative processes or legislation. But decisions on the supply or use of costly technologies, like imaging diagnostics could be made either by the Government or as a result of the competitive market. As we have discussed, competition may result in the decentralization of the decision-making process. This may be advantageous to the system because decisions about rapid and complex scientific advances may prove too difficult for centralized decision making.**

Competition in the delivery of health care services is sometimes associated with the rapid spread of medical technology even beyond the level required by legitimate demand (Luft *et al.* 1986; Robinson and Luft 1987; Culyer and Posnett 1990). This is usually found when competing providers face no serious budgetary constraints. For example, consider the case when the costs of medical treatment are paid by third party insurers. Increases in cost may be passed on by the third party insurers to the insured and to the Government in the form of increases in tax-deductible premiums (Enthoven 1987; Culyer

* My thanks to Ms. Nurit Nirel for this information.

** I am indebted to Dr. Bruce Vladeck for his advice on this point. I am solely responsible for its presentation here.

and Posnett 1990). But if the Government were to place a budget constraint on publicly-funded health programmes, competing providers would allocate medical technology in a more cost-conscious way.

Ironically, for some groups competition can also lead to *under-utilization*. Individuals perceived as bad risks will be excluded by health insurers and providers, and either 'dumped' on the Government or left to their own devices. For example, an insurer may seek to avoid enrolling elderly people who are likely to be costly clients. Health policy analysts have noted that a relatively small group of costly patients account for most health expenditures (Enthoven 1987; Scheffler 1989). Scheffler showed that 7 per cent of the insured in the US Medicare programme account for 70 per cent of the expenditure! Any economically rational insurer would try to discourage enrollment of such cases. This leads to the process known as adverse selection. To eliminate bad risks, insurers in a competitive market use techniques to screen applicants. The price of health insurance for perceived bad risks rises accordingly. Very often such high risk individuals are excluded altogether, which severely curtails their access to health services.

According to some analysts, the problem of adverse selection must be faced by any country considering the introduction of competition into health care delivery and finance (Scheffler 1989; Van de Ven 1990). But until now, analysis of this problem has been grounded largely in micro-economics. Furthermore, it has been assumed those involved will behave as rational, calculating 'economic' men. This assumption may not be equally true for all countries. Differences in culture, particularly in the degree of social solidarity, may alter the degree to which adverse selection becomes a problem. For example, in discussing the introduction of competition into European health systems Glaser (1989) states:

> Competing social insurance carriers would prefer to avoid attracting subscribers who will cause deficits: persons with lower incomes and lower payments (such as pensioners and the poor); and persons with higher morbidity. However, in practice the carriers can only woo the better risks, not screen out the less healthy persons. These are social security programs designed to protect the vulnerable by redistributive financing, and the carriers *are expected to fulfill their duties*. They cannot reject any applicant under social insurance, no matter how poor a risk, and they can do no medical underwriting of rates.
>
> (Author's italics, D. C./A. E.)

Each culture is likely to produce a different tendency to screen applicants and engage in adverse selection. One clue to understanding a health system is its past behaviour. It is clear that in the US, insurers and managed care organizations have attempted to screen out bad risks. It is difficult for the Government to regulate selection bias even in government programmes funded on the basis of open enrollment (Scheffler 1989).

In Israel, on the other hand, the largest sick fund, the General Sick Fund of the Histadrut Labour Federation is committed to accepting any member of the trade union for health insurance. Some of the smaller sick funds do screen applicants. Recent recommendations for social health insurance by the Commission of Inquiry into the Israeli health care system (State of Israel 1990) include legislation mandating open enrollment without screening. It is unclear how this recommendation can be implemented. In the past, the General Sick Fund has been able to allow itself the 'luxury' of open enrolment because the Government has been generous in bailing the sick fund out of financial difficulty. If all the Israeli sick funds must now operate on a cost-conscious basis, they may all want to maintain the right to screen prospective members. On the other hand, the small funds may be compelled to have open enrollment partly because of strong social consensus on this point.

Many analysts in the US and the UK (Scheffler 1989; Barr *et al.* 1989; Henwood 1990) view selection bias as a critical issue for the proposed reforms of the NHS in the UK. This is because according to these reforms, general practitioners (GPs) would receive a fixed capitation budget for each person on their patient lists. To maximize their incomes, GPs could attempt to discourage the enrollment of perceived bad risks. Nevertheless, it may be wrong to assume that the problem will take the same form as it does in the US. As in some countries (Glaser 1989), we may assume that there is a tradition in the UK of universal access to health care and social health insurance. If this tradition can limit adverse selection, then the need for its regulation by the Government will be reduced.

Competition and the organization of the health system: market structure ('If the shoe fits, wear it.')

The health care system reforms discussed here are reforms involving competition and are based on markets. But market structures are often significantly different from the model of perfect competition described earlier. Moreover, market structures in different countries and health systems are likely to vary in ways which make the implementation of competition different for each country.

In the US, with the exception of hospitals in some rural areas, hospitals rarely have a monopoly position in their market. This means that dissatisfied clients can consider competitors. The situation is somewhat different in the NHS in the UK. Within the regionalized structure of the NHS, each health district is responsible for providing hospitalization services to its residents. District hospitals are alloted prospective budgets mostly based on the hospitalization needs of the populations and on the anticipated provision of service to patients from outside the district. For services rendered to non-district patients, hospitals are reimbursed at higher rates than those based on the average cost formulae used to budget districts on a per capita basis. Financial difficulties develop in districts having large outflows of patients to other districts. This situation has created financial incentives for hospitals to treat patients from outside their districts. Also, to avoid paying higher rates, hospitals have an incentive to treat in-district patients only so much as necessary to prevent them from seeking care in other districts (Bevan and Brazier 1987).

This problem of 'cross-boundary flows' and the incentives created by the current methods of resource allocation has contributed to the need for reform of the NHS (Brazier 1987; HMSO 1989). Under the recent NHS reform, regions and districts will be able to purchase services from any provider in the NHS on behalf of their residents. In effect, this would create an internal hospital market within the NHS. Nevertheless, at least for now, the 'monopoly' position of district hospitals within their regions continues to give them a competitive advantage. There are also many problems associated with the costing and pricing of services necessary for the operation of a hospital market (Culyer and Posnett 1990).

Aside from the structural problems in this internal hospital market, it should be noted that the NHS, operating through its districts and regions, constitutes a monopoly both as an insurer and as a purchaser of services. This may interfere with any attempt to adapt to the US competitive model in the situation in the UK. In the US, there are not only competing providers, but also competing insurers, so that a consumer dissatisfied with the price and service offered by one health insurer can chose another. In the UK, even under the terms of the present reform, most individuals will be insured by the health district they live in. The problem is that since each District Health Authority need not fear that its 'insured' will switch to another insurer, its responsiveness to its population may be limited. It has been suggested that the performance of districts in handling health budgets and purchasing services be carefully monitored by the central management of the NHS. But even such monitoring would not result in introducing competition into the NHS since the consumer really has no choice of insurer (Culyer and Posnett 1990).

The problems of combining competition with regional planning in a health system are further illustrated by the dilemmas facing the Israeli Commission of Inquiry for reforming the health care system there. The Commission wanted to retain the advantages of central planning and regionalization. These include restraints on unnecessary duplication of services; the rational allocation of national health budgets; the familiarity of regional health administrators with the special needs of local populations; and continuity of care. At the same time, the Commission wished to maintain and improve the competition among the various sick funds. Its final recommendation was to create health regions within which sick funds and other providers would compete. This solution still does not answer the following problems: assume that the regional authorities receive and control health budgets allocated by the central government; then the cost-consciousness encouraged by market competition could be undermined by political and bureaucratic means for obtaining additional budgets. On the other hand, if the regional authorities do not receive and control health budgets, the power of these authorities to implement the type of planning mentioned above is likely to be limited.

In Chapter 5, we discussed the dimension of accountability in the organization of health care. Our discussion here reveals that each country has a different version of the problem of accountability as connected with the introduction of competition into health care systems. The degree to which a country can successfully reform its health system along competitive lines, will depend on the degree of the consumers' control and on the quality of their decisions. More than one health economist (Evans 1987; Enthoven 1987) have discussed the problem of the weakness of the individual as a health consumer. Enthoven has suggested the notion of sponsors, which are organizations representing the consumers in the health market. In the US, this role has traditionally been played by employers, labour unions, and the Government. In the UK, the assumption in the current NHS reform is that the District Health Authorities are the sponsors for the population within their boundaries. But, we may ask, what mechanism can ensure that the sponsor is truly representative and accountable to the consumer? Accountability may be encouraged by informal peer group mechanisms in small organizations like religious communities, collective settlements, and neighbourhood committees whose members share a clearly articulated set of values. In Worcester, Massachusetts, business and health care leaders have joined in a 'community approach to health care competition' (Bradbury 1987). Such organizations may be potentially good as health sponsors. But it is unlikely that large organizations, and especially governmental divisions, could be held accountable for health service performance. In regional elections, health is unlikely to emerge as a salient enough issue to become a focus for voters. Despite the occasional prominence of health-related issues like abortion and environmental quality, evidence from elections in the US shows that health is not a key issue determining political outcomes (Blendon and Donelan 1990).

In Israel, neither employers nor government units play the role of sponsor for individuals shopping and selecting between health providers. On the other hand, Israel has certain organizational forms, like the kibbutz, which have demonstrated the capacity to play such a role (Chinitz 1988). The kibbutz movement accounts for only about 3 per cent of the population, but there are also neighbourhood committees, for example, which play a prominent role in major government programmes for urban renewal and could act as sponsors for larger portions of the population (Churchman 1985). Sponsorship, and other potential mechanisms for assuring accountability, will take different forms across countries and across cultures. This variation must be taken into account when basing an assessment of competition as an option for health system reform on experience in other countries.

Finally, we must consider the general political culture of a country as an input factor likely to affect the configuration of a country's health system and also the success of any changes introduced in it (Dohler 1990). In the US, competition is traditional in many spheres. This tradition facilitates the refinement of competition in health care and makes it more likely to be adopted than other possible reforms. In Israel, there is already some competition in the health system. However, in many ways the overall political economy of the country is based on centralization, and on government control and service provision (Ben Porat 1986). In Canada, private enterprise is favoured in many spheres of the economy, yet the Government funds health care and controls health care service prices almost exclusively (Iglehart 1990). In the UK, the Thatcher Government strongly supported the market-oriented reforms of the NHS. However, their implementation has encountered significant resistance from the previously existing institutional framework (Dean 1990a, 1990b).

The organization of medical manpower is another cultural aspect of the organization of health systems. Are there unions? How strong are they? In Israel, the unionization of physicians and global wage agreements between the medical unions and large employers like the Government and the sick funds, significantly reduce the system's flexibility in adopting a competitive market (State of Israel 1990; Yishai 1990).

Competition and outcomes: consumer satisfaction and the level of national health expenditure ('You get what you pay for?')

It is most logical to expect that consumer satisfaction would be an outcome (see also our discussion on outcomes in Chapters 7 and 8) of competition in health care delivery and finance. After all, consumers in a free market seek to maximize the utility they obtain from their purchases subject to a budget constraint. In other more centrally-planned health systems, other principle objectives are more important. For example, system administrators may seek to allocate health resources 'rationally' according to particular criteria. These criteria are not derived from the aggregation of individual preferences; rather, they are derived from the planning operations of decision-makers. These planning operations are meant to determine the allocation that will maximize certain health system goals. Health systems are never completely competitive nor completely planned. For those systems moving in the direction of increased competition, it is important to ask how increasing competition may affect satisfaction.

Ironically, there is evidence that even in the US health system, arguably the most competitive of them all, there are still relatively high levels of dissatisfaction. In a comparison of the US, Canada, and the UK, US respondents demonstrated the lowest degree of satisfaction with their health system with 61 per cent indicating a preference for the Canadian system.

Moreover, 89 per cent of the respondents in the US felt the need for fundamental changes in the health system as compared with 44 per cent in Canada and 69 per cent in the UK (Blendon and Taylor 1989). One possible explanation for these results is that a large percentage of the population in the US has little or no access to medical services, especially to personal physicians. Clearly, consumers with no access to the health system would be likely to express dissatisfaction with it. In opposition to this view, people in Canada and the UK consider access to the health system to be 'universal.'

Another problematic aspect of such comparisons is that the baseline of expectations may differ across countries. The higher the expectations the greater the disappointment when they are not met. Blendon and Taylor (1989) presented no data on people's expectations regarding their health systems. As they put it, 'if expectations are higher in one country than another, the same level of service would probably provide different levels of satisfaction.' We further suggest the possibility that the high expectations which cause high levels of dissatisfaction in the US may be caused or at least heightened by the structure of the competitive health system there.

As we mentioned previously, Israelis have high expectations from their health system. As Justice Netanyahu, who chaired the recent Judicial Commission of Inquiry into the health system, stated, Jewish tradition teaches that no effort be spared to save human life, making the idea of rationing care almost a non-starter. It seems that these high expectations have contributed to widespread dissatisfaction with the Israeli health care system. Given their expectation and satisfaction levels, would Israelis look more favourably upon the system in the US than do Canadians and Britons? While some Israelis would vehemently oppose adopting the 'American model', many would probably prefer it to their current system.

The differences in satisfaction levels between the those in the US and those in the UK or Canada are somewhat greater for personal physician care than for hospital care (Blendon and Taylor 1989). In this respect, Israel appears to be closer to the US than to Canada or the UK. In Israel, ambulatory care, especially doctor–patient contacts is the focus of much of the dissatisfaction with the health system (Linder-Pelz *et al.* 1983). But, the reasons for the dissatisfaction with ambulatory care in Israel are likely to be different than those in the US. The Israeli ambulatory system is rife with administrative and organizational problems, more queues than in the US and hurdles the consumer must jump over to get referrals (Yuval 1989).

At present, many health care consumers in the US would prefer the Canadian health system over their own (Blendon and Taylor 1989). However, the introduction of a system of competing HMOs could also lead to increased consumer satisfaction in the US. Early experience with HMOs showed that satisfaction was linked to organizational structure, that is, whether the HMO was open panel or closed panel. In open panel HMOs, the patient can choose his physician quite freely. In closed panel HMOs, the patient's choice of physician is limited. Relative to traditional health insurance programmes like Blue Cross—Blue Shield, satisfaction in open panel HMO's increased at the time of enrollment and over time. At the time of enrollment in closed panel HMOs, there was increased satisfaction, but one year later satisfaction was reduced (Ashcraft *et al.* 1978). Recently, the US Government has been experimenting with the use of capitated competitive health plans (see discussion of capitation in Chapter 5) for the Medicare and Medicaid programmes. In both these programmes, the majority of those enrolled in the experimental competitive plans were satisfied. Nevertheless, for some dimensions like the perceived manner and competence of physicians, persons enrolled in Medicare or Medicaid HMOs were significantly less satisfied than those enrolled in fee-for-service plans. On the other hand, they were more satisfied than those in fee-for-service programmes with the amount of time required to obtain treatment and to process claims. With time, enrollment in HMOs increased and the level of satisfaction of those enrolled was maintained relative to the period before their enrollment (Freund *et al.* 1989; Langwell and Hadley 1989).

In the US, another source of dissatisfaction is the high percentage of the GNP alloted to the health system. Previously, in Chapter 4, we considered the percentage of GNP as an input to a health system; but it can also be considered as an outcome. In fact, that the US spends a high percentage of its GNP on health care is often blamed on the competitive model of health care finance and delivery (Califano 1986; Evans 1987).

Evans and colleagues have compared the US and Canada with respect to expenditures on health care (Evans 1987; Barer *et al.* 1988). In 1971, the Canadian provinces began reimbursing physicians under a universal and comprehensive public medical insurance programme. Since 1971, the rates of health expenditure growth in Canada and the US have diverged. In 1987, Canadian national health expenditures had levelled off at about 8.6 per cent, while expenditure in the US was close to 11.4 per cent of the GNP and showed 'no signs of slowing down'. According to Evans (1987), it is the *collective* purchase of health care which leads to the slower growth in the percentage of GNP allocated to health care. The collective agent could be the Government or a cost-conscious purchaser like an HMO. What is essential, according to Evans, is to avoid the illusion that optimal outcomes will result from individual health consumers operating in a market system.

Enthoven (1987), one of the leading proponents of competition in health care, takes a similar position. He points out that his model of competition is not a traditional free market in which health consumers act as autonomous agents. As we discussed in the section on organization, Enthoven maintains that it is critical that purchasers be organized under the aegis of 'sponsors' which will compensate for some of the deficiencies of individual health consumers (Enthoven 1987; Enthoven and Kronick 1989).

However, Enthoven does not believe that the pecentage of the GNP allocated to health care is necessarily the most important measure of the outcomes of a health system. Equally important is the mechanism used to determine that percentage. If correctly operated, the market will allocate resources to health care at a socially desirable level. Government control over prices as in the Canadian system, or a pre-designated ceiling on national health expenditures need not necessarily encourage efficiency (Enthoven 1987, 1988). We might add, that relying on such methods for controlling health care expenditures also runs the risk of suppressing innovations in health care which may be socially beneficial and cost-effective.

We have considered the overall level of health care expenditure as an important outcome of the health system. It is also important to consider the distribution of that health care expenditure among various inputs to the health system. To understand this better we must refer to some of the issues discussed previously in this book. We discussed problems of comparing national health expenditure across countries in which differing items are included in their national health accounts. For example, a given country may or may not include the costs of transporting patients to the site of medical treatment in its national health accounts (Poullier 1986).

These differences should be taken into account when making such comparisons. We also pointed out that the monetary sums expended on health in different countries may conceal variations in purchasing power. Because of this, it is necessary to weight monetary expenditures according to 'purchasing-power parity.' For example, Israeli economist Ofer (1988) compared the expenditures on health in Israel, Germany, and Denmark during the year 1980. In simple monetary terms, based on foreign currency exchange rates, Israel spent about half of what Germany or Denmark spent on health per capita. However, when the monetary figures are adjusted to take purchasing-power parity in health services into account, the ratio of Israel's per capita expenditure to those of the other two countries rises from one-half to three-fifths. Taking into account that Israel's per capita GNP is lower than Germany's or Denmark's, Israel's health expenditure may be considered similar to that of these more developed countries (Ofer 1988).

Even using purchasing-power parity, however, does not completely solve the problem of international comparisons of health expenditures. For within the health price index of each country are buried weights which alter the relative incomes of various factors of production, especially manpower. As we discussed above, Israeli physicians appear to consider themselves to be underpaid (State of Israel 1990; Rosen 1989). This is likely to affect their level of job satisfaction which in turn may affect their performance. Thus, even if Israel purchases an amount and quality of health resources similar to that purchased by Denmark and Germany, the level of satisfaction emerging in Israel may be very different for both providers and consumers.

Whether competition should be the mechanism for determining the incomes of physicians and other production factors, should not depend only on its short-term impact on national health expenditures. Other considerations include consumer and provider satisfaction, perceived fairness of the mechanism, and the long-term effects of competition on expenditures. Canada has controlled health expenditures through physician fee controls and budget constraints rather than through the market. The US is experimenting with physician fee schedules in the Medicare programme. At the same time, in the US competition is being encouraged among health plans as another avenue for reducing health care expenditures (Ginsburg 1989). In Israel, until recently, physician wages in public hospitals were determined by national wage agreements. Now it has been suggested that these wages be maintained only during the 'normal' working hours of the public system. During 'extra' afternoon sessions, physicians would be paid on a fee-for-service basis, as their hospitals compete for additional patients. Each country must find the blend of policies appropriate to the stage of the development of its health system, the level of satisfaction with the system, and socially acceptable budget constraints. How these factors will be interpreted by each country will vary both across countries and over time.

Conclusion

In this chapter we have applied the modular approach to the analysis of the introduction of competition in health systems. Examination of the meaning and implications of competition within several modules highlighted cross-system differences which should not be overlooked.

For example, in our discussion of medical manpower, we analysed the relationship between the supply of physicians, their background, and their orientation on the one hand, and the likely impact of increased reliance on competition in health care systems on the other. We saw that under conditions of physician-oversupply, unless physicians are encouraged to be cost conscious, competition need not necessarily lead to lower physician wages, lower medical care expenditures, or increased access to health care services.

We have also discussed introducing competition, as a substitute for central planning, as the mechanism for determining which health needs will be met. But while, in some ideal sense, the mechanisms used in different countries may be the same, they may lead to very different results because attitudes toward needs and their measurement differ across countries. In addition, when assessing potential health system reforms, it is important to consider the manner in which competition will blend in with each country's underlying social values.

Cross-system comparisons of satisfaction have revealed a relatively high level of dissatisfaction in the US with the competitive health care system. It may be the competitive nature of that system which contributes to heightened expectations – dooming itself, or its successors to inevitable high levels of dissatisfaction. The Israeli health system is not as competitive as that in the US. Nevertheless, Israelis have high expectations of their health care system. Perhaps these high expectations would make the introduction of increased competition more acceptable to the public in Israel than to the public in Canada or the UK.

Finally, social preferences regarding the mechanism for deciding the level of resources to allocate to health care are likely to vary across countries.

Thus, competition will neither take the same form nor bring about the same results in all systems. This is because:

(1) needs, and the perceptions of needs, differ across countries;

(2) medical manpower and its professional attributes are more conducive to the successful adoption of competition in some countries than in others;

(3) in some countries the introduction of competition into the pre-existing health system structure may cause market failures that are very hard to correct;

(4) the psycho-social bases of satisfaction and social preferences regarding allocations to health care vary across systems and influence the debate about competition and its implementation.

Too often, discussions of health system reforms, like the introduction of increased competition, are focused on a limited number of considerations. In addition, analysts base their conclusions on lessons from a given country without assessing whether the lessons are relevant or meaningful in another. The modular approach enables a more comprehensive, systematic and clarifying assessment of issues related to health system reform.

References

Aaron, H.J. and Schwartz, W.B. (1984). *The painful prescription*. Brookings Institute, Washington, DC.

Altman, L.K. and Rosenthal, E. (1990). Changes in medicine bring pain to healing profession. *New York Times*, 18 February, 1990.

Arrow, K.J. (1963). Uncertainty and the welfare economics of medical care. *American Economic Review*, **53**, 941–73.

Ashcraft, M., Penchansky, R., Berki, S.E., Fortus, R.S., and Gray, J. (1978). Expectations and experience of HMO enrollees after one year: an analysis of satisfaction, utilization, and costs. *Medical Care*, **16**, (1), 14–32.

Barer, M.L., Evans, R.G., and Labelle, R.J. (1988). Fee controls as cost control: tales from the frozen north. *The Milbank Quarterly*, **66**, (1), 1–63.

Barr, N., Glennerster, H., and Le Grand, J. (1989). *Working for patients? The right approach?* Suntory–Toyota International Centre for Economics and Related Disciplines, London.

Ben-Porat, Y. (ed.) (1986). *The Israeli economy: maturing through crisis*. Harvard University Press, Cambridge, Massachusetts.

Bevan, G. and Brazier, J. (1987). Financial incentives of subregional RAWP. *British Medical Journal*, **295**, (6602), 836–8.

Blendon, R.J. and Taylor, H. (1989). Views on health care: public opinion in three nations. *Health Affairs*, **8**, (1), 149–57.

Blendon, R.J. and Donelan, K. (1990). The 1988 election: how important was health? *Health Affairs*, **8**, (3), 6–15.

Bradbury, R.C. (1987). A community approach to health care competition. *Inquiry*, **24**, 253–65.

Brazier, J. (1987). Accounting for cross boundary flows. *British Medical Journal*, **295**, (6603), 898–900.

Califano, J.A. (1986). A corporate Rx for America: managing runaway health costs. *Issues in Science and Technology*, **II**, (3), 81–90.

Chinitz, D.P. (1988). Options for the Israeli health care system: a comparative institutional analysis. Unpublished manuscript JDC-Brookdale Brookdale Institute of Gerontology and Adult Human Development, Jerusalem.

Churchman, A. (1985). *Resident involvement and participation in project renewal.* Technion–Neeman Institute for Advanced Studies, Haifa.

Culyer, A.J. and Posnett, J. (1990). *Hospital behaviour and competition.* Department of Economics, University of York, York.

Dean, M. (1990a). Will the doctors opt out? *The Lancet*, pp. 341–2.

Dean, M. (1990b). Blue and red politics in the NHS. *The Lancet* 844–5.

Dohler, M. (1990). *Policy networks, opportunity structures, and neo-conservative reform strategies in health policy*, Paper presented at the International Sociological Association XIIth World Congress of Sociology, Madrid, 1990.

Enthoven, A. (1986). The US health care economy: from guild to market in ten years. *Health Policy*, **7**, 241–51.

Enthoven, A. (1987). *Theory and practice of managed competition in health care finance.* de Vries Lectures on Economics, Rotterdam School of Economics, Erasmus University, Rotterdam.

Enthoven, A. (1988). Managed competition of alternative delivery systems. *Journal of Health Politics, Policy, and Law*, **13**, (2), 305–21.

Enthoven, A. and Kronick, R. (1989). A Consumer-choice health plan for the 1990s, universal health insurance in a system designed to promote quality and economy. *The New England Journal of Medicine*, **320**, (1) 29–37 and **320**, (2), 94–101.

Evans, R.G. (1987). Public health insurance: the collective purchase of individual care. *Health Policy*, **7**, 115–34.

Evans, R.G., Lomas, J., Barer, M., Labelle, R.J., Fooks, C., Stoddart, G.L., *et al.* (1989). Controlling health expenditures—the Canadian reality. *The New England Journal of Medicine*, **320**, (9), 571–7.

Fay, M. (1987). Why your family doctor is a group. *The New York Times* Magazine 7 June 1987.

Freedman, S.A. (1985). Megacorporate health care, a choice for the future. *New England Journal of Medicine*, **312**, (9), 579–82.

Freund, D.J., Rossiter, L.F., Fox, P.D., Meyer, J.A., Hurley, R.E., Carey, T.S., *et al.* (1989). Evaluation of the Medicaid competition demonstrations. *Health Care Financing Review*, **11**, (2), 81–97.

Ginsburg, P.B. (1989). Physician payment policy in the 101st Congress. *Health Affairs*, **8**, (1), 5–20.

Glaser, W.A. (1989). *Europe's decentralized and semi-private health insurance.* New School for Social Research, New York.

Glasman, D. (1990). Suspicion takes root in the GP surgery. *The Health Service Journal*, **100**, (5188), 232.

Goldfield, N. and Nash, D. (1989). *Physician leaders: past and future challenges*, The American College of Physician Executives, Tampa, Florida.

Greenberg, D. (1990). The doctor glut revisited. *The Lancet*, pp. 902–3.

Haaretz, 16 December 1990, (Hebrew).

Ham, C., Robinson, R., and Benzeval, M. (1990). *Health check, health care reforms in an international context*, King's Fund Institute, London.

Hayek, F. H. (1945). The use of information in society. *American Economic Review*, **35**, 519–30.

Henwood, M. (1990). Undesirable effects of GP budgets. *The Health Service Journal*, **100**, (5186), 153.

HMSO (Her Majesty's Stationery Office) (1989). *Working for patients*. London.

Iglehart, J. K. (1990). Canada's health care system faces its problems. *The New England Journal of Medicine*, **322**, (8), 562–8.

King, N. (1990). Patterns in practice. *The Health Service Journal*, **100**, (5199), 669.

Ku, L. and Fisher, D. (1990). The attitudes of physicians toward health care cost-containment policies. *Health Services Research*, **25**, (1) Part I, 25–42.

Langwell, K. and Hadley, J. P. (1989). Evaluation of the Medicare competition demonstration. *Health Care Financing Review*, **11**, (2), 65–80.

Linder-Pelz, S. Epstein, L., and Tamir, A. (1983). The meaning of patient satisfaction with prepaid primary health care in Israel. *Evaluation and Program Planning*, **6**, (3-4), 385–93.

Luft, H., Robinson, J., Garnick, D., Maerki, S., and McPhee, S. (1986). The role of specialized clinical services in competition among hospitals. *Inquiry*, **23**, 83–94.

Maynard, A. (1986). Public and private sector interactions: an economic perspective. *Social Science and Medicine*, **22**, (11), 1161–6.

Modan, B. (1985). *Medicine under siege: the physicians' strike/crisis in the health care system*. Adam Publishers, Israel, (Hebrew).

Ofer, G. (1988). National expenditure on health. In *Allocation of resources to social services* (ed. Y. Kop), Chapter 3. Centre for Social Policy Studies, Jerusalem.

Poullier, J-P. (1986). Levels and trends in the public–private mix of the industrialized countries' health systems. In *Public and private health services, complementarities and conflicts* (ed. A. J. Culyer, and B. Jonsson), Chapter 2. Basil Blackwell, New York.

Robinson, J. C. and Luft, H. S. (1987). Competition and the cost of hospital care, 1972-1982. *Journal of the American Medical Association*, **257**, (23), 3241–5.

Rosen, B. (1989). Physician reimbursement in Israel: an analysis of selected policy proposals. *Economics Quarterly*, **139**, 556–76.

Saltman, R. B. and von Otter, C. (1989). Public competition versus mixed markets: an analytic comparison. *Health Policy*, **11**, 43–55.

Saltman, R. B. and von Otter, C. (1990). Implementing public competition in Swedish county councils: A Case Study. *International Journal of Health Planning and Management*, **5**, 105–16.

Scheffler, R. (1989). Adverse selection: the achilles heel of the NHS reforms. *The Lancet*, pp. 950–2.

Schulz, R., Scheckler, W. E., Girard, C., and Barker, K. (1990). Physician adaptation to health maintenance organizations and implications for management. *Health Services Research*, **25**, (1), Part I, 43–64.

Starr, P. (1982). *The social transformation of American medicine*. Basic Books, New York.

State of Israel (1990). *Report: The State Commission of Inquiry into the performance and effectiveness of the health care system*. Government Printing House, Jerusalem (Hebrew).

Van de Ven, W.P.M.M. (1988). *A future for competitive health care in the Netherlands*, NHS White Paper Occasional Paper 9, Centre for Health Economics, Health Economics Consortium, University of York, York.

Van de Ven, W.P.M.M. (1990). *How can we prevent cream skimming in a competitive health insurance market?* Paper presented at the Second World Congress on Health Economics, Zurich.

Welch, H.G. and Larson, E.B. (1988). Dealing with limited resources, the Oregon decision to curtail funding for organ transplantation. *New England Journal of Medicine*.

Yishai, Y. (1990). *The power of expertise*. Israel Medical Association, Jerusalem Institute for Israel Studies Jerusalem. (Hebrew).

Yuval, D. (1989). Consumer satisfaction with regard to health care services; conceptual framework. Unpublished manuscript, JDC-Brookdale Institute of Gerontology and Adult Human Development, Jerusalem.

13. The sky is the limit—prospects for the future

For those looking for ways to simplify the study of health systems and to benefit from easy comparisons, this book brings no salvation. Perhaps a typology classifying health systems into a few prototypes would be more appealing. However, as we noted before, in our view the application of such typology is not realistic. Health systems simply are not adaptable to simplistic presentations based on a small number of descriptive dimensions. Based on our understanding that there is little sense in comparing *health systems* as such, we have suggested that *modules* be compared instead, since—according to our model—the modules make up the health system. Now, a crucial question remains unanswered: Can we still predict the future development of a health system based on our partial knowledge of these components called modules? Well, the answer is definitely yes. In this concluding chapter, we shall examine the effects of trends in health systems and seek to understand their implications for the future of these systems. We shall discuss these trends in relation to each separate module of our model and in the order dictated by our discussion in previous chapters.

Population needs

The future of population needs will be different for developed and developing countries. For the developed countries, the process of ageing will determine needs for health services in the next decades. For the developing countries, the eradication of communicable disease, the elimination of malnutrition, and an increase in life expectancy will still be regarded as major concerns. In developed countries, the WHO projects at 12 per cent population increase between the years 1980 and 2000. The greatest increase, 30 per cent will be in the age group 65 and older (UN 1985). Consequently, even more than their already significant impact on today's health systems, the most alarming future health problems in developed countries are likely to be the health problems of the elderly. The needs of the greying population will be reflected by a higher volume of patients with chronic disease in ambulatory settings, an increased admission rate to medical and surgical departments in acute care hospitals, and more nursing and rehabilitation units. More preventive care and health educational activities for the elderly will also be needed.

In developing countries, unfortunately the economies continue to deteriorate as seen by the lower growth rate of the economy with respect to population growth in a large number of developing countries (UNICEF 1990). Because of this, the prospects for eradicating communicable diseases in these countries seems gloomier than ever. However, some encouraging findings help lighten this dark picture. Consider the 30 countries with the highest mortality rates for children under 5 years of age. Between 1981 and 1988, these mortality rates have all been decreased. It appears that this decrease is a result of improved immunization programmes. For example, in 1981, only 26 per cent of infants less than 1 year old were immunized against tuberculosis, and 14 per cent against DPT. By 1988, these rates rose to 53 and 30 per cent respectively. Similarly, for these same 30 countries, the percentage of children under 4 years of age suffering from moderate to severe malnutrition decreased from 36 per cent in 1980 to only 8 per cent in 1987 (UNICEF 1990).

Resources at the system's command

In contrast to the popular belief supported by the vociferous proponents of cost-containment, resources are not becoming scarcer: they are just not growing fast enough to satisfy the requirements of modern health systems. In fact, for industrialized countries, the *real* per capita expenditure on health is growing everywhere as shown in Fig. 13.1. Countries differ with respect to the growth *rate* and not to growth itself (Schieber 1990). Expressing this increase in terms of volumes of manpower resources or physical resources available to health systems, reveals steady increases in modern health systems in both health workers and beds per capita.

Of course there are intra-system adjustments and also change in emphasis within subsystems. For example, in most industrialized countries, there is a shift of beds from the acute care sector into the needy long-term care sector. This kind of transfer of resources is an immediate consequence of the ageing process described above. In addition to transfers of physical resources, there is also a shift in health manpower. This is a vertical shift reflected by the growing proportion of better trained health workers in health systems. From a qualitative manpower perspective, the impetus to achieve a higher professional status is a universal phenomenon in developed countries. In the case of nurses, it is reflected by the increasing number of academically trained nurses at the expense of non-academic nursing manpower. For other professions, it is reflected by the legalisation of several of paramedical professions including paramedics, assistant physicians, and physiotherapists. More and more requirements for formal and increased intensive training accompany the process of the licensure of these professionals.

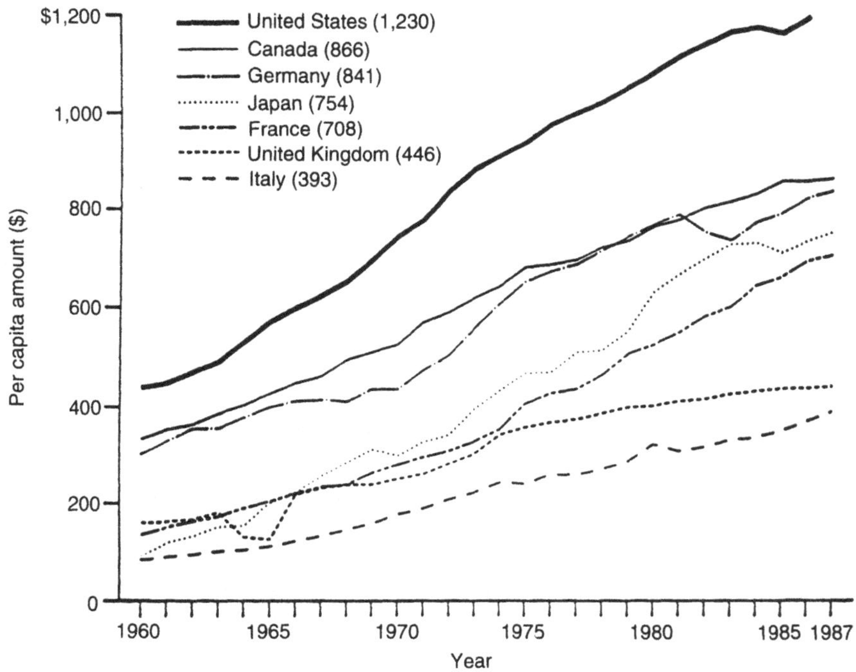

Fig. 13.1 Real per capita health expenditures in US dollars: selected countries, 1960–1987. (Data from OECD; HCFA (US Health Care Financing Administration) (1989).)

For physicians, when emerging specialities and subspecialities require extra training, transitions are vertical. Typically, in many countries the need for more qualified physicians in ambulatory care resulted in the establishment of specialist training programmes in family or community medicine.

The general trends for developing countries are different. The main focus is on curative care. In developing countries, the public often perceives health care as synonymous with hospital care. Thus, the scarcity of resources in some countries is amplified by the skewed distribution of manpower and physical resources. In Ghana, for instance, 40 per cent of the national health budget goes to the 2 leading teaching hospitals which benefit only 1 per cent of the population (Ghana Ministry of Health 1988). Another concern is that while several Third World countries like India, Pakistan, and Nigeria have been able to respond to the needs of medical education by training large numbers of physicians, they cannot maintain their health manpower reservoir. Some of their expensively trained medical graduates prefer to migrate to more developed countries. This migration of professional manpower from developing to developed countries further exacerbates the shortage of professional manpower in the developing world (Colledge *et al.* 1986).

Socio-economic development

In Chapter 2 we referred to Roemer (1977) who noted that health systems are determined by politics, economics, and societal values. The ways that these three sets of concepts interact may vary across health systems. However, operationally, their overall effect may be seen as the conflict between regulation and competition. As we have described in Chapter 12, both regulation and competition may be variously interpreted in different health systems. However, it is still possible to generalize to some degree. From the point of view of society, we can summarize the conflict by asking: which is more viable: a planned and regulated health system heavily financed by the public sector or a competitive system motivated by private financial incentives? For any given country or society, the choice will be determined by the relative ability of the public or the private sectors to produce effective health care efficiently and equitably. Earlier in this century, the idea of the Welfare State emerged as a possible solution to ineffective and inequitable modern social systems. As Titmuss (1963) put it, social welfare consists of:

> states of dependency that have been defined and recognized as collective responsibilities, and more differential provision has been made in respect to them.

Democratic societies have been particularly attracted to assuming collective responsibility for social issues. Furthermore, in such democratic societies, politicians are generally unable or unwilling to confront public pressures aimed at achieving social equity. In general, the achievement of collective responsibility implies that governments are empowered to intervene and regulate issues of social concern. However, recently a variety of factors have combined, gradually changing governments' attitudes towards regulatory mechanisms contained within this collective responsibility. From the supply side, decreased economic growth in the 1980s and increasing concerns about a deficit in public budgets have lowered the expectations for expanding the public funding of social programmes (Culyer and Jonsson 1986). From the demand side, two factors have negated the ability of governments to support health services. First, the ageing of the population has overburdened the public sector and catalysed the failing attempt of health systems to maintain equitable services. Second, the demand for advanced medical technology by consumers could not be met by the financially-constrained public sector. As a result, in recent years the shrinking financial leverage of the public sector has led to the decline in regulatory mechanisms and to the fast growth of a competitive market. Rather than full privatization, different types of a private–public mix have emerged in various countries. For example, the experience of many countries in the European continent was that centrally-mandated systems need not include a bureaucratic central administration. Within such systems, regulation is only required to encourage competition. In Germany this regulation takes the form of a federal law requiring that persons whose income is below a certain level receive mandatory health insurance. However, such individuals are free to select their insurers, and the entire insurance market is competitive (Henke 1989). In the Netherlands, the Government has proposed fundamental changes to strengthen market elements and to reduce government intervention in the health care system. According to this proposal, in the market-oriented system, insurers will be able to select among providers and will also be free to set premiums competitively (Elsinga 1989).

In England too, the White Paper (HMSO 1989) proposes to increase competition between hospitals and other providers who would have to compete for the limited resources available to them in the health district. In Canada, as we noted in Chapter 11, the decrease in federal funding may lead to the reinstitution of market mechanisms, particularly extra-billing of patients by physicians. In Israel, the health care system is moving in the direction of increased private ownership of health institutions, particularly of chronic care hospitals and of clinics (Rosen 1989). Free selection of providers by patients has even been proposed in Sweden, (Lindgren 1989).

The only major exception is the US where the share of the expenditure on health spent by the public sector is relatively small. In spite of this, both the Republican administrations of Reagen and of Bush swept into office proclaiming the virtues of competition and de-regulation. Such a policy is far removed from the regulatory cost-containment policies made by the Carter administration in the 1970s. The trend to increased competition in the US was twofold:

(1) constraints in budgetary support of federally funded programmes like Medicaid (Baldwin 1987);

(2) encouragement of competition, as by the development of new models for the provision of health care (managed care).

Two examples of such competitive models in the US are Preferred Provider Organizations (PPOs) and Health Maintenance Organizations (HMOs). A PPO is an arrangement in which a group of health providers agree to provide services to a defined group of consumers under special agreements. The concept of PPO was created as a competitive mechanism to maintain or expand the market share of health care providers (de Lissovoy *et al.* 1986). Increased competition in the US health care system is also seen in the extensive growth in health maintenance organizations (HMOs). Since 1970, the number of HMOs has grown nearly twenty fold, and HMOs now compete vigorously for their share in the employer-based insurance market (Mayer and Mayer 1985). While the 1980s can be seen as a decade of increasing competition in the US, growing competition has also caused problems for cost control. As a result, some analysts (Altman and Rodwin 1988) have predicted that the failure of cost-controlling will bring a return of stronger regulatory mechanisms in the US in the 1990s.

In summary, except in the US perhaps, it seems that industrialized societies are tending more and more to establish new balances in health care. Currently, governments in many countries have chosen to liberalize health systems so as to allow the private sector to compete with the publicly-owned services in the provision of health care. The establishment of free-market elements and the decline in government involvement in the provision of health care need not preclude some role for the Government in health systems. While in the past, the main role of governments was to control the *process* of care, the governments are now developing capacities for assessing the effectiveness of the health service *outcomes*. This focus on effectiveness is based on the recognition that enhanced efficiency in health care systems would be achieved only if some level of public intervention were to be preserved. Comparative analyses of spending and efficiency in health systems supports this recognition. It has been shown that health systems with substantial levels of public intervention are more efficient than those with less, as seen in a recent analysis comparing Canada, Germany, and the US (Pfaff 1990).

The organization of the health system

In Chapter 2 we discussed the issue of universal trends of convergence or divergence in health systems. We concluded that there is not enough evidence to support either the contention that health systems show converging trends or the contention that health systems are diverging. Nevertheless, over the last decades there have been universal trends across systems; these trends were undoubtedly caused by the communications breakthrough. MacBride, who presided over the UNESCO commission on Communication Problems, chose a highly significant title for the book reporting the Commission's findings, *Many voices, one world* (MacBride *et al.* 1980). This title represents the essence of current and future developments in the structure of health systems. While policies and trends may differ, the flow of information among systems allows them to draw important lessons from each other and to co-operate on an international scale. A recent example of this phenomenon is currently taking place in Europe where the post-socialist governments in Hungary and Poland intend to reform their health services.

Indeed, a project funded by the WHO and carried out by the European Health Care Management Association (EHMA) is focused on reshaping Hungarian health management teams into a competitive configuration. This kind of configuration, suggested by the US economist Enthoven (1988), is known as managed competition. In Enthoven's model, 'collective agents' representing consumers would contract competing health providers thus ensuring better quality and efficiency in health care. This phenomenon of the transfer of knowledge and expertise from one environment to a totally different one could only have happened with the advent of developed communication networks.

The changes in the health care systems of developed countries are geared towards new managerial structures based on increased competition. The opposite trend is seen in developing countries where the attempt is to increase public sponsorship of health programmes. Over the last decade, in many countries, national and local governments have gradually increased their participation in the health sector. Operationally, government participation involves the transfer from the private health care sector to public sponsorship of the responsibility for a large variety of health services (Kleczkowski *et al.* 1984, Chapter 5).

Decentralization has also been an issue in studying the organizational aspects of health systems. Decentralization in health systems involves the delegation of power and authority to distinct geographical units. Decentralization is not new and has been seen in many health systems for many years. However, health systems have been decentralized for opposite reasons in developed and developing countries.

For developing countries decentralization was promoted by colonial administrations as part of their philosophy of power; for developed countries decentralization surged because historically local governments were often stronger than central governments (Mills *et al.* 1990). Recently, both in developed and developing countries, there have been new efforts to ensure more autonomy to peripheral managements of the health care systems. In England, the White Paper (HMSO 1989) for example, proposes that the health districts should have more autonomy in their choices of personnel and resource acquisitions. In Spain, after 1978 the very centralized structure of the health system was replaced by 17 autonomous communities each assuming total responsibility for public health and partial responsibility for hospitals and health centres (Antigas 1990). Currently, in the western and southern areas of the Netherlands, regional planning is being carried out experimentally. Within the experimental design, regions have been defined, block grants given to regional authorities, and regional plans have been developed. Their overall goal is to respond to both population needs and institutional units and targets (Schrijvers 1990). In Israel, decentralization is a cornerstone of the proposed health reform (State of Israel 1990). According to this reform, the Israeli health scene will be dominated by regionalized insurance agencies, independent hospitals, and regional management teams of the Government.

Regionalization is also re-emerging in developing countries. In several developing countries regionalization is now possible because the central governments managed to establish a sufficient basis of power so that they now feel secure enough to relinquish part of their tight control to local governments (Mills *et al.* 1990). Indeed, in many countries including: Mexico, Senegal, Papua New Guinea, and Sri Lanka the health systems have recently been successfully regionalized (Mills *et al.* 1990).

Utilization

Health policy-makers and researchers in many countries continue to be interested by findings on substantial geographic variations in the use of medical care, as we discussed in Chapter 6. These findings suggest that health services may be over-utilized in some professional domains or geographic areas and under-utilized in others. While there are no easy global solutions to these questions, there have been several proposals for determining appropriate volumes of utilization. For example, the DRG system in the US is perhaps the most sophisticated approach to standardizing hospital utilization and curtailing hospital costs. However, the DRG system may also have caused a sharp rise in physicians' services so that the net benefits of the DRG system with respect to costs and utilization are questionable (Kinzer 1990). Another approach, appealing to policy-makers in a number of countries, is outcome measurement. The rationale is to determine whether or not there is over-utilization by evaluating outcomes. This resurgence of interest in measuring outcomes has led to various types of activities. For example, large computerized databases are being used more and more frequently. In Canada several provinces already have a database including all the data on medical procedures (for example, Roos and Shapiro 1981). In the US, the introduction of national insurance plans for selective populations has led to the construction of large data sets, like those for Medicare beneficiaries (Ellwood 1988).

There is also a steady effort in many countries to develop explicit guidelines and criteria for appropriate care. On the one hand, these guidelines can help physicians to make clinical decisions. On the other hand, they support the managements of health services or funding agencies in controlling the appropriateness of care rendered by physicians and other providers to their patients. As we mentioned in Chapter 8, there are now explicit criteria for the appropriateness of use of many different medical procedures and therapies (Relman 1988). The level of appropriateness of care could potentially be used to explain variations in utilization cross-regionally and cross-nationally. With the existing criteria, only modest success has been reported among small areas (Leape *et al.* 1990). However, perhaps, in the future, with improved criteria for the appropriateness of several procedures and therapies, this approach will prove useful.

In summary, whichever approach is followed, it seems that governments in developed countries are becoming increasingly committed to curtailing unnecessary utilization. Thus, more than ever before, they are willing to interfere with physician autonomy. However, the prospects of success should be considered carefully. On the one hand, governments in some countries like France, West Germany, and the UK have been able to marshal the physicians so that they would accept health care reforms restricting their professional autonomy (Godt 1987). On the other hand, several factors beyond government control like the country's economic level or its population morbidity-profile have an even stronger influence on physicians' behaviour (Sandier 1989).

Problems in utilization are different for the developing countries. In those countries, the main problem is under-utilization. But under-utilization of health services is not evenly distributed over the whole population. For those with access to health services, levels of utilization are surprisingly similar to those in developed countries (Gish 1990). Thus, for the non-privileged, who may have *no access to modern health services at all*, the problem is essentially to secure access. Perhaps in the near future, the principal challenge of health planners in developing countries would be to switch from their *input*-related planning (e.g. more doctors, beds etc.) to *process*-related planning, that is to eliminate the barriers to access prevailing for substantial proportions of the population (Gish 1990).

Issues of effectiveness, efficiency, and quality

We have mentioned previously that health care expenditures in developed countries grow at *different* rates. Which socio-economic factors may be responsible for these different rates? In effect, the percentage of a country's GNP expended on health care is not really determined by socio-economic or organizational factors. In both Sweden and the US, there are quite a high levels of expenditure on health. Yet Sweden has an organized health system and the US has a mixed private and public system. Although in both Sweden and Britain there are organized public health care systems, when expressed as a percentage of GNP, Britain's expenditure is quite low compared with Sweden's. So, if socio-economic factors and organizational patterns are not responsible for the differences in the initial levels of expenditures, or for the differences in the increases in the growth rates of these expenditures, what does cause these differences? It seems that stronger *control* mechanisms have provided increased efficiency in health systems; two typical examples can be cited. First, Britain fares better in managerial efficiency than other industrialized countries because it constantly controls the level of resources. Considering the ratio between outcomes and costs, levels of general health outcomes in Britain are roughly similar to those in other industrialized countries, while at the same time, the British health system maintains a relatively low level of expenditure on health – about 6 per cent of the GNP. In Canada, our second example, controls on the levels of the process of care are achieved by restricting hospital budgets and by imposing limits on global reimbursement for physician services. These two restrictions have kept the growth rate of health expenditures lower in Canada than in the US (Evans *et al.* 1989). However, this successful cost-containment in Britain, and to a lesser extent in Canada, has not yielded the expected benefits. Particularly in Britain, there is consumer-dissatisfaction with the health system and a tendency towards a move to a public–private mix based on competition, rather than a tendency towards regulation. Perhaps the role of politics in the health care system in the UK may help to explain this. The process of privatization may be seen as part of the emergence of neo-conservatism in many industrialized countries in the 1980s. However, another dimension beyond the political scene may also help to explain this phenomenon. Several systems, including the British system, are just not doing well enough with respect to both the physical accessibility to care and the quality of care. As a result, the public has become less satisfied with health care and is seeking alternative sources of care in the private market. To respond to these pressures, competition has been introduced in several countries. This reliance on competition may be only a temporary fashion characteristic of the late 1980s and the 1990s. It may, however, also reflect the decline of the Welfare State as a viable concept with the concomitant emergence of health systems of the new era dominated by a public–private mix (Culyer and Jonsson 1986).

Health outcomes

When measured by classical indicators like mortality and communicable morbidity, there is no doubt that health outcomes are constantly improving globally. In 1900, in most industrialized countries, a child's chance of living to age 65 was less than 50 per cent; today it is 78 per cent. The usual explanations for this dramatic improvement were discussed in previous chapters, and included better medical care, nutrition, sanitation, and water supplies. What are the future trends? Will life expectancy lengthen indefinitely? There are two opposing scenarios in the biological literature. Fries and Carpo (1981), for example, envision the rectangularization of survival curves. According to their scenario, maximum life expectancy will converge in all developed countries at approximately age 85. With the advent of new technologies, people will not only live longer but also the dispersion of mortality by age will become narrower so that more people will die closer to the population mean of age 85. If this scenario would hold true, then the decrease in mortality at early ages would not be accompanied by the outcome of similar decreases in morbidity, disability, nor by increased well-being!

That people would live longer does not necessarily mean that they would become healthier. Rather, it could mean that sophisticated health technologies may provide them with better chances to survive at the expense of higher morbidity and disability at later ages. Recent evidence, however, hints that even for morbidity, there could be a compressed pattern emerging at later stages of life (Fries 1989).

According to the other scenario, there is no 'biological wall' either at age 85 or at any other age. Rather it is hypothesized that there is no biological limit for life. With the increase in medical technology there would be a flattening rather than a rectangularization of the survival curve (Schneider and Brody 1983; Grundy 1984). Unfortunately, extending life would undoubtedly cause outcomes like those predicted by the first scenario. As Verbrugge (1984) put it, 'there is evidence that shows rising morbidity for middle-aged and older people since 1957.' That is, whichever scenario will prevail, the improvement in mortality would not be followed by similar improvements in morbidity and disability. Thus, as life expectancy is extended beyond its present level, we may expect a decrease in the 'utility' of life at advanced ages. From a global perspective, and particularly for developed countries, this may be the most important 'message' about health outcomes in the years to come.

Health outcome goals are more modest for the developing countries. Of course, the general environmental conditions affecting health, including sanitation and water supplies, will continue to be improved. Also, health education campaigns aimed at educating mothers or reducing addiction to tobacco, alcohol, and drugs, must be strengthened. However, the greatest efforts should probably be to modify utilization patterns so as to increase health coverage and to distribute preventive and curative health services equitably over whole populations (Gish 1990). As Gish points out, health outcomes at large may be improved only if a well-distributed utilization level of three to four annual physician contacts per capita can be established. He suggests that at such a level of care, most preventive and curative health goals may be reached in the developing countries.

Conclusions

Little, perhaps too little, can be said about the fate of health systems. The trends of the multidimensional complex of causes and effects operating in health systems may sometimes converge and sometimes diverge. All in all, it seems certain that there is no way to make clear cut generalizations across all modules for all health systems. The future of health systems is closely linked to their past. It will be turbulent, undecisive, and strongly affected by external factors influencing inputs, processes, and outcomes. Understanding this strengthens our belief that even in the future it will be crucial to use the modular approach to reach rational conclusions about health systems. From our observations on the behaviour and dynamics of health systems in this book, we learned that understanding the complex trends of health systems depends first on the conceptualization of issues and then on their operationalization. Since the rules governing the health care scenario were not changed, there is no reason to believe that, even in the future, understanding health systems will require an instrument other than the modular approach. This is why we hope that future analysts of the complex array of health system dynamics will find the modular approach as promising as it seems today.

References

Altman, S. H. and Rodwin, M. A. (1988). Halfway competitive markets and ineffective regulation: the American health care system. *Journal of Health Politics, Policy and Law*, **13**, (2), 323–40.

Artigas, J. (1990). Health services decentralization in spain. In *Health system decentralization* (ed. A. Mills, J.P. Vaughan, D.L. Smith, and I. Tabibzadeh). WHO, Geneva.

Baldwin, M.F. (1987). Who will pay indigent's bill? *Modern Health Care*, 16 January, pp. 26–9.

Colledge, M., van Geuns, H.A., and Svensson, F.G. (ed.) (1986). *Migration and health*, WHO Regional Office for Europe, Copenhagen.

Culyer, A.J. and Jonsson, B. (1986). Introduction. In: *Public and private health services. Complementarities and conflicts*. Basil Blackwell, Oxford.

de Lissovoy, G., Rice, T., Ermann, D. and Gabel, J. (1986). Preferred provider organization: today's models and tomorrow's prospects. *Inquiry*, **23**, (1), 7–15.

Ellwood, P.M. (1988). Outcome management. A technology of patient experience. *New England Journal of Medicine*, **318**, 1549–56.

Elsinga, E. (1989). Political decision-making in health care: the Dutch case. *Health Policy*, **11**, 243–55.

Enthoven, A. (1988). Managerial competition of alternative delivery systems. *Journal of Health Politics, Policy, and Law*, **13**, (2), 305–21.

Evans, R.G., Lomas, J., Barer, M.L., Labelle, R.J., Fooks, C., Stoddard, G.L., *et al.* (1989). Controlling health expenditures—the Canadian reality. *New England Journal of Medicine*, **320**, (9), 571–7.

Fries, J.P. (1989). The compression of morbidity—near or far? *The Milbank Quarterly*, **67**, (2), 208–32.

Fries, J.P. and Carpo, L.M. (1981). *Vitality and ageing: implications of the rectangular curves*. W.H. Freeman, San Francisco.

Ghana Ministry of Health (1988). *Issues, problems and priorities of the health system in Ghana*. Background Paper, Ministry of Health Accra, 31 May.

Gish, O. (1990). Some links between successful implementation of primary care interventions and the overall utilization of health services. *Social Science and Medicine*, **30**, 401–5.

Godt, P.J. (1987). Confrontation, consent and corporatism: State strategies and the medical profession in France, Great Britain and West Germany. *Journal of Health Politics, Policy and Law*, **12**, (3), 459–80.

Grundy, E. (1984). Mortality and morbidity among the old. *British Medical Journal*, **288**, 663–4.

Henke, K.D. (1989). What can Americans learn from Europeans, (Respondent.) *Health Care Financing Review*, Annual Supplement, pp. 93-6.

HMSO (Her Majesty's Stationery Office) (1989). *Working for patients*. London.

Kinzer, D.M. (1990). Universal entitlement to health care. *New England Journal of Medicine*, **322**, 467-70.

Kleczkowski, B.M., Roemer, M.I., and van der Werff, A. (1984). *National health systems and their reorientation towards health for all*, Public Health Papers No. 77. WHO, Geneva.

Leape, L.L., Park, R.D., Solomon, D.H., Chassin, M.R., Kosecoff, J., and Brook, R.H. (1990). Does inappropriate use explain small area variations in the use of health care services? *Journal of the American Medical Association*, **263**, 669-72.

Lindgren, B. (1989). Symposium: What Can Americans Learn from Europeans, (Respondent.) *Health Care Financing Review*, Annual Supplement, pp. 67-71.

MacBride, S. (ed.) (1980). *Many voices, one world*. Kogan Page, London; Unipub, New York; Unesco, Paris.

Mayer, T.R. and Mayer, G.G. (1985). HMOs: origins and development. *New England Journal of Medicine*, **312**, 590-4.

Mills, A., Vaughan, J.P., Smith, D.L., and Tabidzadeh, I. (1990). *Health system decentralization – concepts, issues and country experience*. WHO, Geneva.

Pfaff, M. (1990). Differences in health care spending across countries: statistical evidence. *Journal of Health Politics, Policy and Law*, **15**, 1-68.

Relman, A.S. (1988). Assessment and accountability. The third revolution in medical care. *New England Journal of Medicine*, **319**, 1220-2.

Roemer, M.I. (1977). *Comparative national policies on health care*. Marcel Dekker, New York.

Roos, N.P. and Shapiro, E. (1981). The Manitoba Longitudinal Study on Ageing. *Medical Care*, **19**, (6), 644-57.

Rosen, B. (1989). *The public-private mix in Israeli health care*, Research Report RR-13-89. The Brookdale Institute, Jerusalem.

Sandier, S. (1989). Health service utilization and physician income trends. *Health Care Financing Review*, Annual Supplement, pp. 33-48.

Schieber, G.J. (1990). Health expenditures in major industrialized countries 1960-1987. *Health Care Financing Review*, **11**, (4), 159-67.

Schneider, E.L. and Brody, J.A. (1983). Ageing, natural death and the compression of morbidity: another view. *New England Journal of Medicine*, **309**, 854-6.

Schrijvers, G. (1990). The decentralization of the Netherlands health services. In *Health system decentralization* (ed. A. Mills, J.P. Vaughan, D.L. Smith, and I. Tabibzadeh). WHO, Geneva.

State of Israel (1990). *Report: The State Commission of Inquiry on the performance and effectiveness of the health care system*. Government Printing House, Jerusalem (Hebrew).

Titmuss, R.M. (1963). *Essays on 'The Welfare State'*, (2nd edn), p. 42. Unwin Books, London.

UN (United Nations) (1985). *World population prospects – estimates and projections as assessed in 1982*, Population Studies No. 86. United Nations, New York.

UNICEF (United Nations Children's Fund) (1990). *The state of the world's children 1990*. Oxford University Press, Oxford.

Verbrugge, L. (1984). Longer life but worsening health. Trends in health and mortality of middle aged and older persons. *Milbank Memorial Fund Quarterly*, **62**, 475-519.

Appendix—Concepts and indicators

Module	Concept	Indicators
Population needs (Chapter 3)	Population needs	Basic set of Indicators (income, education, type of residence, ethnicity, etc.)
		Compound methods (1) *Z*-score additive model (2) Socio-economic Status (SSI) (3) Multivariate regression
		Qualitative comparisons (1) Social Indicators Approach (2) Rates Under Treatment (RUT)
Input resources: Manpower (Chapter 4)	Quantitative aspects of manpower	Rates of manpower per population
	Qualitative aspects of manpower	Age
		Gender
		Family and dependents
		Culture and socialization
	Quality assurance of manpower	Comprehensiveness of licensure requirements
		Depth of licensure/certification
Inputs: Physical resources (Chapter 4)	Quantitative aspects of physical resources	Rates of physical resources per capita (e.g. beds, CT-scanners etc.)
	Qualitative aspects of physical resources	Determination of levels of resources available (the Rand curve, see Chapter 4)
	Quality assurance of physical resources	Comprehensiveness of the requirements for accreditation/certification
		Depth of the requirements for accreditation/certification
		Control of capital investment

Module	Concept	Indicators
Inputs: Socio-economic development (Chapter 4)	Direct influences	Size of health expenditure Per capita expenditure on health Structure of expenditures Income of health professionals
	Indirect influences	Demographic structures (1) Yearly birth-rate (2) Life expectancy at given ages (3) Age/sex distribution (4) Death rates (5) General and specific infant mortality (6) Type of residence (7) Migration (8) Dependency ratio
		Socio-political variables (1) Public expenditure on health (2) Health sector structure
		General economic variables (1) GNP per capita (2) Income distribution
		Individual achievements (1) Levels of education (2) Employment/unemployment (3) Distribution of professions/ occupations
Organization of health care (Chapter 5)	Organizational classification	Control and governance
		Planning and evaluation (1) Resource allocation (a) Type of resource allocation (b) Autonomy of health planners (c) Centralized/decentralized resource allocation (2) Strategic planning (a) Type of planning

Module	Concept	Indicators
		(b) Content of implementation
		Financial process (1) Financial process (2) Type of reimbursement; individual providers (3) Type of reimbursement; institutional providers
	Centralization or decentralization	Decentralization Index Democratization Index
	Coordination and continuity	Horizontal coordination Vertical coordination Use of information systems Use of group coordination
	Configuration of professional teams	Work teams in primary care (1) Distribution of physicians (2) Ratio of physicians to non physicians
		Work team in institutional care (1) Types of institutional arrangements (2) Intra institutional configuration (3) Employment status
	Equity	Descriptive evaluation of equity (distribution of manpower, physical resources, sanitary installations, etc.) Analytical evaluation of equity—Gini Index
	Appropriateness of care	Extent of coverage Comprehensiveness of coverage Ratio of health professionals per capita Balance between health professionals
	Accountability of a health system	Structural accountability (1) Frequency of data reporting

Module	Concept	Indicators
		(2) Consistency (reliability) of data reporting
		Action accountability. Investigation of controlled processes
		Consumer accountability
The process of health care delivery (Chapter 6)	Utilization	Utilization: primary care
		(1) Physician contacts
		(2) Population not seeing a physician
		(3) Referrals to laboratory or X-rays
		(4) Consumption of medicines
		Utilization: hospital care
		(1) Admissions/discharge rate
		(2) Hospital days
		(3) Average length of stay
		(4) Occupancy rates
		(5) Bed turnover
		Utilization: long-term care, same as hospital care
	Accessibility	Physical accessibility
		(1) Ratios of resources to population
		(2) Attraction rates
		(3) Continuity of care
		(4) Time-based indicators
		Economic accessibility
		(1) Coverage of health care
		(2) Range of health care
		(3) Cost-sharing
		Social accessibility (acceptability)
		(1) Age distribution
		(2) Proportion of females
		(3) Educational status
		(4) The use of non-urgent services
		(5) Continuity of care

Module	Concept	Indicators
	Ethical issues in utilization	Barriers to resource allocation Regulatory mechanisms
	Indirect attributes constraints on utilization	Method of rationing
	Quality assurance (related to process)	Utilization review
	Labour unrest	Frequency of industrial disputes Volume of industrial disputes Working days lost
General health outcomes (Chapter 7)	Mortality	Basic set of mortality indicators (see Tables 7.2, 7.3) Composite indices (1) Standardized Mortality Ratio (SMR) (2) Years of Life Lost (YLL) (3) Excess Mortality Ratio (EMR)
	Morbidity	Prevalence and incidence rates (see Table 7.4) Morbidity list
	Disability	Universal disability indicators (see Table 7.5)
	Positive health (well being)	General well-being indicators (1) Life expectancy (2) Levels of health awareness Lifestyle indicators (1) Death rates from accidents (2) Alcohol consumption (3) Daily calorie intake (4) Cigarette smoking Environmental influences (1) Water supply (2) Adequate sanitary facilities (3) Suicide rate

Module	Concept	Indicators
Health system outcomes (Chapter 8)	Effectiveness	List of key questions for reviewing the effectiveness of a system (see Table 8.1)
	Efficiency	Allocative efficiency: cost–benefit analyses
		Distributive efficiency
		(1) Supply-oriented: determination of longitudinal trends in health systems
		(2) Equity based: same as equity in the 'organization of health care' module
		Dynamic efficiency
		(1) Static comparisons: rate of technological units or procedures
		(2) Dynamic comparisons: rates of technological diffusion
		Managerial efficiency: cost-effectiveness analyses
	Outcome-related quality of care	QALYs
		Success rates (tracer method)
	Outcome-related equity	Indicators similar to those at the 'organization of health care' module

Index

The manufacturer's authorised representative in the EU for product
safety is Oxford University Press España S.A. of El Parque Empresarial
San Fernando de Henares, Avenida de Castilla, 2 - 28830 Madrid
(www.oup.es/en or product.safety@oup.com). OUP España S.A. also acts
as importer into Spain of products made by the manufacturer.
Printed and bound by CPI Group (UK) Ltd, Croydon, CR0 4YY
14/09/2026
02216286-0006